Preventing and Mitigating AIDS in Sub-Saharan Africa

Research and Data Priorities for the Social and Behavioral Sciences

Barney Cohen and James Trussell, editors

Panel on Data and Research Priorities for Arresting AIDS in Sub-Saharan Africa

Committee on Population

Commission on Behavioral and Social Sciences and Education

National Research Council

NATIONAL ACADEMY PRESS
Washington, D.C. 1996

NATIONAL ACADEMY PRESS • 2101 Constitution Avenue, N.W. • Washington, D.C. 20418

NOTICE: The project that is the subject of this report was approved by the Governing Board of the National Research Council, whose members are drawn from the councils of the National Academy of Sciences, the National Academy of Engineering, and the Institute of Medicine. The members of the committee responsible for the report were chosen for their special competences and with regard for appropriate balance.

This report has been reviewed by a group other than the authors according to procedures approved by a Report Review Committee consisting of members of the National Academy of Sciences, the National Academy of Engineering, and the Institute of Medicine.

The project that is the subject of this report was funded principally by the Bureau for Africa of the U.S. Agency for International Development (USAID) through a cooperative agreement administered by USAID's Office of Health and Nutrition. The Andrew W. Mellon Foundation also provided funding to the Committee on Population for this project.

Library of Congress Cataloging-in-Publication Data

National Research Council (U.S.). Panel on Data and Reseach
Priorities for Arresting AIDS in Sub-Saharan Africa.
Preventing and mitigating AIDS in Sub-Saharan Africa : research and data priorities for the social and behavioral sciences / Barney Cohen and James Trussell, editors ; Panel on Data and Research Priorities for Arresting AIDS in Sub-Saharan Africa, Committee on Population, Commission on Behavioral and Social Sciences and Education, National Research Council.
p. cm.
Includes bibliographical refererences and index.
ISBN 0-309-05480-X
1. AIDS (Disease)—Africa, Sub-Saharan. I. Cohen, Barney, 1959- .
II. Trussell, James. III. Title
RA644.A25N264 1996
614.5′993—dc20 96-11347
CIP

Additional copies are available for sale from
National Academy Press
2101 Constitution Avenue, N.W.
Box 285
Washington, D.C. 20055.
Call 800-624-6242 or 202-334-3313 (in the Washington Metropolitan Area).

Printed in the United States of America

PANEL ON DATA AND RESEARCH PRIORITIES FOR ARRESTING AIDS IN SUB-SAHARAN AFRICA

JANE MENKEN (*Cochair*), Population Studies Center, University of Pennsylvania
JAMES TRUSSELL (*Cochair*), Office of Population Research, Princeton University
KOFI AWUSABO-ASARE, University of Cape Coast, Cape Coast, Ghana
JOHN G. CLELAND, Center for Population Studies, London School of Hygiene and Tropical Medicine
CARL KENDALL, Department of International Health and Development, Tulane School of Public Health and Tropical Medicine
PETER R. LAMPTEY, Family Health International, Arlington, Virginia
EUSTACE P.Y. MUHONDWA, The Population Council, Dar es Salaam, Tanzania
A. MEAD OVER, The World Bank, Washington, D.C.
THOMAS C. QUINN, Infectious Disease Division, Johns Hopkins University
DEBORAH L. RUGG, Centers for Disease Control and Prevention, U.S. Department of Health and Human Services, Atlanta, Georgia
DANIEL TARANTOLA, François-Xavier Bagnoud Center for Health and Human Rights, Harvard School of Public Health
JUDITH WASSERHEIT, Centers for Disease Control and Prevention, U.S. Department of Health and Human Services, Atlanta, Georgia
MARIA J. WAWER, Center for Population and Family Health, Columbia University
PETER O. WAY, International Programs Center, Bureau of the Census, U.S. Department of Commerce
DEBREWORK ZEWDIE, The World Bank, Washington, D.C.

National Research Council Staff

BARNEY COHEN, *Study Director*
TRISH DeFRISCO, *Senior Project Assistant*

Liaison Representatives to the Panel

BENOIT FERRY, World Health Organization, Global Programme on AIDS
DEAN T. JAMISON, Board on International Health, Institute of Medicine

Consultants to the Panel

BETSY ARMSTRONG, Population Studies Center, University of Pennsylvania
LORNA EDWARDS, Harare, Zimbabwe
JENNIFER JOHNSON-KUHN, Department of Anthropology, Northwestern University
SAHR KPUNDEH, National Research Council
ALEXIS KUATE, Ministry of Health, Yaoundé, Cameroon
ANNICK MADY, Association de Soutien à L'Autopromotion Sanitaire et Urbaine, Côte d'Ivoire
DECLARE MUSHI, Tanzania AIDS Project, Dar es Salaam, Tanzania
RICHARD ODINDO, Medical Education Department, Nairobi, Kenya
ELIZABETH PISANI, Center for Population Studies, London School of Hygiene and Tropical Medicine
CHRISTINE SOLOMON, Family Health International, Arlington, Virginia
LAURA ZANINI, François-Xavier Bagnoud Center for Health and Human Rights, Harvard School of Public Health

COMMITTEE ON POPULATION

RONALD D. LEE (*Chair*), Departments of Demography and Economics, University of California, Berkeley
CAROLINE H. BLEDSOE, Department of Anthropology, Northwestern University
JOSE-LUIS BOBADILLA, World Bank, Washington, D.C.
JOHN BONGAARTS, The Population Council, New York
JOHN B. CASTERLINE, The Population Council, New York
LINDA G. MARTIN, RAND, Santa Monica, California
MARK R. MONTGOMERY, The Population Council, New York
ROBERT A. MOFFITT, Department of Economics, Brown University
ANNE R. PEBLEY, RAND, Santa Monica, California
RONALD R. RINDFUSS, Carolina Population Center, University of North Carolina, Chapel Hill
JAMES P. SMITH, RAND, Santa Monica, California
BETH J. SOLDO, Department of Demography, Georgetown University
MARTA TIENDA, Population Research Center, University of Chicago
AMY O. TSUI, Carolina Population Center, University of North Carolina, Chapel Hill

JOHN G. HAAGA, *Director*
BARNEY COHEN, *Program Officer*
TRISH DeFRISCO, *Senior Project Assistant*
KAREN A. FOOTE, *Program Officer*
JOEL A. ROSENQUIST, *Project Assistant*
JOYCE E. WALZ, *Administrative Associate*

Acknowledgments

This report is the product of the efforts of many people. The panel was established under the auspices of the Committee on Population. The committee, chaired by Ronald Lee, was responsible for establishing the panel and for reviewing the final report.

We are most grateful to the organizations that provided financial support for the work of the panel: The Bureau for Africa of the U.S. Agency for International Development and the Andrew W. Mellon Foundation. Besides providing funding, the representatives of these organizations were a valuable source of information and advice in the development of the panel's overall work plan.

Special thanks are due to Claude Cheta, Hortense Deffo, Jean-Pierre Edjoa, Zakariaou Njoumeni, and others on the staff of the Institut de Recherche et des Etudes de Comportements (IRESCO) in Cameroon, who prepared two very useful background papers for the panel.

Thanks are also due to Lorna Edwards, Alexis Kuate, Annick Mady, Declare Mushi, and Richard Odindo for their help implementing a questionnaire to nongovernmental organizations in various sub-Saharan African countries; to Jeff O'Malley and Ioanna Trilivas, who participated in the design of the survey; and to Sahr Kpundeh, who managed its implementation.

We are very grateful to the numerous researchers and policy makers in Africa who made time in their busy work schedules to talk to members of the panel during their mission to Africa in January and February 1995.

We are especially indebted to Betsy Armstrong for her many hours of thoughtful editing, to John Belanger and Joanna Sadowska for checking and rechecking of the references, and to Claire Del Medico and Amy Worlton for preparation of the manuscripts. We are also grateful to Elizabeth Pisani and Christine Solomon for their substantial contributions to Chapters 4 and 5, respectively. Special thanks are due as well to Trish DeFrisco for her superb administrative and logistical support to the panel, to Jennifer Johnson-Kuhn for her valuable research assistance on Chapter 6, to Rona Briere for her skillful editing of the report, and to André Lux for his excellent translation of the Summary into French.

We owe the greatest debt to Barney Cohen, who managed the entire process and ensured that we met our deadlines and whose intellectual contributions can be found in every chapter of the report, especially Chapters 1, 2, 6, and 7.

We close by expressing our heartfelt appreciation to the members of the panel who contributed long hours and their special expertise to the crafting of this report. Kofi Awusabo-Asare and Daniel Tarantola prepared the initial draft of sections of Chapter 2; Thomas Quinn, Maria Wawer, and Peter Way prepared the initial draft of Chapter 3; John Cleland prepared the initial draft of Chapter 4; Peter Lamptey, Deborah Rugg, and Carl Kendall prepared the initial draft of Chapter 5; and Mead Over prepared the initial draft of Chapter 6.

James Trussell and Jane Menken, *Cochairs*
Panel on Research and Data Priorities for
Arresting AIDS in Sub-Saharan Africa

Contents

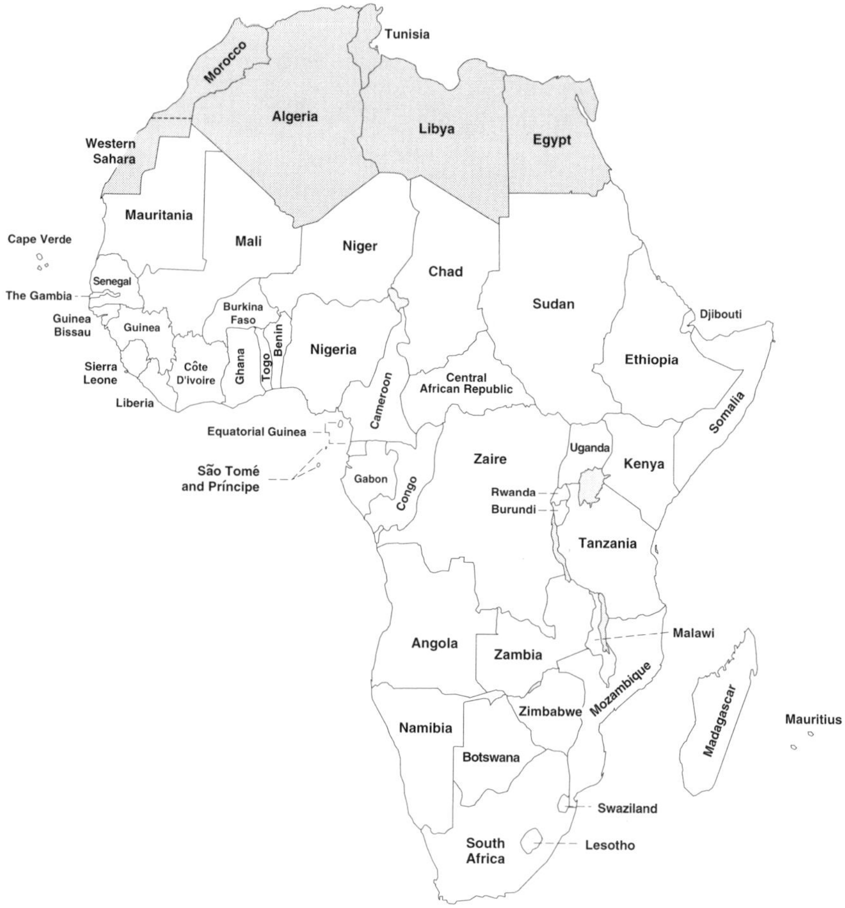

NOTE: This map, which has been prepared solely for the convenience of readers, does not purport to express political boundaries or relationships. The scale is a composite of several forms of projection.

Summary

The official number of acquired immune deficiency syndrome (AIDS) cases worldwide since the start of the epidemic passed the 1 million mark near the end of 1994—a fact that was covered in a six-sentence story on an inside page of *The New York Times* (January 4, 1995). Moreover, given the chronic underreporting and under-diagnosis in developing countries, the actual number of AIDS cases may be four times as high. The official statistics also do not reflect the millions of people who are infected with the human immunodeficiency virus (HIV) but have yet to develop symptoms of AIDS. The situation is critical in sub-Saharan Africa, where the World Health Organization (WHO) estimates that approximately 11 million adults and as many as 1 million children have been infected with HIV, and where basic infrastructure, financial, and managerial resources, as well as health-care personnel to deal with the catastrophe, are all extremely scarce.

Sub-Saharan Africa is geographically, demographically, socially, and culturally heterogeneous, and the extent and spread of HIV infection and AIDS have accordingly been heterogeneous as well. Thus, it is difficult to generalize about the AIDS epidemic in the region. There have been only a few nationally or regionally representative seroprevalence studies conducted to date in sub-Saharan Africa, and information is available predominantly on the groups with the highest risk of HIV infection. Yet some overall characteristics and trends can be seen. The most afflicted countries are geographically concentrated: other than Côte d'Ivoire in West Africa, they lie in a region of East and Southern Africa that stretches from Uganda and Kenya southward to include Rwanda, Burundi, Tanzania, Malawi, Zambia, Zimbabwe, and Botswana.

Patients seeking treatment today probably contracted the virus years ago. Thus, no matter how serious the situation currently appears, there will be very large increases in the number of AIDS deaths in sub-Saharan Africa in the future. By the year 2010, demographers project that life expectancy will fall from 66 to 33 years in Zambia, from 70 to 40 years in Zimbabwe, from 68 to 40 years in Kenya, and from 59 to 31 years in Uganda.

NEED FOR IMMEDIATE ACTION

There is encouraging evidence that intervention programs to change behavior can be effective in preventing the spread of HIV. Public awareness of the AIDS epidemic is extremely high throughout Africa, and condom sales have risen dramatically across the continent in the past few years. Other promising findings include a recent reduction in the prevalence of HIV-1 infection among young males in rural Uganda and evidence that treating sexually transmitted diseases (STDs) in rural Tanzania may reduce the spread of HIV. But many interventions have been experimental and small scale and so are not sufficient to reverse the course of the epidemic. At the same time, discovery of an effective vaccine or treatment shows little promise. Furthermore, even if a vaccine or cure were developed, it would probably not be sufficient to bring a speedy end to the epidemic—because of imperfect effectiveness, cost, and less than universal distribution and acceptance. In addition, many of the millions of people already infected with HIV are unaware of their status and so represent a pool capable of passing the virus to new cohorts. Thus, changing human behavior to slow the speed or limit the extent of transmission will remain for the foreseeable future the first and probably the most important line of defense against HIV/AIDS in sub-Saharan Africa. More and better social and behavioral research is needed to develop more effective and acceptable preventive strategies and to find more effective ways of mitigating the negative effects of the epidemic.

Perhaps the most important argument for immediate action to slow the further spread of HIV is that, as suggested above, in many parts of the region the epidemic has not yet peaked. HIV tends to spread quickly among individuals whose behaviors place them at high risk of infection, such as commercial sex workers and their clients; it spreads thereafter—at first slowly and then at an accelerated pace—into the general population. In many sub-Saharan African countries the disease has already spread widely, but in others it has not. Because the cost-effectiveness of prevention efforts declines rapidly as the epidemic spreads, the timing of interventions is crucial. Failure to control the epidemic now will mean that far more costly and difficult interventions will be necessary in the future.

Another important reason for acting now to revitalize programs to combat

HIV and AIDS is that the region's governments are facing a critical turning point in prevention efforts. Since their inception in the late 1980s, national prevention programs often have operated on the assumption that traditional health education about HIV/AIDS would be sufficient to induce widespread behavior change. This has not proved to be the case. The most optimistic reading of the results of these prevention efforts is that they have been less successful than was at first hoped. At the same time, leadership of the global effort to fight AIDS is changing hands, creating an important opportunity to review what has been achieved to date and to develop a coherent global strategy for the foreseeable future. In response to a recommendation by the executive board of WHO, and with firm commitments to AIDS activities from other United Nations organizations, a joint United Nations Programme on AIDS (UNAIDS) is being created to improve coordination among the various organizations and to boost the global response.

Finally, for a number of reasons, current AIDS-prevention efforts may be reaching a plateau. Agencies and governments in developed countries are beginning to suffer from "donor fatigue," induced partly by the realization that the epidemic is unlikely to affect the developed world as badly as was first feared, and partly by an inability to see how the money and effort expended on prevention thus far have affected the course of the epidemic. Furthermore, international donors do not want to commit themselves to providing care for the growing number of AIDS patients in countries where expenditures on health averaged less than US $15 per capita in 1990. The most visible consequence of donor fatigue in Africa is the withdrawal of resident advisers of WHO's Global Programme on AIDS from national AIDS control programs. This reduction in assistance has had enormous costs, in both human and economic terms. It also increases the urgency for action by Africans and their governments.

We recommend research and data in the social and behavioral sciences to improve and extend existing successful programs and devise more effective strategies for preventing HIV transmission, as well as support efforts to mitigate the impact of the AIDS epidemic. Our recommendations cover five areas: the monitoring of the epidemic, information on sexual behavior and HIV/AIDS, primary HIV-prevention strategies, mitigation of the impacts of the epidemic, and the building of an indigenous capacity for AIDS-related research. Both our five key recommendations and our other recommendations are offered with full acknowledgment of the importance of the economic, political, and societal context of the HIV/AIDS epidemic in Africa. Our five key recommendations are numbered separately from our other recommendations, which are numbered by chapter in the order in which they appear.

SOCIETAL CONTEXT OF HIV/AIDS IN AFRICA

The societal context within which people are born and raised, are initiated to sexuality, and lead their lives strongly influences their perceptions of risk and their sexual behavior. Social, cultural, and economic factors can act either to speed or to retard the spread of infection. Planners and policy makers must be cognizant of the societal context and attempt to modify it in ways that are conducive to and supportive of change. Effective interventions must target not only individual perceptions and behavior, but also their larger context.

Among the salient factors that affect the size and shape of the HIV/AIDS epidemic in sub-Saharan Africa are the age and gender composition of the population; the pattern of sex roles and expectations within society; inequities in gender roles and power; sexual access to young girls and the acceptance of widespread differentials in the ages of sexual partners; rapid urbanization under conditions of high unemployment; poverty; considerable transactional sex fostered by limited earning opportunities for women; and lack of access to health care, particularly treatment for various STDs. These factors are often exacerbated by social upheavals related to economic distress, political conflicts, and wars. Of course, there is enormous variation in the situation from country to country; particularly noteworthy are the differences between West Africa and East and Southern Africa.

EPIDEMIOLOGY OF THE HIV/AIDS EPIDEMIC

The global HIV/AIDS epidemic consists of many separate, individual epidemics, each with its own distinct characteristics that depend on geography, the specific population affected, the frequencies of risk behaviors and practices, and the timing of the introduction of the virus. No single factor, biological or behavioral, determines the epidemiologic pattern of HIV infection. Instead, a complex interaction among several variables determines how and where HIV spreads in a population. The primary mode of HIV transmission is sexual, with heterosexual transmission accounting for at least 80 percent of adult HIV infections in sub-Saharan Africa.

Biological factors also influence the spread of the epidemic by increasing or decreasing susceptibility to the virus, altering the infectiousness of those with HIV, and hastening the progression of infection to disease and death. Such biological factors include the presence of classical STDs, male circumcision, and the viral characteristics of both HIV-1 and HIV-2 and their multiple genetic strains.

A growing body of data suggests that HIV cannot be considered in isolation from other STDs because it shares with them modes of transmission and behavioral risk factors. More important, there is evidence that other STDs may increase susceptibility to and transmission of HIV, so that treatment and prevention of STDs may serve as an important weapon in curbing the HIV/AIDS epidemic.

Although HIV infection rates are high among many populations and subgroups in sub-Saharan Africa, there is much variation in incidence and prevalence, both geographically and by population subgroups. The probable causes of this heterogeneity in seroprevalence include behavioral, biological, and societal factors. As suggested above, trying to explain the phenomenon by a single factor—such as civil war, male circumcision, STDs, or rate of partner change—is simplistic. Instead, it appears that the simultaneous occurrence of several risk factors for HIV transmission determines how rapidly and to what level HIV spreads among a population and who becomes infected. This epidemiologic diversity not only reflects differences in sexual and other behaviors, but also suggests that the epidemic has not reached an equilibrium in most areas.

The HIV epidemic and the demographic structure of the population of sub-Saharan Africa will have complex interactions over time. The population is predominantly young, in sharp contrast with the age structure in developed countries, and many of the behavioral factors associated with HIV transmission are common among young people. Accordingly, the large number of people under age 15, who will soon enter their sexual and reproductive lives, represent a priority group for AIDS and STD prevention.

KEY RECOMMENDATION 1. Basic surveillance systems for monitoring the prevalence and incidence of STDs and HIV must be strengthened and expanded.

Good social science research is as dependent as public health and medical research on reliable and valid HIV/AIDS surveillance data. With the implementation of various interventions aimed at controlling HIV transmission, periodic monitoring of STD and HIV prevalence and incidence among selected populations is essential both for assessment of the impact of these programs and for decision making on program design and implementation.

Recommendation 3-1. More emphasis must be placed on HIV incidence studies for monitoring trends in HIV infection rates.

Although seroprevalence provides important information regarding currently infected individuals in an area, measuring incidence is also critically important for estimating the rate of change in the spread of HIV infection in a given population. In particular, data on current incidence provide the most direct and immediate information regarding the potential effects of a given intervention. Together, prevalence and incidence studies can provide information regarding the current status of the epidemic in terms of numbers of infected individuals and the rate of spread within a given population on an annual basis.

Recommendation 3-2. STD and HIV prevalence and incidence data should be combined with behavioral and demographic information.

Current surveillance systems are often limited, incomplete, and inconsistent, and they rarely measure behavioral or demographic variables. Given new, noninvasive techniques for the collection and analysis of biological specimens (including blood, urine, vaginal secretions, and saliva), accurate assessment of STD and HIV prevalence and incidence can readily be combined with behavioral and demographic information.

In conjunction with periodic serosurveys, demographic information is needed to elucidate the differential spread of STD and HIV infection in rural and urban settings and variations in seroprevalence and incidence by gender, educational level, profession, income level, age, and other demographic factors. This type of information is critical for targeting prevention messages to selected groups at risk of acquiring and transmitting HIV and for projecting the effects of HIV and other STDs on a population over time.

SEXUAL BEHAVIOR AND HIV/AIDS

Patterns of sexual behavior—both partner selection and particular practices—are clearly the primary determinant of the spread of the HIV/AIDS epidemic in sub-Saharan Africa. Information on sexual behavior is needed to help project the future course of the epidemic, to develop more effective prevention strategies, and to provide baseline data for evaluating the effectiveness of alternative preventive strategies.

Several studies have begun to address how sexual networks channel and potentially amplify HIV transmission in sub-Saharan Africa. Such networking studies encompass the role of migration, transportation systems, and local markets. Asymmetric age matching, where young women have sexual contact with older men, results in a young cohort of women who have been exposed to older male partners with higher HIV prevalence; this pattern creates a chain of infection that passes from generation to generation.

Heterogeneity in the composition of sexual networks may have strong implications for the speed or direction of viral transmission. Patterns of mixing between people in high-risk core groups and others in the general population observed in sub-Saharan African settings (in contrast to pairings confined within well-defined core groups) can result in substantial spread of STDs and HIV among the general population. Although much emphasis has been placed on "high-risk" behaviors associated with multiple, sequential, short-term relationships, there is a growing body of research suggesting that concurrent multiple partnerships, including those that are stable and long term (common in many African settings), may contribute substantially to HIV transmission.

At the same time, however, networks also serve as bases of social support and the development of behavioral norms. Networks are a potential natural resource for behavioral interventions. Support for behavioral change, such as acceptance of condoms among peers, can enable individuals to negotiate these matters more effectively when confronted with a resistant partner. Conversely, the absence of support networks can make behavioral change more difficult to achieve.

Recommendation 4-1. Research on sexual networks is critical.

Population-based research is needed to collect and analyze data on both the variables that describe individual sexual behavior and the possible socioeconomic determinants of the decision to have sex with a new partner or forgo protection. Since the details of interconnected sexual networks are difficult to deduce from the answers to individual questionnaires, there is also an important role for social network research.

Recommendation 4-2. Researchers need to develop more reliable ways of collecting information on sexual behavior and to find ways of testing its validity.

There appears to be a much greater willingness to report sexual behavior than was believed until recently, but this field of research requires sensitivity. The challenge is to develop definitions and appropriate vocabulary, such as for categories of relationships, that are both specific enough to be clear to respondents and generalizable enough to be useful to analysts and program planners. The challenge is likely to grow as information about high-risk behavior spreads, increasing the likelihood that respondents will seek to give the "right" answers on questionnaires and in interviews. Hybrid research strategies involving both qualitative and quantitative approaches are essential. Where appropriate, and when both privacy and confidentiality can be ensured, biological markers of sexual activity (such as HIV or STD status) should periodically be incorporated into behavioral surveys to allow assessment of the validity of questionnaire responses and the extent to which the latter provide adequate information on risk.

Recommendation 4-3. Research is needed on patterns of sexual initiation and on the formation of sexual norms and attitudes.

The sexual habits of a lifetime may well be influenced by a socialization process that starts at or before puberty, often before sexual activity begins. A better understanding of the early influences on sexual norms and attitudes and of patterns of sexual initiation may prove essential to promoting safer behavior. For this recommended research to be successful, studies must include children and prepubescent youths, as well as sexually active adolescents and their partners. Recognition that sexuality is socially constructed and changing rapidly is essential to broadening the research agenda and improving interventions.

Recommendation 4-4. More work is needed to clarify the frequency of specific sexual practices.

Because the epidemic in sub-Saharan Africa is being sustained by heterosexual transmission, information on sexual behavior is needed to help develop more effective prevention strategies, as well as to provide baseline data to evaluate their effectiveness. Specific sexual practices—dry sex, oral sex, and anal sex being but a few examples—may impede the success of particular interventions, yet information about such practices is necessary for encouraging behavioral change.

Recommendation 4-5. Research on coercive sex, especially among adolescents, is critical.

The magnitude of the problem of coercive sex is all but unknown, as are the circumstances under which forced sex or rape takes place. How frequently does it happen and why? Do the aggressors or the victims share characteristics that might suggest a path for preventive or protective interventions? Research on community attitudes, mores, and gender expectations that may serve to encourage or inhibit coercive sex is urgently needed in order to determine how to enlist community support for the curtailment of such practices.

Recommendation 4-6. Research aimed at achieving a better understanding of perceptions about the dual roles of condoms is required.

Condoms help prevent the spread of HIV/AIDS; they also prevent pregnancy. How aware are people of these dual roles, and what weight do they give each when deciding whether to use condoms? How often are these roles in concord and how often in conflict? Do partners discuss this issue, and if so, what are the negotiating mechanisms used?

Recommendation 4-7. Research on attitudes and beliefs about and behavioral responses to sexually transmitted diseases is required.

To develop effective strategies for the treatment of STDs, understanding is needed about social and cultural responses to STDs, including stigmatization. Much more knowledge about the health-seeking behaviors of people infected with STDs, and whether their sexual habits are altered by knowledge of infection, is also needed.

Recommendation 4-8. Research on acceptance of and behavioral responses to HIV vaccination is urgently needed.

Because vaccine trials are likely to begin with vaccines of limited efficacy, there is an urgent need to learn whether individuals who are vaccinated increase their exposure to HIV through riskier behavior, and if so, to determine how to mitigate this response.

PRIMARY HIV-PREVENTION STRATEGIES

As suggested earlier, despite the many limitations inherent in attempting to evaluate the effectiveness of interventions aimed at HIV prevention, clear evidence is emerging that such efforts can be successful, particularly among higher-risk groups. At the same time, however, data from various surveillance systems indicate that current interventions are probably not yet having a significant impact on the epidemic at the subcontinent or even the country level. Despite the fact that levels of AIDS awareness are extremely high in sub-Saharan Africa, getting people to change their behavior is difficult. Denial, fear, external pressures, social and sexual norms, other priorities, or simple economics can keep people from adopting healthier life-styles.

Yet getting people to change their behavior is not impossible. Indeed, health educators in sub-Saharan Africa have had a fair amount of success in recent years. For example, broad-based education campaigns have persuaded large numbers of people to have their children immunized against various childhood diseases and have educated mothers to give their children oral rehydration formula during episodes of diarrhea. Of course, attempting to modify more personal behavior, such as sexual practices, is more challenging. Yet family planning programs have been successful even in some of the most disadvantaged countries of the world. Even the most cautious reviews of behavioral interventions aimed at slowing the spread of HIV conclude that although most have not been rigorously evaluated, some approaches do seem to work. At the same time, it is important to have realistic expectations about what can be achieved. Behavior change will never be 100 percent: some individuals will never choose to protect themselves, while others will lapse into old patterns of behavior after a short period of time.

To increase the likelihood of success, interventions need to be culturally appropriate and locally relevant, reflecting the social context within which they are embedded. They should be designed with a clear idea of the target population and the types of behaviors to be changed. In turn, recognized impediments in the social environment to behavior change probably need to be specifically addressed. Behavior-change interventions should include promotion of lower-risk behavior, assistance in development of risk-reduction skills, and promotion of changes in societal norms. It must be noted that in sub-Saharan Africa, there is an urgent need to design ways of targeting women and adolescents for prevention messages.

Basic principles of successful intervention programs include the following:

- learning about and adapting to local conditions,
- ensuring community participation,
- carefully targeting the audience,
- identifying effective strategies and messages,

- building local capacity,
- evaluating results, and
- using the results from evaluation studies for improvement.

Successful intervention programs should also be multidisciplinary and multifaceted and involve multiple contacts with targeted populations. In sub-Saharan Africa, as elsewhere, HIV-prevention messages have included promotion of partner reduction, postponement of sexual debut, alternatives to risky sex, mutually faithful monogamy, consistent and proper use of condoms, better recognition of STD symptoms, and more effective health-seeking behavior.

Numerous interventions are being implemented throughout Africa, but most are still information-based health education campaigns. Many of the messages communicated are generic or vague and do not address specific risk behaviors. Innovative approaches are typically small scale and lack rigorous evaluation. Furthermore, it is not easy to demonstrate the success of a particular intervention because it is difficult to define and measure such outcome variables as "better health status" and to determine whether the intervention in question was the reason for a desired change. Consequently, the need for solid evaluation research is still urgent.

KEY RECOMMENDATION 2. An increase in research funding for the development of social and behavioral interventions aimed at protecting women and adolescents, especially girls, from infection deserves highest priority.

An important step in arresting the spread of AIDS in sub-Saharan Africa is to recognize that, although African women have relatively high autonomy by the standards of developing countries, their low and separate status remains a major obstacle to HIV prevention. In many societies, the presence of unmarried, postpubertal girls is a new phenomenon. Guidelines for their sexual behavior and that of others toward them are not well established; their low social status makes them particularly vulnerable. Moreover, in many areas of sub-Saharan Africa, high HIV incidence has been detected among adolescents and young adults, especially girls. Research on which to base the design of culturally relevant programs targeted to adolescents and to adults who might be their sexual partners is an important priority.

KEY RECOMMENDATION 3. More evaluation research is needed to correlate process and outcome indicators—such as reported condom sales and behavior change—with reductions in HIV incidence or prevalence.

Rigorous designs, such as controlled intervention studies to assess the effectiveness of different prevention approaches, are needed. To date, few rigorous evaluations of intervention programs in sub-Saharan Africa have been conducted. Evaluations that have been reported often lack precision in their measurement of risk behaviors and are therefore not very informative. As a result, few strategies can demonstrate whether they are effective. Barriers to rigorous evaluation research include lack of human resources, expertise, financial resources, and equipment. Overcoming these barriers requires major changes in research infrastructure. Nevertheless, it is a priority to begin now a few large-scale behavioral interventions, including adequate baseline surveys, multiround surveys, and longitudinal studies with comparison cohorts, even if these interventions are relatively expensive. It is only with these types of studies that more definitive information on the effectiveness of various interventions, which is so desperately lacking for most studies in sub-Saharan Africa, can be obtained. The longer such studies are delayed, the longer will exist the uncertainty about which HIV-prevention strategies work best, for whom, and under what circumstances. In the interim, basic program evaluation and some formative and operational research can be completed, and such work should be required by donors as part of program implementation awards.

Recommendation 5-1. Interventions that promote gender equality deserve high priority as AIDS-prevention strategies in every country.

Women's primary source of risk is their society-wide subordination, not their lack of knowledge. Governments can effect change in many ways to empower women: reducing the financial necessity for multiple partnerships by changing laws to give women equal access to training and jobs, equal rights of inheritance and property ownership, equal access to education, and equal wage scales; enacting and enforcing laws against rape; building the capacity of women for collective action; and educating everyone about women's rights. Enhancing the status of women is a long-term strategy that would have many beneficial effects for development, in addition to the likely effect of reducing the transmission of HIV and other STDs.

Recommendation 5-2. In the short term, a female-controlled vaginal microbicide that would allow women to protect themselves without their partner's participation is an urgent research and development priority for international donors.

A microbicide is not a quick-fix substitute for the fundamental structural reforms necessary to achieve gender equality, but rather a temporary and partial response to this problem as it influences HIV transmission. Yet in the same way that the use of spermicides by women can reduce fertility, the use of a microbicide could, in and of itself, help arrest the spread of HIV.

Recommendation 5-3. Research is needed to address the HIV-prevention needs of several other populations with marked vulnerability, particularly the mobile and the disenfranchised.

There is a need to reach mobile individuals and groups with comprehensible and acceptable programs, particularly where linguistic and cultural barriers exist between migrants and the local population. Ways of effectively providing preventive services to the disenfranchised populations in the ever-growing urban slums and in refugee camps need to be developed; a major challenge to such programs is the lack of resources and social support for individuals in such settings.

Recommendation 5-4. Additional research should be conducted to determine the impact of specific STD interventions on the incidence of HIV infection within defined populations.

Research is needed to determine the extent to which STDs help cause HIV infection, to examine the importance of the behavioral synergy of STD and HIV transmission, and to design more effective intervention programs. There is a need for assessment of the relative efficacy and feasibility of various interventions for STD treatment and sexual behavior change in reducing HIV transmission. This research includes assessing the effects of programs that target individuals at high risk of acquiring and transmitting STDs, as well as the effects of community-based STD programs. The interventions themselves could comprise STD education, condom distribution, increased STD screening, and mass antibiotic therapy. Data on the effectiveness of these interventions, particularly those focused on decreasing STD prevalence, are essential for evaluating the impact of STD reduction on the spread of HIV. Behavioral research on ways of ensuring acceptance of various STD control strategies should be directly integrated into the epidemiological research.

Recommendation 5-5. Research is needed to assess the effectiveness and cost-effectiveness of the syndromic approach to STD diagnosis and treatment.

Clinical testing for STDs is expensive and not widely accessible. Therefore, research is needed on better ways to identify STDs more accurately through symptoms. In addition, new screening methods, including urine-based assays for chlamydia and gonorrhea and self-administered vaginal swabs for trichomonas culture and bacterial vaginosis gram stain, should be incorporated into research. Efforts are needed to make these techniques available and affordable in developing-country settings for surveillance, diagnosis, and validation.

Recommendation 5-6. For long-term program planning and resource allocation, cost-effectiveness studies should be incorporated in donor research work and the cost-effectiveness of HIV prevention compared with that of other health interventions.

Few intervention evaluations have adequately assessed effectiveness in terms of behavior change or seroincidence declines, much less cost-effectiveness. Results of evaluation studies currently in progress in several countries in sub-Saharan Africa are expected to provide data on the cost-effectiveness of various HIV-prevention strategies. However, determining the effectiveness of HIV-prevention strategies is methodologically complex and will take several more years to complete. In the meantime, since resources are insufficient and may well decline further, efficient resource utilization is paramount. Thus, basic analysis of overall program costs and specific intervention costs is critical. Simple cost analyses and cost-effectiveness estimates could provide data that would be helpful for public health decision making and program design.

Recommendation 5-7. Operations research should be a high priority.

The growth of the HIV/AIDS pandemic in the past 20 years in sub-Saharan Africa has led to the development of institutional and community-based responses and a corresponding need for operations research to improve the effectiveness, cost-effectiveness, and quality of these responses. Primary research needs include scaling up successful experimental interventions, improving the effectiveness and reducing the cost of existing programs, examining the cost-effectiveness of linking HIV prevention with HIV/AIDS care, and improving the sensitivity and specificity of criteria for targeting interventions.

Recommendation 5-8. Research should be undertaken to measure the impact of female-controlled barrier contraceptive use on HIV transmission.

Studies should be undertaken to determine the effectiveness against STDs and HIV of female-controlled barrier contraceptives such as female condoms and spermicides. This research should encompass field-based studies of the acceptability of these methods. Moreover, greater efforts need to be made to integrate appropriate HIV/AIDS-prevention messages and programs for STD diagnosis, referral, and treatment into family planning programs.

Recommendation 5-9. Behavioral research is needed to develop effective pregnancy-related HIV counseling programs.

Given the rapid spread of HIV among women in sub-Saharan Africa, perinatal transmission continues to have a major impact on infant and child morbidity and mortality among populations with a high HIV seroprevalence. Studies using modified treatment regimens with Zidovudine (AZT), hyperimmune gammaglobulin, vitamin A, vaginal washes, and other means of intervention should be undertaken to determine their overall effectiveness and cost-effectiveness in decreasing HIV perinatal transmission.

MITIGATING THE IMPACT OF THE EPIDEMIC

AIDS will have a large social, psychological, demographic, and economic impact on both individuals and societies. In addition to the physical suffering and grief caused by the disease, AIDS can lead to social and economic hardship, isolation, stigmatization, and discrimination.

As noted above, even if transmission of HIV were halted today, millions of Africans who are currently infected would still develop AIDS and die over the next 10 to 20 years. But transmission has not ceased. To the contrary, evidence from a variety of populations in Africa suggests that seroprevalence either is continuing to climb or has leveled off at discouragingly high levels. For at least the next several decades, the HIV/AIDS epidemic will continue to ravage African prime-age adults and their children with death rates as much as 10 times higher than they would otherwise have been.

Although not immediately visible, the cumulative mortality effects of this "slow plague" will be substantial. Increases in infant and child mortality will be accompanied by increases in adult mortality and reductions in life expectancy. Population growth will decline more rapidly than expected, and the populations in sub-Saharan Africa in the year 2000, particularly among the countries in the main AIDS belt, will be somewhat smaller than those projected in the absence of AIDS. In many of the worst-afflicted countries, deaths will more than double during the 1990s as compared with the number estimated without AIDS. These additional deaths will put increasing strains on already overburdened health-care systems and on individual households trying to manage with limited economic resources. Care and support for orphans will be a growing concern, and traditional inheritance and other legal rights will be challenged.

Relatively little research has been conducted on the economic consequences of adult morbidity and mortality. AIDS is one of several diseases with potentially great economic significance for developing countries. Diseases such as malaria and measles are far more prevalent in Africa, yet there are reasons to believe that the economic impact of AIDS will be greater. The long incubation period of HIV implies that the economic impact of existing levels of infection would be felt for 10 years or more even if all infection were to cease today. The benefits of averting a case of HIV are very high relative to other diseases.

Whether directed at individuals with AIDS and their households or at other levels of social organization, mitigation interventions divert scarce resources from other uses, including efforts to prevent transmission. Thus, the value to society of any mitigation intervention should be as least as great as the cost of the resources devoted to the effort. Research on this issue might improve the efficiency of current expenditures, as well as justify a case for or against additional spending.

KEY RECOMMENDATION 4. Research on mitigating the impact of the disease should focus on the needs of people with HIV/AIDS.

A great deal more is known about designing and implementing HIV-prevention programs than is known about providing care to the millions of people in sub-Saharan Africa already infected with the virus. Simple, cost-effective solutions to daily living problems faced by persons with AIDS, such as palliative care, part-time home care, and group counseling, may make larger, more expensive interventions unwarranted.

Recommendation 6-1. Research efforts to evaluate the impact of HIV/AIDS on individuals, households, firms, economic sectors, and nations are badly needed.

Research on impact should incorporate both qualitative and quantitative approaches to data collection and should evaluate both short- and long-term effects. Of particular interest is research that would permit an understanding of the impact of HIV/AIDS on poverty and on individual decision making. Research is needed to ascertain whether decreased life expectancy reduces willingness to save or invest in financial and real assets, in human capital, and in the relationships necessary to maintain social interactions. In the long term, the impact of HIV/AIDS on sub-Saharan Africa will depend on the strength and malleability of social and economic networks in accommodating the changes that are occurring.

Recommendation 6-2. Since the attempt to assist directly every affected household would be financially nonsustainable, research is needed on criteria for determining which households and communities should be targeted for assistance and which institutions should deliver that assistance.

The epidemic has already affected millions of households in sub-Saharan Africa and will continue to do so for at least the next 20 years. Efforts to mitigate the effects of the disease have been uncoordinated and poorly targeted, and their ability to provide solutions for those infected and their families remains to be proven.

Recommendation 6-3. Discovering the optimal roles of government, nongovernmental organizations, and donors in HIV/AIDS prevention and mitigation is critical and requires further study.

Governments are now moving to decentralize and privatize AIDS programs by contracting, licensing, or franchising activities to various types of nongovernmental institutions. Research is needed on the determinants of the effectiveness of nongovernmental organizations, including those not devoted primarily to AIDS prevention and mitigation, in a variety of AIDS prevention and mitigation activities. Care is needed in defining the technical assistance needs and the absorptive capacities of nongovernmental organizations, to enhance their roles in research and prevention and to avoid overload and inefficient use of scarce resources.

BUILDING CAPACITY FOR AIDS-RELATED RESEARCH

If useful research on HIV/AIDS is to be undertaken and its results are to be applied appropriately and effectively, the necessary infrastructure must be in place, a prerequisite that is often lacking in sub-Saharan Africa. As a result, virtually all research undertaken to date has been possible only with technical cooperation and foreign assistance from the international community. Thus, beyond the immediate challenge of identifying the critical research questions, there remain enormous practical challenges of actually obtaining the answers.

Key aspects of a basic infrastructure for conducting effective research include access to adequate funding, skilled labor, and appropriate technology, as well as sufficient managerial and administrative capacity to plan, execute, monitor, and evaluate studies. Even in developed countries, amassing the resources required to undertake complex research endeavors is difficult, and these difficulties are multiplied many-fold in sub-Saharan Africa. Many of the region's universities have been badly neglected in recent years. The poor preparedness of matriculating students, entirely inadequate salaries for all levels of professional and support staff, neglect of buildings and libraries, and a lack of core funds necessary to move institutions into the technological age have contributed to the universities' slow demise and the widespread departure of their faculties to the private sector.

Many of the findings from the research that has been conducted have not been adequately disseminated, so that results are not widely known across the continent. As a consequence, the contributions of social and behavioral scientists have not been fully utilized. In addition, inadequate coordination of research efforts has resulted in duplication and the need to "reinvent the wheel."

These structural problems are compounded by donor policies and practices that result in short-term studies that do not allow sufficient time for local capacity building, the predominance of expatriate personnel in most projects, and at least the perception among the recipients of donor assistance that projects address donor rather than local priorities. Yet the dominance of international donors in AIDS research in Africa is the result of a lack of domestic funding for such research in the region: many of the region's governments appear complacent about the magnitude of the epidemic and have so far contributed little to HIV/AIDS research.

In the long run, it is essential to help sub-Saharan African countries develop their own research capacity by strengthening their universities and augmenting the technical skills of their researchers. There is considerable debate and controversy, however, about how best to achieve this goal. Regardless of what the best mechanisms may be, no significant progress is likely to be made until the region's governments understand that they must put AIDS more squarely on their own research and policy agendas. Clearly, a major constraint on the amount of HIV/AIDS research that is undertaken is inadequate funding. Potential sources of funding include communities, private-sector firms, the public sector, and international donors. Because it is unlikely that donors are going to increase significantly their levels of funding in the near future, the governments will have to find additional resources. Given the weak economic position of most sub-Saharan African countries, however, it will be difficult to persuade their governments to pursue more vigorous research agendas in the near future.

KEY RECOMMENDATION 5. Linkages between sub-Saharan African institutions and international research centers must be established on a wide range of activities, including teaching, research, and faculty and student exchanges. International donors should seriously consider establishing a sub-Saharan African AIDS research institution with a strong behavioral and social science element.

There is a critical need to strengthen research institutions in sub-Saharan Africa. Linkages with international organizations, especially if built on an evolving and well-defined research agenda, can help local institutions develop and assist local researchers by providing relatively secure long-term funding, offering support for the preparation of data and manuscripts for publication and dissemination, and providing in-country technical assistance and research training. Experience in a number of settings has demonstrated that such long-term collaboration, in addition to contributing significantly to understanding of the HIV/AIDS epidemic, is mutually beneficial to all institutions involved; it could be very successful in providing highly skilled African researchers with support and the possibility of remaining in their country of origin.

Recommendation 7-1. The number of African scientists well trained to conduct research on HIV and AIDS must be increased.

Research capacity in sub-Saharan Africa cannot be improved without an increase in the number of well-trained local researchers. Four possible ways to introduce and keep more researchers in the field are to (1) integrate more graduate students and young professionals into all new AIDS-related research initiatives; (2) establish small grants programs to fund the projects of young researchers; (3) adjust pay scales to attract and retain talented professionals; and (4) provide other incentives for researchers to remain in their home institutions, including small-scale research grants, fewer teaching or administrative responsibilities, and more opportunities for international travel. Providing technical assistance to local researchers is an important priority. Local researchers could benefit from workshops that would help them design research projects, prepare research proposals, identify potential sources of funding, write reports describing interim results, and prepare final manuscripts for submission to peer-reviewed journals.

Recommendation 7-2. Each national AIDS control program should establish a local AIDS-information center that would develop and maintain a database of all AIDS-related research conducted in the country.

These centers should be linked via available technology, such as the Internet. They should also have AIDS databases on CD-ROM (CD-ROM-equipped computers are available in most national AIDS control program offices.) In addition, national and regional conferences should be held to provide forums at which researchers can discuss their research plans and present their results to a larger group of local researchers than those that attend international conferences.

Recommendation 7-3. There is an urgent need for sub-Saharan African countries to establish and periodically update research priorities at the regional and national levels, providing a basis for discussions with donors on AIDS-related research.

It is important to reduce the proportion of donor-driven research taking place in the region.

Recommendation 7-4. International organizations and donors should utilize existing local resources to the fullest extent possible.

It is paradoxical that donors underutilize existing talent in the region. Utilizing local expertise can strengthen local institutions, generate employment, and create opportunities for talented researchers in sub-Saharan Africa.

Recommendation 7-5. Greater dialogue between researchers and policy makers is necessary.

Not only is there an urgent need to increase indigenous capacity to conduct research, but there is also a need to better synthesize and translate research findings into effective prevention and control programs and policies. Otherwise, prevention programs will be only marginally based on local needs or tailored to local conditions, and research will be even more undervalued and underfunded. Researchers need to do a better job of drawing out the policy implications of their work, and planners and policy makers need to articulate more clearly to researchers what information they need for effective planning and programs.

Recommendation 7-6. If more effective strategies for AIDS prevention and mitigation are to be developed in the future, better coordination among donors is needed, particularly sharing of information about which prevention and control efforts work and which do not.

The role of the new cosponsored United Nations Programme on AIDS (UNAIDS) will be critical to future work. Success will also require greater political will and commitment on the part of the governments of sub-Saharan Africa and other countries.

CONCLUSION: THE NEED FOR BETTER BEHAVIORAL AND SOCIAL SCIENCE RESEARCH

Because AIDS is an epidemic firmly rooted in human behavior, driven by economic, cultural, and social conditions, the behavioral and social sciences are essential to identifying solutions for its control. Yet to date, most funding for HIV/AIDS research has been devoted to biomedical studies of the nature of the virus as a logical starting point for identifying a vaccine or a cure. All too often it has been implicitly assumed that behavioral and social science research should take place only because there are currently no effective vaccines or treatments for the disease, as if the discovery of a vaccine or a cure would eliminate any further need for such research. This assumption that the availability of treatment solves all problems is simply not true. For example, the resurgence of tuberculosis has become one of the world's most serious health problems, even though a cure that is 95 percent effective has been available for almost 50 years.

Effective prevention of HIV/AIDS will require enormous and continued commitment in order to achieve lasting changes in human behavior. No one set of interventions—behavioral or medical—will be sufficient by itself to combat the epidemic. More behavioral and social research is needed to develop effective and acceptable preventive strategies to refine successful programs and to help find more effective ways of mitigating the negative impacts of the epidemic.

The interpretation and utility of much epidemiological, behavioral, and social research have been limited by the lack of a multidisciplinary approach. Data on reported behavior change may be difficult to assess in the absence of biological validation that such change is reducing STD/HIV infection. Efforts to model the demographic effects of the HIV/AIDS epidemic are hindered by a paucity of data sets that combine fertility, mortality, migration, and other sociodemographic information with HIV serology. Conversely, serological studies that fail to collect adequate behavioral data miss an important opportunity to assess the effects of key factors in the spread of HIV, such as sexual practices and sexual networks within given populations. The design, execution, and analysis of clinical trials for STD control, HIV vaccines, antiretroviral drugs, and genital barrier methods and virucides all depend on appropriate behavioral research to guide enrollment; ensure adherence to trial protocols; and permit adequate interpretation of epidemiological results, including the very basic need to control for differential behavioral change between study groups.

Until new research is available, it is critical to keep trying the existing strategies that are believed to be most effective, as well as designing new and innovative ones. The epidemic is forcing people to rethink their values and behavior, and is changing the social context. Strategies and policies must be responsive to the ever-changing situation, as well as receptive to the findings of research being carried out throughout the region. An effective partnership between research and program interventions will be key to lessening the spread and impact of the HIV/AIDS epidemic in sub-Saharan Africa.

Resumé

Depuis le début de l'épidémie du syndrome d'immunodéficience acquise (SIDA), le nombre de cas enregistrés à l'échelle mondiale a franchi le seuil du million vers la fin de l'année 1994, un fait que *The New York Times* a signalé en six petites phrases d'une page intérieure de son édition du 4 janvier 1995. En fait, comme beaucoup de cas survenant dans le tiers monde échappent couramment à l'enregistrement et au diagnostic, le chiffre réel de cas de SIDA peut bien être quatre fois supérieur. Les statistiques officielles ne tiennent pas non plus compte des millions de gens qui sont séropositifs sans avoir encore développé la maladie au grand jour. La situation est critique en Afrique subsaharienne, car selon les estimations de l'Organisation mondiale de la santé (OMS), environ onze millions d'adultes et près d'un million d'enfants y sont contaminés par le virus d'immunodéficience humaine (VIH), alors que les infrastructures de base, les ressources en matière de finances, de gestion, ainsi que de personnel sanitaire capable d'affronter cette catastrophe y sont toutes extrêmement rares. L'Afrique subsaharienne affiche une hétérogénéité géographique, démographique, sociale et culturelle qui explique l'hétérogénéité de l'étendue et de la propagation du VIH et du SIDA, de sorte qu'il est malaisé de dresser un tableau général de cette épidémie dans l'ensemble du continent. Jusqu'à présent, on n'a fait que quelques études de séropositivité représentatives à l'échelle nationale ou régionale, et l'information disponible concerne en grande partie les groupes qui courent le plus de risques d'infection VIH. Certaines caractéristiques et tendances générales

---

Traduit de l'anglais par André Lux.

émergent cependant. On observe une concentration géographique des pays les plus atteints: à l'exception de la Côte d'Ivoire en Afrique occidentale, on les retrouve dans une région d'Afrique orientale et méridionale qui s'étend de l'Ouganda et du Kénya vers le sud pour inclure le Rwanda, le Burundi, la Tanzanie, Le Malawi, la Zambie, le Zimbabwé et le Botswana.

Les patients actuellement en quête de soins ont probablement contracté le virus il y a plusieurs années. C'est pourquoi, indépendamment de la gravité de la situation telle qu'elle apparaît actuellement, l'avenir nous réserve une augmentation très sensible du nombre des décès par SIDA en Afrique subsaharienne. A en croire les projections des démographes, l'espérance de vie tombera en l'an 2010 de 66 à 33 ans en Zambie, de 70 à 40 au Zimbabwe, de 68 à 40 au Kénya et de 59 à 31 en Ouganda.

IL FAUT AGIR SANS TARDER

Nous disposons de données encourageantes sur l'efficacité possible des programmes d'intervention visant à modifier les comportements en vue de prévenir la propagation du VIH. Partout en Afrique, la prise de conscience du danger est très vive, avec en conséquence une poussée spectaculaire de la vente de condoms depuis quelques années. Comme autres constatations prometteuses, citons la réduction récente de la prévalence de l'infection par le VIH-I chez les jeunes hommes en Ouganda et la preuve que le traitement des maladies transmises sexuellement (MTS) en Tanzanie peut réduire la propagation du VIH. Cependant, beaucoup de ces interventions avaient un caractère expérimental à petite échelle et ne suffisent donc pas à renverser la tendance de l'épidémie. En attendant, les chances de découvrir un vaccin ou un traitement efficace sont bien minces. Il faut ajouter que même si ces chances devenaient réalité, cela ne suffirait pas pour vaincre rapidement cette épidémie; en effet, l'efficacité de ces vaccins serait imparfaite, leurs coûts élevés et leur distribution loin d'être généralisée. En outre, un grand nombre parmi les millions de personnes déjà porteuses du VIH n'ont pas conscience de leur état et forment dès lors un bassin capable de transmettre le virus à de nouvelles cohortes. C'est pourquoi la première et probablement la plus importante ligne de défense contre le VIH/SIDA en Afrique subsaharienne sera dans un avenir prévisible de changer les comportements humains de manière à ralentir le rythme ou à limiter la propagation de ce fléau. Il nous faut accentuer et améliorer les recherches en matière sociale et comportementale pour mettre au point des stratégies préventives plus efficaces et plus acceptables, et pour découvrir des procédés capables de mieux atténuer les effets négatifs de cette épidémie.

Le meilleur argument en faveur de l'urgence d'une action immédiate destinée à ralentir à l'avenir l'extension du VIH, est peut-être de souligner, conformément à la suggestion faite plus haut, qu'en beaucoup de régions du continent l'épidémie n'a pas encore atteint son plafond. Le VIH tend à se répandre comme une traînée de poudre auprès des personnes à qui leurs comportements font courir des risques élevés d'infection, notamment celles qui font commerce de leur corps et leurs clients; il se répand ensuite dans l'ensemble de la population, d'abord lentement, ensuite à un rythme accéléré. Cette maladie s'est déjà installée solidement dans beaucoup de pays d'Afrique subsaharienne, mais pas dans tous. Puisque l'efficacité des dépenses engagées dans la prévention diminue rapidement avec la propagation de l'épidémie, le calendrier des interventions est un facteur crucial. Si les efforts d'endiguement échouent maintenant, cela voudra dire qu'il faudra entreprendre à l'avenir des interventions beaucoup plus coûteuses et difficiles.

Il y a une autre raison d'agir maintenant pour rendre leur force de frappe aux programmes de lutte contre le VIH et le SIDA; en effet, les gouvernements du continent sont arrivés à une croisée des chemins décisive en ce qui regarde leurs efforts de prévention. Depuis leur lancement à la fin des années 80, les programmes nationaux de prévention ont fonctionné sur la base de l'hypothèse voulant que l'éducation sanitaire traditionnelle au chapitre du VIH/SIDA suffirait à enclencher des changements de comportement à grande échelle. Cela ne s'est pas avéré exact. La façon la plus optimiste d'interpréter les résultats de ces programmes est de constater qu'ils n'ont pas répondu aux espoirs placés en eux. Au même moment, la direction générale de l'effort global de lutte contre le SIDA change de mains, ce qui offre l'occasion rêvée de passer en revue les résultats obtenus jusqu'à présent et de mettre en oeuvre une stratégie d'ensemble cohérente pour un avenir prévisible. En réponse à une recommandation du Bureau de direction de l'OMS et avec des engagements fermes de la part d'autres organismes des Nations Unies en faveur de la lutte contre le SIDA, un programme conjoint des Nations Unies sur le SIDA (UNAIDS) s'est créé dans le but d'assurer une meilleure coordination entre ces différents organismes et de renforcer leur capacité de prise en charge globale de ce problème.

Enfin, diverses raisons font que les efforts actuels de prévention contre le SIDA souffrent peut-être d'essoufflement. Une certaine «lassitude à financer» se fait jour chez des organismes et gouvernements des pays développés, en partie parce que ces pays réalisent que l'épidémie ne les frappera probablement pas autant qu'ils ne l'avaient d'abord craint, en partie aussi parce qu'ils sont incapables de voir comment l'argent dépensé et les efforts de prévention consentis jusqu'à présent ont influencé le cours de cette épidémie. De plus, les donateurs internationaux ne veulent pas s'engager à prendre en charge de plus en plus de sidatiques dans des pays qui ne consacraient en moyenne à la santé que 15 dollars U.S. par habitant en 1990. En Afrique, la conséquence la plus visible de la «lassitude à financer» est le fait que les conseillers résidants du Programme global de l'OMS sur le SIDA ont été retirés des programmes nationaux de contrôle du SIDA. Les coûts tant humains que financiers de cette réduction de l'aide sont énormes, ce qui augmente l'urgence pour les Africains et leurs gouvernements de passer à l'action.

Nous recommandons la production de recherches et de données dans le champ des sciences sociales et comportementales en vue d'améliorer et d'essaimer les programmes existants qui ont connu du succès, ainsi que pour appuyer les efforts destinés à atténuer l'impact de l'épidémie du SIDA. Nos recommandations portent sur cinq champs: la surveillance de l'épidémie, l'information en matière de comportements sexuels et de VIH/SIDA, les stratégies préventives de base contre le SIDA, l'atténuation des impacts de cette épidémie, et la mise sur pied d'un potentiel autochtone de recherche sur le SIDA. En présentant nos cinq recommandations clés ainsi que nos autres recommandations, nous reconnaissons sans réserves l'importance du contexte économique, politique et sociétal de l'épidémie du VIH/SIDA en Afrique. Nous numérotons nos cinq recommandations clés séparément des autres recommandations, qui portent un numéro par chapitre selon l'ordre de leur apparition.

CONTEXTE SOCIETAL DU VIH/SIDA EN AFRIQUE

Le contexte sociétal dans lequel les gens naissent, sont élevés, s'initient à la sexualité et mènent leur vie, exerce une forte influence sur leur perception du risque et sur leur comportement sexuel. Des facteurs sociaux, culturels et économiques peuvent soit accélérer soit ralentir la propagation de la contamination. Les planificateurs et les décideurs doivent être au fait de ce contexte sociétal et trouver des façons de l'infléchir dans un sens qui encourage le changement. Pour être efficaces, les interventions doivent viser non seulement les perceptions et les comportements individuels, mais aussi leur contexte ambiant.

Voici quelques-uns des facteurs saillants qui influencent l'ampleur et la forme de l'épidémie de VIH/SIDA: la composition par âge et par sexe de la population, le modèle des rôles et des attentes selon le sexe dans la société, les manques d'équité dans les rôles et les pouvoirs entre hommes et femmes, l'accès sexuel aux adolescentes et le large éventail des âges entre partenaires sexuels, l'urbanisation accélérée en situation de chômage aigu, la pauvreté, l'ampleur du commerce sexuel encouragée par la pénurie d'autres sources de revenu chez les femmes, et le peu d'accès aux soins de santé, surtout en matière de maladies transmises sexuellement (MTS). L'impact de ces facteurs est souvent exacerbé par des révoltes sociales, des conflits politiques et des guerres. La situation varie certes énormément d'un pays à l'autre, comme c'est le cas, notons-le, entre l'Afrique occidentale et l'Afrique orientale et méridionale.

EPIDEMIOLOGIE DU VIH/SIDA

Sous l'appellation globale de VIH/SIDA se cachent beaucoup d'épidémies distinctes dont chacune présente ses caractéristiques propres en fonction de la géographie, des populations spécifiques qu'elle frappe, de la fréquence des comportements et pratiques à risque, et du rythme auquel le virus s'introduit. Il n'y a pas de facteur unique, biologique ou comportemental, qui détermine la configuration épidémiologique de l'infection par le VIH. C'est au contraire de l'interaction complexe entre plusieurs variables que dépend le moment et la façon dont le virus se répand dans une population. Le principal canal de propagation est la transmission sexuelle, qui est à plus de 80 pour cent hétérosexuelle chez les adultes d'Afrique subsaharienne.

Des facteurs biologiques exercent aussi une influence dans la propagation de l'épidémie en augmentant ou diminuant la sensibilité au virus, en modifiant l'état septique des personnes atteintes par le virus et en accélérant le passage de l'infection à la maladie et au décès. Citons parmi ces facteurs la présence des MTS classiques, la circoncision masculine et les caractéristiques virales tant du VIH-1 que du VIH-2 avec leurs multiples souches génétiques.

Les données s'accumulent qui suggèrent de ne pas considérer le VIH à l'exclusion des autres MTS parce qu'ils partagent les mêmes canaux de transmission et les mêmes facteurs comportementaux à risque. Mieux encore, on dispose de preuves que d'autres MTS peuvent accroître la sensibilité au VIH et sa transmission, de sorte que le traitement et la prévention des MTS peuvent servir d'arme importante pour ralentir l'épidémie de VIH/SIDA.

Les taux élevés d'infection par VIH chez beaucoup de populations et de sous-groupes en Afrique subsaharienne n'empêchent pas la présence de variations sensibles dans l'incidence et la prévalence à la fois par région et sous groupe. Les causes probables de cette hétérogénéité dans la séroprévalence sont d'ordres comportemental, biologique et sociétal. Comme nous l'avons déjà laissé entendre plus haut, il serait simpliste d'essayer de privilégier un seul facteur—comme la guerre civile, la circoncision masculine ou le taux de mobilité des partenaires—dans l'explication de ce phénomène. Il apparaît au contraire que c'est la survenance simultanée de plusieurs facteurs de risque de transmission du VIH qui détermine la rapidité et l'ampleur de la dissémination de ce virus dans une population ainsi que les individus qu'il contamine. Non seulement cette diversité épidémiologique reflète-t-elle les différences dans les comportements sexuels et autres, mais encore suggère-t-elle que l'épidémie n'a pas encore atteint son point d'équilibre dans la plupart des zones.

L'épidémie du VIH et la structure démographique de la population d'Afrique subsaharienne développeront avec le temps des interactions complexes. La structure par âge de cette population est très jeune, tout au contraire de celle des pays développés; or, beaucoup de facteurs de comportement reliés à la transmission du VIH sont communs chez les jeunes. Par conséquent, la classe nombreuse des jeunes de moins de 15 ans, qui sont à la veille d'entamer leurs activités sexuelles et de reproduction, constitue le groupe à qui s'adresse par priorité l'action préventive contre le SIDA et les MTS.

RECOMMANDATION-CLE N°1: Nécessité de renforcer et de multiplier la présence de systèmes de surveillance pour suivre à la trace l'incidence et la prévalence des MTS et du VIH.

La recherche de qualité en sciences sociales dépend autant que la recherche en santé publique et en médecine de statistiques fiables et valides sur la surveillance du VIH/SIDA. En même temps que se réalisent diverses interventions destinées à contrôler la transmission du VIH, il est essentiel d'assurer une surveillance périodique de l'incidence et de la prévalence des MTS et du VIH parmi une sélection de populations à la fois pour évaluer l'impact de ces programmes et prendre des décisions concernant la conception et la mise en oeuvre de programmes.

Recommandation 3-1. Il faut mettre davantage l'accent sur les études d'incidence du VIH en vue de surveiller les tendances qu'empruntent ses taux d'infection.

Bien que la séroprévalence fournisse une information importante sur les individus atteints à un moment donné par le VIH dans une région, la mesure de l'incidence du VIH est également d'importance vitale dans l'estimation du taux auquel change l'infection par ce virus. En particulier, les données sur l'incidence en cours fournissent l'information la plus directe et immédiate sur les effets potentiels d'une intervention donnée. Une fois combinées, les études de prévalence et d'incidence nous éclairent sur la situation courante de l'épidémie en termes de nombre de personnes infectées et du taux annuel auquel le virus se répand dans une population donnée.

Recommandation 3-2. Il s'agit de combiner les données relatives à la prévalence et à l'incidence des MTS et du VIH avec l'information sur les comportements et la démographie.

Les systèmes courants de surveillance sont souvent limités, incomplets, peu cohérents et ne mesurent que rarement les variables comportementales et démographiques. Grâce aux nouvelles techniques, non invasives, de prélèvement et d'analyse de spécimens biologiques (sang, urines, sécrétions vaginales et salive), on peut facilement combiner l'évaluation précise de la prévalence et de l'incidence des MTS et du VIH avec les informations de nature comportementale et démographique.

De concert avec les enquêtes sérologiques périodiques, on a besoin d'informations démographiques pour mettre en lumière les différences de propagation des MTS et du VIH dans les habitats ruraux et urbains, et les variations de séroprévalence et d'incidence selon le sexe, le niveau d'instruction et de revenu, l'âge et autres facteurs démographiques. Ce type d'information est vital pour qui veut que ses messages de prévention atteignent exactement les groupes choisis parmi ceux qui sont à risque d'attraper et de transmettre le VIH, et pour projeter dans le temps les effets du VIH et d'autres MTS sur une population donnée.

COMPORTEMENT SEXUEL ET VIH/SIDA

Il est clair que les modes de comportement sexuel—tant la sélection des partenaires que les pratiques particulières—sont le déterminant prédominant de la dissémination de l'épidémie du VIH/SIDA en Afrique subsaharienne. Nous avons besoin d'informations sur le comportement sexuel pour nous aider à projeter le cours à venir de cette épidémie et à mettre au point des stratégie de prévention plus efficaces, et pour fournir des données de base permettant d'évaluer l'efficacité de stratégie préventives de remplacement.

Plusieurs études se sont attelées à la tâche de dépister la manière dont les réseaux de partenaires sexuels servent de canaux de transmission, voire d'amplification potentielle du VIH/SIDA en Afrique. De telles études de réseaux englobent le rôle joué par les migrations, les systèmes de transports et par les marchés locaux. Les accouplements asymétriques entre jeunes femmes et hommes plus âgés font en sorte d'exposer les jeunes cohortes de femmes à des partenaires masculins plus âgés, chez qui la prévalence du HIV est plus forte; ce processus crée des infections en chaîne qui se transmettent de génération en génération.

L'hétérogénéité dans la composition des réseaux sexuels peut avoir des répercussions majeures sur la vitesse et l'orientation de la propagation du virus. Les manières dont se font les rencontres entre individus appartenant aux groupes les plus à risque et d'autres provenant de la population en général, telles qu'on les observe dans des contextes africains (par contraste avec les appariement confinés à des groupes cibles bien définis) peuvent déboucher sur une extension substantielle des MTS et du VIH dans l'ensemble de la population. Bien qu'on ait insisté beaucoup sur les comportements à haut risque associés avec des relations multiples, successives et passagères, de plus en plus de recherches suggèrent que des relations conjointes multiples, y compris celles qui sont stables et de longue durée (ce qui est habituel en milieu africain), peuvent contribuer de manière substantielle à la diffusion du VIH.

En même temps cependant, les réseaux peuvent aussi servir de base à l'encadrement social et au développement de normes de comportement. Ils peuvent être une ressource naturelle pour l'intervention dans les comportements. Leur appui à des changements de comportement tels que, par exemple, l'acceptation des condoms entre pairs, peut permettre à des individus de négocier plus efficacement ces choses avec un partenaire réticent. Inversement, l'absence d'un réseau de support peut rendre la réalisation de changements de comportement plus difficile.

Recommandation 4-1. La recherche sur les réseaux sexuels est vitale.

Il faut une recherche à base démographique pour collecter et analyser des données portant à la fois sur les variables décrivant le comportement sexuel des individus et sur les éventuels déterminants socio-économiques commandant la décision d'avoir une relation sexuelle avec un nouveau partenaire ou de ne pas se protéger. Etant donné qu'on peut difficilement dégager les détails relatifs aux interconnexions entre réseaux sexuels à partir des réponses figurant sur des questionnaires individuels, la recherche sur les réseaux sociaux doit également jouer un rôle important.

Recommandation 4-2. Il faut que les chercheurs mettent au point des procédés plus fiables de collecte d'informations sur les comportements sexuels et trouvent le moyen d'en tester la validité.

Contrairement à ce qu'on avait cru jusqu'à récemment, les gens s'avèrent beaucoup plus disposés à parler de leur comportement sexuel, mais voilà un champ d'investigation à ne pénétrer qu'avec délicatesse. Le défi porte sur l'élaboration de définitions et d'un vocabulaire approprié concernant notamment des catégories de relations qui soient à la fois suffisamment claires aux yeux des répondants et assez généralisables pour répondre aux besoins des analystes et des bâtisseurs de programmes. C'est un défi qui a toute chance de s'amplifier à mesure que se répand l'information sur les comportements à haut risque, puisque la probabilité augmentera de voir les répondants chercher à donner la «bonne» réponse dans le questionnaire ou en entrevue. Il est essentiel d'avoir des stratégies de recherches hybrides, combinant les approches qualitative et quantitative. Dans la mesure où la chose est appropriée et que l'intimité et la confidentialité peuvent être garanties, il faudrait incorporer périodiquement dans les enquêtes de comportement des marqueurs biologiques de l'activité sexuelle (tels que le statut en matière de VIH ou de MTS), de manière à permettre l'évaluation des réponses aux questionnaires et de la mesure où celles-ci fournissent une information adéquate sur le risque encouru.

Recommandation 4-3. Il faut des recherches sur les modes d'initiation sexuelle et de formation des normes et attitudes sexuelles.

Les habitudes sexuelles d'une vie entière peuvent avoir subi l'influence d'un processus de socialisation enclenché au moment ou avant la puberté, souvent avant le début de l'activité sexuelle. Il peut s'avérer essentiel de mieux comprendre les influences précoces modelant les normes et attitudes sexuelles, et les modes d'initiation sexuelle en vue de promouvoir un comportement plus sécuritaire. Pour que cette recherche qui est recommandée obtienne du succès, les études doivent inclure des enfants et des adolescents prépubères ainsi que des adolescents sexuellement actifs et leurs partenaires. Pour élargir l'agenda des recherches et améliorer les interventions, il est essentiel de reconnnaître que la sexualité est socialement construite et qu'elle change rapidement.

Recommandation 4-4. Il faut investir plus de travail dans l'élucidation de pratiques sexuelles spécifiques.

Etant donné que c'est la transmission hétérosexuelle qui alimente l'épidémie du VIH/SIDA en Afrique subsaharienne, il importe de disposer d'informations sur les comportements sexuels de manière à mettre au point des stratégies préventives plus efficaces tout en fournissant des données de base permettant d'évaluer leur efficacité. Des pratiques sexuelles spécifiques—dont les rapports secs, oraux et anaux ne sont que quelques exemples—peuvent faire obstacle au succès d'interventions particulières; cependant il est nécessaire d'être informé de telles pratiques pour encourager les changements de comportement.

Recommandation 4-5. Il est vital de faire des recherches sur les rapports sexuels sous contrainte, en particulier parmi les adolescentes.

L'ampleur du problème des abus sexuels reste largement inconnue, tout comme le sont les circonstances dans lesquelles se déroulent ces abus et les viols. Quelles en sont la fréquence et les causes? Les agresseurs et leurs victimes partageraient-ils des caractéristiques qui entr'ouvriraient la porte à des interventions préventives ou protectrices? Il y a un besoin urgent de mener des recherches dans le milieu sur les attitudes, les moeurs et les attentes selon le sexe qui peuvent encourager ou réfréner les abus sexuels de manière à déterminer comment gagner l'appui de ce milieu pour mettre fin à de telles pratiques.

Recommandation 4-6. On a besoin d'une recherche visant à mieux comprendre la perception de la dualité des rôles des condoms.

Les condoms aident à prévenir la propagation du VIH/SIDA; ils empêchent aussi les grossesses. Dans quelle mesure les gens sont-ils conscients de ces deux rôles séparés et quel poids accordent-ils à chacun d'eux en décidant d'utiliser des condoms? Combien de fois ces rôles sont-ils concordants et combien de fois entrent-ils en conflit? Les partenaires discutent-ils de cette question et, si oui, de quels mécanismes de négociations se servent-ils?

Recommandation 4-7. On a besoin de recherches sur les attitudes et croyances relatives aux maladies transmises sexuellement et sur les comportements adoptés en réponse à ces maladies.

Pour mettre en route des stratégies efficaces de traitement des MTS, il faut comprendre quelles sont les réactions sociales et culturelles à ces maladies, incluant leur stigmatisation. Il faut aussi en savoir beaucoup plus sur les comportements des personnes atteintes de MTS et qui veulent en guérir, et sur l'influence que peut avoir leur connaissance de leur contamination sur le changement éventuel de leurs habitudes sexuelles.

Recommandation 4-8. Il y a un besoin urgent de recherches sur l'acceptation de la vaccination contre le VIH et sur les comportements que cette vaccination engendrerait.

Comme les vaccinations expérimentales débuteront probablement avec des vaccins d'efficacité limitée, il est urgent de découvrir si les personnes vaccinées augmentent leur exposition au VIH par des comportements à risque accru, et dans l'affirmative, de déterminer comment réfréner leur réaction.

STRATEGIES PREVENTIVES DE BASE CONTRE LE VIH

Comme nous l'avons déjà suggéré, malgré les nombreuses limitations inhérentes aux tentatives d'évaluer l'efficacité des interventions destinées à prévenir le VIH, il apparaît clairement que de tels efforts peuvent être payants, en particulier parmi les groupes à risque élevé. En même temps cependant, les données tirées de divers systèmes de surveillance montrent que les interventions courantes n'exercent probablement pas encore d'impact significatif sur cette épidémie à l'échelle du sous-continent, voire à celle des pays. Malgré que les habitants d'Afrique subsaharienne aient une conscience aiguë de la présence du SIDA, ils se laissent difficilement convaincre de changer leurs comportements. Le refus, la peur, des pressions externes, d'autres priorités ou de simples considérations économiques sont autant de facteurs qui peuvent empêcher les gens d'adopter des styles de vie plus sains.

Il n'est pourtant pas impossible d'amener ces gens à modifier leurs comportements. Les éducateurs en matière de santé ont en effet récolté pas mal de succès depuis quelques années en Afrique subsaharienne. A titre d'exemple, ils ont réussi, grâce à de vastes campagnes d'éducation, à persuader un grand nombre de gens de faire vacciner leurs enfants contre diverses maladies enfantines et ont amené les mères à administrer à leurs enfants des potions de réhydratation orale en périodes de diarrhée. Certes, chercher à modifier des comportements plus personnels, comme le sont les pratiques sexuelles, représente un plus grand défi. Les programmes de planification familiale ont néanmoins connu du succès même dans certains des pays les plus démunis de la planète. Même les évaluations les plus prudentes des interventions visant les comportements en vue de ralentir la propagation du VIH aboutissent à la conclusion que malgré l'absence d'une évaluation rigoureuse de la plupart de ces interventions, certaines approches semblent fonctionner. Il importe en même temps d'avoir des attentes réalistes quant aux résultats possibles. Les comportements ne se modifieront jamais à 100 pour cent: certains individus ne choisiront jamais de se protéger, tandis que d'autres le feront très temporairement avant de retomber dans leurs vieilles habitudes de comportement.

Pour augmenter leurs chances de réussite, les interventions doivent s'harmoniser avec la culture et les conditions locales et traduire de la sorte le contexte social dans lequel elles s'inscrivent. Il faut les concevoir en ayant clairement à l'esprit les populations visées et les types de comportement à changer. Il faut probablement prendre spécifiquement en charge à leur tour les éléments du contexte social en qui l'on voit des obstacles au changement des comportements. Les interventions visant à changer les comportements devraient inclure la promotion des comportements à risque réduit, l'appui à la formation de qualifications dans l'art de réduire les risques, ainsi que la promotion des modifications aux normes sociétales. Il faut souligner le besoin urgent qui existe en Afrique subsaharienne de concevoir des moyens d'atteindre les femmes et les adolescents pour leur transmettre les messages de prévention.

Les principes de base du succès des programmes d'intervention sont les suivants:

- se mettre au courant des conditions locales et s'y adapter,
- s'assurer la participation du milieu,
- prendre soin de bien choisir l'auditoire visé,
- identifier les stratégies et les messages efficaces,
- former des compétences locales,
- évaluer les résultats, et
- apporter des amélioration à l'aide des résultats des études d'évaluation.

Pour avoir du succès, les programmes d'intervention devraient aussi être multidisciplinaires et multidimensionnels, et favoriser la multiplication des contacts avec les populations cibles. En Afrique subsaharienne comme ailleurs, les messages des programmes de prévention contre le VIH portent sur la promotion de la réduction du nombre de partenaires, l'ajournement du début des activités sexuelles, les substituts aux rapports sexuels à risque, la fidélité mutuelle des époux monogames, l'utilisation régulière et correcte des condoms, une meilleure reconnaissance des symptômes des MTS, et des comportements pro-santé plus efficaces.

De nombreuses interventions ont lieu partout en Afrique, mais la plupart sont des campagnes d'information visant l'éducation à la santé. Les contenus de beaucoup de ces messages sont génériques et ne visent pas des comportements à risque spécifiques. Les approches innovatrices se font typiquement à petite échelle et sans évaluation rigoureuse. En outre, il n'est pas aisé de faire la preuve de la réussite d'une intervention particulière à cause de la difficulté de définir et mesurer ses résultats sous la forme de variables telles que «meilleur état de santé», et de déterminer si c'est bien cette intervention qui a suscité le désir de changement. C'est pourquoi subsiste l'urgence de mener de solides recherches évaluatives.

RECOMMANDATION-CLE N°2. L'accroissement du financement de la recherche visant le développement des interventions socio-comportementales en faveur de la protection des femmes et des adolescents, des filles en particuliers, contre la contamination, mérite la toute première priorité.

Pour enrayer la progression du SIDA en Afrique subsaharienne, un pas important est de reconnaître que malgré l'autonomie relativement grande dont jouissent les femmes africaines à l'aune des pays du tiers monde, leur statut inférieur et séparé reste un obstacle important à la prévention du HIV. Dans beaucoup de société, la présence d'adolescentes postpubères non mariées est un phénomène nouveau. Il n'y a pas de lignes directrices bien établies au sujet de leur comportement sexuel et de celui des autres à leur égard; leur statut social inférieur les rend particulièrement vulnérables. Ajoutons qu'on a détecté dans beaucoup de régions d'Afrique subsaharienne une forte incidence du VIH parmi les adolescents et les jeunes adultes, particulièrement chez les jeunes filles. D'où la forte priorité en faveur de recherches servant à concevoir des programmes de prévention destinés aux adolescentes et à leurs éventuels partenaires adultes.

RECOMMANDATION-CLE N°3. Il faut plus de recherches évaluatives pour corréler les indicateurs d'activités en cours et de résultats obtenus—comme les déclarations de ventes de condoms et les changements de comportement—avec les réductions dans l'incidence et la prévalence du VIH.

On a besoin d'études conçues avec rigueur, comme celles qui portent sur des interventions contrôlées, en vue d'évaluer l'efficacité des différentes approches préventives. Jusqu'à ce jour, on a fait peu d'évaluations rigoureuses des programmes d'intervention en Afrique subsaharienne. Celles qui ont été publiées manquent souvent de précision dans leur mesure des comportements à risque de sorte qu'on ne peut pas en tirer beaucoup d'informations. Le résultat en est que peu de stratégies peuvent faire la preuve de leur efficacité. Les obstacles à une recherche évaluative rigoureuse proviennent d'une pénurie de ressources humaines et fiscales, d'un manque d'expertise et d'équipements. Il faudra changer en profondeur l'infrastructure de recherche pour renverser ces obstacles. Il faut néanmoins entamer dès maintenant et en priorité quelques interventions à grande échelle dans le champ des comportements, avec des enquêtes de base adéquates, des enquêtes à passages répétés et des études longitudinales incluant des cohortes témoins même si ces interventions sont relativement coûteuses. Ce n'est qu'avec ces types d'études qu'on pourra se procurer une information plus définitive sur l'efficacité d'interventions variées; cette information fait désespérément défaut dans la plupart des études en Afrique subsaharienne. Plus de telles études se font attendre, et plus longtemps subsistera l'incertitude quant aux stratégies préventives du VIH qui fonctionnent le mieux et pour qui et dans quelles circonstances. Dans l'intervalle, on peut mener à terme l'évaluation de programmes de base et certaines recherches formatives et opérationnelles, travaux que les bailleurs de fonds devraient exiger comme partie des programmes à réaliser et à financer.

Recommandation 5-1. Les interventions pour promouvoir l'égalité entre les sexes méritent un rang élevé dans les priorités en tant que stratégies de prévention contre le VIH dans chaque pays.

Le risque que courent les femmes provient non pas de leur manque de connaissances, mais de leur subordination à l'échelle de la société. Les Etats peuvent introduire des changements de plusieurs façons pour donner plus de pouvoirs aux femmes: ils peuvent alléger la contrainte financière qui force les femmes à multiplier leurs partenaires par l'instauration de lois favorisant l'égalité d'accès à l'instruction, à la formation professionnelle et aux emplois avec des échelles de salaires communes, et leur donnant des droits de propriété et d'héritage identiques; ils peuvent promulguer et renforcer des lois contre le viol, fournir aux femmes les outils d'une action collective et faire connaître à tous les droits des femmes. La promotion du statut des femmes représente une stratégie à long terme qui aurait beaucoup d'effets favorables au développement en plus de réduire probablement la transmission du VIH et d'autres MTS.

Recommandation 5-2. Une priorité urgente s'impose à court terme aux donateurs internationaux en matière de recherche et de développement: procurer aux femmes un microbicide vaginal dont elles auraient le contrôle et qui leur garantirait une protection sans la participation de leur partenaire.

Ce microbicide n'est pas un substitut-gadget aux réformes de structure fondamentales qui sont nécessaires à l'obtention de l'égalité entre les sexes, mais plutôt une réponse temporaire et partielle à ce problème dans la mesure où celui-ci influence la transmission du VIH. Cependant, de la même façon que l'emploi de spermicides par les femmes peut réduire leur fécondité, l'utilisation d'un microbicide pourrait, en soi et par soi-même, aider à contenir la propagation du VIH.

Recommandation 5-3. Des recherches sont nécessaires pour répondre aux besoins de prévention anti-VIH provenant de diverses populations très vulnérables, en particuliers les personnes mobiles et celles qui vivent en marge de la société.

Le besoin se fait sentir de rejoindre les individus et les groupes mobiles avec des programmes compréhensibles et acceptables, particulièrement lorsqu'existent des barrières linguistiques et culturelles entre les migrants et la population locale. Il faut mettre au point des procédés efficaces de fourniture de services préventifs aux populations marginalisées des bidonvilles en pleine croissance et des camps de réfugiés; le principal défi qu'affrontent ces programmes tient au manque de ressources et d'appui du public pour des individus vivant dans de tels environnements.

Recommandation 5-4. Il faudrait mener des recherches additionnelles pour déterminer l'impact que des interventions anti-MTS spécifiques ont sur l'incidence de l'infection par VIH au sein de populations définies.

Il faut faire de la recherche pour déterminer dans quelle mesure les MTS contribuent à l'infection par le VIH, pour examiner l'importance de la synergie comportementale de la transmission des MTS et du VIH, et pour concevoir des programmes d'intervention plus efficaces. Le besoin se fait sentir d'évaluer avec quelles efficacité et faisabilité relatives les différentes interventions portant sur le traitement des MTs et le changement des comportements sexuels réduisent la transmission du VIH. Cette évaluation porte à la fois sur les effets des programmes destinés aux individus à haut risque de contracter et de transmettre des MTS, et sur les effets des programmes communautaires de lutte contre ces MTS. Quant aux interventions elles-mêmes, elles pourraient prendre la forme d'éducation sur les MTS, de distribution de condoms, de dépistage accru des MTS et de thérapie de masse par antibiotiques. Il est essentiel de disposer de données sur l'efficacité de telles interventions, particulièrement de celles qui visent à réduire la prévalence des MTS, en vue d'évaluer l'impact de ces réductions sur la propagation du VIH. Les recherches comportementales sur les moyens de rendre acceptables les différentes stratégies de contrôle des MTS devraient faire partie intégrante de la recherche épidémiologique.

Recommandation 5-5. On a besoin de recherche pour évaluer l'efficacité et le rapport coût-rendement de l'approche syndromique du diagnostic et du traitement des MTS.

Les tests cliniques des MTS coûtent cher et leur accessibilité est géographiquement réduite. D'où le besoin de recherches sur les moyens d'identifier les MTS de façon plus précise à l'aide de leurs symptômes. Il faut incorporer dans ces recherche des méthodes de dépistage, incluant des tests d'urine pour la chlamydia et la gonorrhée, et des tampons vaginaux auto-administrés pour la culture de la trichomonas et des colorations gram de la vaginose bactérielle. Il faudra faire les efforts nécessaires pour rendre ces techniques disponibles et abordables en vue de la surveillance, du diagnostic et de la validation dans le contexte des pays en développement.

Recommandation 5-6. Dans la planification des programmes de longue durée et l'allocation des ressources, les bailleurs de fonds devraient inclure dans leur travail de recherche des études de coût-rendement et comparer à son sujet la prévention du HIV à d'autres interventions en matière de santé.

Rares sont les évaluations des interventions à en avoir estimé l'efficacité en termes de changements de comportement, de baisse de séro-incidence et encore moins de coût-rendement. On s'attend à voir les études evaluatives actuellement en cours dans plusieurs pays d'Afrique subsaharienne fournir des données sur les coûts-rendements de diverses stratégies d'intervention contre le VIH. Cependant, la détermination de l'efficacité. de la prévention du VIH pose des problèmes de méthode complexes, de sorte qu'elle n'aboutira pas avant plusieurs années. En attendant, l'utilisation efficiente des ressources est de prime importance, compte tenu de leur pénurie qui pourrait bien s'aggraver encore. D'où l'importance vitale d'une analyse de base de l'ensemble des coûts des programmes et des coûts spécifiques reliés aux interventions. De simples analyses de coûts et des estimations des coûts-rendements pourraient apporter des données qui aideraient à prendre des décisions et à concevoir des programmes en matière de santé publique.

Recommandation 5-7. Il faudrait accorder une nette priorité à la recherche opérationnelle.

L'expansion de la pandémie du VIH/SIDA ces vingt dernières années en Afrique subsaharienne a entraîné la multiplication des réponses de la part des institutions et au niveau des collectivités locales, avec un besoin correspondant de mener des recherches opérationnelles pour améliorer l'efficacité, le coût-rendement et la qualité de ces réponses. En première ligne des besoins de recherche figurent l'augmentation des réussites rattachées aux interventions expérimentales, l'amélioration de l'efficacité et la baisse des coûts des programmes existants, l'examen du coût-rendement d'une liaison entre prévention anti-VIH et soins des personnes atteintes du VIH/SIDA, ainsi que l'amélioration de la sensibilité et de la spécificité des critères servant à cibler les interventions.

Recommandation 5-8. Il faudrait entreprendre des recherches mesurant l'impact des contraceptifs féminins d'occlusion sur la transmission du VIH.

Il faudrait faire des études qui déterminent l'efficacité préventive anti-MTS et anti-VIH des contraceptifs sous contrôle des femmes, tels que le diaphragme et les spermicides. Elles devraient inclure des recherches de terrain sur l'acceptabilité de ces méthodes. Il faudrait en outre intensifier les efforts pour intégrer des messages et des programmes appropriés de prévention contre le VIH/SIDA dans les programmes de planification familiale au chapitre du diagnostic, du transfert et du traitement des malades.

Recommandation 5-9. Des recherches comportementales sont requises à l'élaboration de programmes efficaces de consultations prénatales sur le VIH.

Compte tenu de sa propagation rapide parmi les femmes d'Afrique subsaharienne, le VIH continue, par sa transmission périnatale, d'avoir un impact important sur la morbidité et la mortalité des jeunes enfants dans les populations à forte séroprévalence du VIH. Il faudrait entreprendre des études à base de traitements modifiés recourant à la Zidovudine (AZT), à la globuline gamma hyperimmunisante, à la vitamine A, aux douches vaginales et autres moyens d'intervention, dans le but de déterminer leur efficacité d'ensemble et leur coût-rendement comme moyens de réduire la transmission périnatale du VIH.

L'ALLEGEMENT DE L'IMPACT DE L'EPIDEMIE

Le SIDA aura tant sur les individus que sur les sociétés un lourd impact social, psychologique, démographique et économique. En plus des souffrances physiques et des dommages qu'elle infligera, cette maladie peut entraîner des épreuves sociales et économiques, l'isolement, la réprobation et la discrimination.

Comme déjà dit, même si l'on arrêtait aujourd'hui la transmission du VIH, des millions d'Africains actuellement séropositifs développeraient quand même le SIDA et mourraient dans les dix à vingt prochaines années. Sa transmission n'a cependant pas cessé, bien au contraire. En effet, les informations en provenance de diverses populations africaines suggèrent soit une progression continue de la séroprévalence, soit un plafonnement à des niveaux d'une hauteur décourageante. Pendant plusieurs décennies au moins, l'épidémie du VIH/SIDA poursuivra ses ravages chez les jeunes adultes et leurs enfants avec des taux de mortalité pouvant décupler par rapport à ce qu'ils seraient sinon.

Bien que pas immédiatement visibles, les effets cumulatifs de cette «peste lente» sur la mortalité sont substantiels. Il y aura des hausses de mortalité en bas âges et aux âges adultes avec une réduction de l'espérance de vie. La croissance démographique déclinera plus rapidement que prévu, et la taille des populations en l'an 2000, surtout dans le bassin principal du SIDA, restera quelque peu inférieure aux projections faites en l'absence du SIDA. Parmi les pays les plus affligés, beaucoup verront leurs décès plus que doubler au cours des années 90 par rapport aux estimations en l'absence de cette maladie. Ces décès additionnels créeront des pressions accrues sur des services de santé déjà surchargés et sur des ménages individuels qui cherchent à s'en tirer avec des ressources limitées. La prise en charge des orphelins causera des préoccupations croissantes, et les modes traditionnels d'héritage et autres droits légaux seront mis à l'épreuve.

Relativement peu de recherches se sont intéressées à la morbidité et à la mortalité des adultes. Le SIDA fait partie d'une série de maladies susceptibles d'avoir une grande signification économique dans le tiers monde. Des maladies telles que la malaria et la rougeole ont beau être beaucoup plus fréquentes en Afrique, on a des motifs de croire que le SIDA y aura un impact économique plus grand. La longue période d'incubation du VIH fait en sorte que l'impact des niveaux actuels d'infection se ferait sentir pendant au moins dix ans même après l'arrêt immédiat de toute nouvelle infection. Dès lors, il y a beaucoup plus de bénéfices à tirer d'un cas de VIH évité que de tout autre maladie.

Les interventions atténuantes, qu'elles s'adressent aux malades du SIDA et à leur ménage ou à d'autres paliers de l'organisation sociale, exercent une ponction sur des ressources rares au détriment d'autres affectations, parmi lesquelles les efforts de prévention contre la transmission. C'est pourquoi de telles interventions devraient avoir pour la société une valeur au moins égale au coût des ressources qu'elles y consacrent. Des recherches sur cette question pourraient améliorer l'efficience des dépenses courantes tout en justifiant une décision favorable ou non à des dépenses supplémentaires.

RECOMMANDATION CLE N°4. Les recherches ayant pour but d'atténuer l'impact du VIH/SIDA devraient mettre l'accent sur les besoins des personnes souffrant de cette infection.

On en sait beaucoup plus sur la conception et la mise en oeuvre des programmes de prévention anti-VIH que sur la manière d'assurer des soins aux millions de personnes déjà contaminées par ce virus. Il se peut que des solutions rentables aux problèmes que rencontrent les sidatiques dans leur vie quotidienne, comme les soins palliatifs, les soins à temps partiel à domicile et les consultations en groupe, puissent enlever leur raison d'être à des interventions plus coûteuses.

Recommandation 6-1. Il y a un grand besoin de recherches permettant d'évaluer l'impact du SIDA sur les individus, les ménages, les firmes et les secteurs économiques.

Ces recherches d'impact devraient combiner les collectes de données tant qualitatives que quantitatives, et évaluer autant les effets à court qu'à long terme. Il y aurait un intérêt particulier à mener une recherche qui permettrait de comprendre l'impact du VIH/SIDA sur la pauvreté et sur les processus décisionnels des individus. Des recherches sont nécessaires pour s'assurer si la baisse de l'espérance de vie affaiblit la volonté d'épargner et d'investir dans des actifs financiers et réels, dans le capital humain et dans les relations nécessaires au maintien des interactions sociales. A long terme, l'impact du VIH/SIDA sur l'Afrique subsaharienne dépendra de la force et de la malléabilité avec lesquelles les réseaux sociaux et économiques assimileront les changements qui se produiront.

Recommandation 6-2. Puisqu'il n'est financièrement pas possible de tenter d'aider directement chaque ménage atteint, il faut étudier quels critères utiliser pour déterminer vers quels individus et communautés orienter l'aide, et quelles institutions devront fournir cette aide.

Cette épidémie a déjà frappé des millions de ménages d'Afrique subsaharienne et continuera sur sa lancée au moins pendant les vingt prochaines années. Les efforts pour en alléger les effets ont manqué de coordination et d'orientation précise sans avoir fait la preuve de leur capacité d'apporter des solutions aux malades et à leurs familles.

Recommandation 6-3. Il est de la plus haute importance de découvrir la manière optimale pour les gouvernements, les ONG et les donateurs d'intervenir dans la prévention contre le VIH/SIDA; d'où le besoins de plus d'études à ce sujet.

Les gouvernements se lancent maintenant dans la décentralisation et la privatisation des programmes SIDA en les confiant à divers types d'organisations non gouvernementales (ONG) par voie de contrats, de licences et de franchises. Il faut étudier les déterminants de l'efficacité de ces ONG dans la prévention et l'atténuation du SIDA, y compris chez celles dont ce n'est pas là l'objectif premier. Il faut définir avec grand soin les besoins d'assistance technique et la capacité d'absorption des ONG pour accroître leurs rôles en recherche et prévention et ne pas les surcharger ni faire mauvais usage de ressources rares.

MISE SUR PIED D'UNE CAPACITE DE RECHERCHE SUR LE SIDA

Il n'est pas question d'entreprendre une recherche utile sur le VIH/SIDA et d'en tirer des applications appropriées et efficaces sans mettre au préalable en place l'infrastructure nécessaire; c'est un prérequis qui fait souvent défaut en Afrique subsaharienne. C'est pourquoi, pratiquement toutes les recherches entreprises jusqu'à présent n'ont été possibles qu'avec la coopération technique et l'aide extérieure de la communauté internationale. Dès lors, mis à part le défi immédiat que représente l'identification des sujets vitaux de recherche, les réponses à leur apporter effectivement forment un énorme ensemble de défis qui restent à relever.

Les aspects clés d'une infrastructure de base permettant de faire de la bonne recherche portent sur un financement adéquat, un personnel qualifié, une technologie appropriée, ainsi que sur des capacités suffisantes de direction et d'administration pour planifier, exécuter, surveiller et évaluer les études. Même les pays développés éprouvent des difficultés à réunir les ressources nécessaires au lancement d'entreprises complexes de recherche; le coefficient de ces difficultés est beaucoup plus élevé en Afrique subsaharienne. Beaucoup d'universités y sont très négligées depuis plusieurs années. La mauvaise préparation des étudiants qui s'y inscrivent, les salaires tout à fait inadéquats des cadres et du personnel de soutien à tous les niveaux, le délabrement des bâtiments et des bibliothèques, ainsi que le manque de fonds nécessaires à l'entrée de ces universités dans l'âge technologique, expliquent leur lente agonie et le départ de leurs professeurs vers le secteur privé.

Une bonne partie des résultats des recherches achevées n'a pas été diffusée adéquatement, de sorte que ces résultats restent mal connus à travers le continent. Ajoutons qu'un défaut de coordination des efforts de recherche s'est traduit par des répétitions et par le besoin de «réinventer la roue».

Les politiques et pratiques des bailleurs de fonds viennent aggraver ces problèmes structurels avec, comme résultat, des études à court terme qui ne laissent pas aux capacités locales le temps de s'édifier, la prédominance d'un personnel expatrié dans la plupart des projets et, à tout le moins, la perception, de la part des récipiendaires de l'aide étrangère, que les projets répondent plutôt aux priorités des donateurs qu'à celles du pays concerné. Cependant, la place dominante qu'occupent les bailleurs de fonds internationaux dans la recherche sur le SIDA en Afrique découle du manque de financement domestique pour de telles recherches: beaucoup de gouvernements de ce continent apparaissent ne pas prendre au sérieux la gravité de cette épidémie et n'ont versé que des miettes à la recherche dans ce domaine.

A long terme, il est essentiel d'aider les pays d'Afrique subsaharienne à se doter de leur propre capacité de recherche en consolidant leurs universités et en augmentant les compétences techniques de leurs chercheurs. Il y a cependant beaucoup de débats et de controverses sur la meilleure façon d'y parvenir. Quoi qu'il en soit de cette meilleure façon, des progrès significatifs ont peu de chance de se produire tant que les gouvernements de ce sous-continent ne comprendront pas qu'ils doivent inscrire tout de go le SIDA dans les agendas de leurs recherches et politiques. Le manque de fonds constitue sans conteste un frein important à la quantité de recherches entreprises sur le VIH/SIDA. Comme sources de financement, il y a les collectivités locales, les firmes du secteur privé, le secteur public et les donateurs internationaux. Comme il est peu probable que les donateurs augmentent de façon substantielle leurs contributions à court terme, les gouvernements devront trouver des ressources supplémentaires. La position de faibless économique de la plupart des pays d'Afrique subsaharienne n'aidera cependant pas à convaincre leurs gouvernements de gonfler leur agenda de recherche dans un proche avenir.

RECOMMANDATION-CLE N°5. Il faut relier les institutions d'Afrique subsaharienne et les centres de recherche internationaux dans un vaste réseau d'activités incluant enseignement, recherche et échanges de professeurs et d'étudiants. Les donateurs internationaux devraient envisager sérieusement la création dans ce sous-continent d'une institution de recherche sur le SIDA avec une section solide de sciences sociales et comportementales.

Il y a un besoin urgent de consolider les institutions de recherche en Afrique subsaharienne. Les jumelages avec des organismes internationaux, surtout s'ils reposent sur un agenda de recherche progressif et bien défini, peuvent aider les institutions locales à se développer et à encadrer leurs chercheurs, en leur attribuant un financement à long terme relativement sûr, en leur offrant un support pour le traitement des données et pour la publication et la diffusion de manuscrits, et en procurant sur place une assistance technique et un entraînement à la recherche. L'expérience tirée d'un certain nombre de situations a démontré que cette collaboration à long terme non seulement apporte une contribution significative à la compréhension de l'épidémie du VIH/SIDA, mais est encore mutuellement bénéfique pour toutes les institutions concernées; elle pourrait s'avérer un franc succès en assurant un encadrement à des chercheurs africains très qualifiés et en leur permettant de rester dans leur pays d'origine.

Recommandation 7-1. Il faut augmenter le nombre de scientifiques africains bien formés pour faire des recherches sur le VIH.

La capacité de recherche ne peut pas s'améliorer en Afrique subsaharienne sans une augmentation du nombre de chercheurs locaux bien formés. Il y a quatre moyens d'introduire et de maintenir plus de chercheurs sur le terrain: 1° intégrer plus d'étudiants diplômés de second cycle et plus de jeunes professionnels dans toutes les initiatives de recherche reliées au SIDA; 2° créer des programmes avec subventions à montants réduits pour financer les projets de jeunes chercheurs; 3° ajuster les échelles de rémunération pour attirer et retenir des professionnels de talent; et 4° offrir aux chercheurs d'autres incitations à rester dans leur institution d'origine, sous forme de subventions de recherches à petite échelle, moins de charges d'enseignement et d'administration, et plus d'occasions de voyages internationaux. La fourniture d'une assistance technique à ces chercheurs est une priorité importante. Ils pourraient tirer profit d'ateliers de travail qui leur prêteraient main forte dans la conception et l'élaboration de projets de recherche, dans la détection de sources potentielles de financement, dans la rédaction de rapports décrivant leurs résultats intérimaires, et dans la préparation de manuscrits terminaux à soumettre à des revues avec évaluation par leurs pairs.

Recommandation 7-2. Chaque programme national de contrôle du SIDA devrait installer un centre national d'information sur cette maladie, qui mettrait sur pied et tiendrait à jour une banque de données sur toutes les recherches menées dans le pays en rapport avec le SIDA.

Il faudrait relier ces centres entre eux grâce à l'internet ou toute autre technique disponible. Ils devraient également disposer de banques de données de type CD-ROM (La plupart des bureaux nationaux des programmes de contrôle du SIDA disposent d'ordinateurs équipés en CD-ROM). Il faudrait en outre organiser des conférences nationales et régionales qui donneraient aux chercheurs l'occasion de discuter de leurs plans de recherche et de présenter leurs résultats à un groupe de chercheurs plus nombreux que ceux qui fréquentent les congrès internationaux.

Recommandation 7-3. Les pays d'Afrique subsaharienne doivent de toute urgence établir et mettre à jour périodiquement leurs priorités de recherche aux niveaux national et régional, offrant ainsi à leurs donateurs une base de discussion de leurs recherches sur le SIDA.

Il est important de réduire la proportion des recherches faites sur place qui sont commandées par les bailleurs de fonds.

Recommandation 7-4. Les organismes internationaux et les donateurs devraient utiliser le plus possible les ressources disponibles dans le pays.

Il est paradoxal de voir les donateurs sous-utiliser les talents disponibles dans la région. Le recours aux talents de la place peut solidifier les institutions locales, créer de l'emploi et offrir des débouchés aux chercheurs de talent en Afrique subsaharienne.

Recommandation 7-5. Il faut intensifier le dialogue entre chercheurs et décideurs.

Non seulement y a-t-il un besoin urgent d'accroître la capacité des pays à mener des recherches, mais il faut aussi en synthétiser mieux les résultats et les traduire en des programmes et politiques efficaces de prévention et de supervision. Sinon, les programmes de prévention ne répondront aux besoins locaux et ne seront taillés à la mesure des conditions locales que de façon marginale, et la recherche n'en sera que plus dévaluée et sous-financée. Les chercheurs doivent améliorer leur performance au chapitre de la rédaction des implications politiques de leurs travaux, tandis que les planificateurs et décideurs doivent faire savoir plus clairement aux chercheurs quelles informations leur sont nécessaires pour une planification efficace et pour l'élaboration de leurs programmes.

Recommandation 7-6. Si l'on veut promouvoir à l'avenir des stratégies plus efficaces de prévention du SIDA et d'allègement de ses effets, il faudra assurer une meilleure coordination entre donateurs, et particulièrement partager l'information sur les actions de prévention et de contrôle qui fonctionnent et celles qui ne fonctionnent pas.

Le nouveau programme conjoint des Nations Unies sur le SIDA (UNAIDS) jouera un rôle clé dans le travail à venir. Son succès exigera aussi une volonté politique plus ferme de la part des gouvernements d'Afrique subsaharienne et d'autres pays.

CONCLUSION: BESOIN DE MEILLEURES RECHERCHES EN SCIENCES SOCIALES ET COMPORTEMENTALES

Puisque le SIDA est une épidémie bien enracinée dans les comportements humains et activée par l'environnement économique, culturel et social, les sciences sociales et comportementales sont essentielles dans l'identification des solutions permettant sa mise sous contrôle. Jusqu'à présent, cependant, la part du lion dans le financement de la recherche sur le VIH/SIDA est allée aux études biomédicales centrées sur la nature du virus comme point de départ logique de la mise au point d'un vaccin ou d'un traitement curatif. Trop souvent prévaut la supposition implicite voulant que la recherche en sciences sociales et comportementales n'a sa place qu'en l'absence actuelle de vaccins ou de traitements efficaces contre cette maladie, comme si la découverte de ces derniers éliminerait à l'avenir tout besoin de poursuivre une telle recherche. Cette supposition n'est tout simplement pas vraie. A titre d'exemple, la résurgence de la tuberculose est devenue un des problèmes de santé les plus sérieux au monde, bien que nous disposions depuis près de 50 ans d'un remède efficace à 95 pour cent.

Pour prévenir efficacement le VIH/SIDA, il faudra fournir de façon continue d'énormes efforts visant à modifier durablement les comportements humains. Une seule dose d'interventions—comportementales ou médicales—ne suffira pas par elle-même à combattre cette épidémie. Nous avons besoin de plus de recherches sociales et comportementales pour mettre au point des stratégies préventives efficaces et acceptables qui affineront les programmes qui fonctionnent bien, et pour aider à trouver des moyens efficaces d'atténuer les impacts négatifs de cette épidémie.

L'absence d'une approche interdisciplinaire a limité l'interprétation et l'utilité de beaucoup de recherches épidémiologiques, comportementales et sociales. Il peut être difficile d'évaluer les données relatives aux déclarations de changements de comportement en l'absence d'une validation biologique du fait qu'un tel changement réduit l'infection par MTS/VIH. Les efforts pour modéliser les effets démographiques du VIH/SIDA se heurtent à la rareté d'ensembles de données combinant fécondité, mortalité, migration et autres informations socio-démographiques avec la sérologie VIH. Réciproquement, des études sérologiques qui ne prennent pas soin de récolter des données adéquates sur les comportements perdent une belle occasion d'estimer les effets qu'ont sur la propagation du VIH des facteurs clés tels que les pratiques sexuelles et les réseaux sexuels dans une population donnée. La conception, l'exécution et l'analyse des essais cliniques portant sur le contrôle des MTS, les vaccins VIH, les médicaments antirétroviraux, les méthodes contraceptives par barrière génitale et les virucides, toutes dépendent d'une recherche comportementale appropriée pour guider le choix des individus à tester, garantir la conformité au protocole de l'essai clinique et permettre une interprétation adéquate des résultats épidémiologiques; cette dernière inclut le besoin fondamental de neutraliser les différences observées dans les changements de comportement selon les groupes étudiés.

En attendant que de nouvelles recherches soient disponibles, il est crucial de continuer à employer les stratégies jugées les plus efficaces tout en en concevant de nouvelles qui soient innovantes. Le SIDA force les gens à revoir leurs valeurs et leurs comportements, et il modifie le contexte social. Les stratégies et les politiques doivent être à la fois capables de s'adapter à une situation en changement continuel, et réceptives aux découvertes des recherches qui se déroulent partout dans la région. Une collaboration effective entre la recherche et les interventions est la clé permettant de ralentir la propagation et l'impact de l'épidémie du VIH/SIDA en Afrique subsaharienne.

1

Introduction

PURPOSE OF THE REPORT

The human immunodeficiency virus (HIV) causes significant morbidity and ultimately death by destroying the immune system. The rapid spread of HIV has become one of the major health challenges of our time. The situation is particularly bleak in parts of sub-Saharan Africa, despite the fact that HIV-prevention programs have been initiated in every country in the region (Mann et al., 1992). The number of people infected with the virus, and with its attendant constellation of morbidity known as acquired immune deficiency syndrome (AIDS), continues to rise. Prevention efforts to date have included attempting to ensure a safe blood supply, launching massive public awareness campaigns about HIV and AIDS in an attempt to induce widespread behavior change, and instituting extensive marketing and distribution of condoms.

There is encouraging evidence that behavior-change interventions can be effective. Public awareness of the AIDS epidemic is extremely high throughout Africa, and condom sales have risen dramatically across the continent in the past few years. Other promising findings include a recent reduction in the prevalence of HIV-1 infection among young males in rural Uganda and evidence that treating sexually transmitted diseases (STDs) in rural Tanzania may reduce the spread of HIV (Mulder et al., 1995; Grosskurth et al., 1995). But many interventions have been experimental and small scale and so are not sufficient to reverse the course of the epidemic (Lamptey et al., 1993). At the same time, discovery of an effective vaccine or treatment is hindered by a variety of scientific, economic, ethical, and logistical obstacles, and neither is likely to be developed soon (International Ad Hoc Scientific Committee on HIV Vaccines, 1994a, 1994b; Cohen, 1993, 1994a, 1994b). As discussed further below, even if a vaccine or cure were developed, it would probably not be sufficient to bring a speedy end to the epidemic because of imperfect effectiveness, cost, and less than universal distribution and acceptance. In addition, many of the millions of people already infected with HIV are unaware of their status and so represent a pool capable of passing the virus to new cohorts. Therefore, with or without a vaccine, behavior change is necessary.

The purpose of this report is to consider the needs for research and data in the social and behavioral sciences that could help improve and extend existing successful programs and devise more effective strategies for preventing HIV transmission. We do so while recognizing that were such strategies to stop transmission tomorrow, a formidable burden of disease would remain because of the number of current infections. Thus the report also focuses on research and data that could support efforts to mitigate the impact of the AIDS epidemic.

BACKGROUND

Extent of the Epidemic

With little fanfare, the official number of AIDS cases worldwide since the start of the epidemic passed the 1 million mark near the end of 1994. By December 31, governments had notified the World Health Organization's (WHO) Geneva headquarters of 1,025,073 cases of the disease since the start of record keeping in 1980—a fact that was covered in a six-sentence story on an inside page of *The New York Times* (January 4, 1995). Moreover, given the chronic underreporting and under-diagnosis in developing countries, the actual number of AIDS cases may be four times as high (World Health Organization, 1995). The official statistics include people who have died, but they do not reflect the millions of people who are already infected with HIV but have yet to develop the symptoms of AIDS.

The situation is critical in sub-Saharan Africa, where WHO estimates that approximately 11 million adults and as many as 1 million children have been infected with HIV and where basic infrastructure, financial, and managerial resources, as well as health-care personnel to deal with the catastrophe, are all extremely scarce (World Health Organization, 1994, 1995). The magnitude of the epidemic varies widely across the continent. All of the most seriously afflicted countries are geographically concentrated in sub-Saharan Africa. With the exception of Côte d'Ivoire in West Africa, they all lie in a region of East and Southern Africa that stretches from Uganda and Kenya southward to include Rwanda, Burundi, Tanzania, Malawi, Zambia, Zimbabwe, and Botswana (U.S. Bureau of the Census, 1994; Stanecki and Way, 1994). In certain cities such as Kampala, Uganda; Lusaka, Zambia; Blantyre, Malawi; and Francistown,

Botswana, as many as 1 in 3 sexually active women is infected. In others, such as Niamey, Niger, and Bamako, Mali, fewer than 1 in 100 sexually active women may be affected (see Chapter 3). HIV infection and AIDS have been documented as the leading cause of adult death in Abidjan, Côte d'Ivoire; Kinshasa, Zaire; rural southwest Uganda; and various urban and rural parts of Tanzania (De Cock et al., 1990; Nelson et al., 1991; Kitange et al., 1994; Sewankambo et al., 1994; Mulder et al., 1994a, 1994b). A substantial proportion of many African governments' health budgets is now spent on the treatment and care of those with AIDS, and there are reports that half of some hospitals' medical-ward beds are occupied by AIDS patients (e.g., Hassig et al., 1990, for Mamo Yemo Hospital, Kinshasa, Zaire; Tembo et al., 1994, for Rubaga Hospital, Kampala, Uganda). More detailed HIV/AIDS statistics are presented in Chapter 3.

Patients seeking treatment today probably contracted the virus years ago. Thus no matter how serious the situation currently appears, it is only the tip of the iceberg. For those countries most severely affected by the epidemic, projections of the number of AIDS deaths in sub-Saharan Africa indicate that there will be very large increases in years to come. In many African countries, demographers expect adult and child mortality to increase enormously as a result of the epidemic. By the year 2010, if present trends in the growth of the epidemic continue, life expectancy is expected to fall from 66 to 33 years in Zambia, from 70 to 40 years in Zimbabwe, from 68 to 40 years in Kenya, and from 59 to 31 years in Uganda (Way and Stanecki, 1994; see also Chapter 6).

Need for Immediate Action

Perhaps the most important argument for immediate action to slow the further spread of HIV is that in many parts of the region, the epidemic has not yet peaked: not only is it bad, but it is getting worse. HIV tends to spread quickly among individuals at high risk of infection, such as commercial sex workers and their clients; it spreads thereafter—at first slowly and then at an accelerated pace—into the general population. In many sub-Saharan African countries the disease has already spread widely, but in others it has not. Because the cost-effectiveness of prevention efforts declines rapidly as the epidemic spreads, the timing of interventions is crucial. Failure to control the epidemic now will mean that far more costly and difficult interventions will be necessary in the future (Potts et al., 1991; World Bank, 1993). Prevention is considerably more cost-effective than "treatment" in the future, because "treatment" is limited solely to caring for the sick, burying the dead, and mitigating the economic impact of sickness and premature death. Lessons learned in those countries where the epidemic occurred early may help slow the further spread of HIV there and perhaps have an even greater impact in areas where HIV is not yet widespread.

A second reason for acting now to revitalize programs to combat HIV and AIDS is that African governments are facing a critical turning point in prevention efforts. Since their inception in the late 1980s, national prevention programs have operated on the assumption that traditional health education about HIV/AIDS would be sufficient to induce widespread behavior change. The most optimistic reading of the results of these prevention efforts is that they have been less successful than was at first hoped. While targeted behavioral interventions are undoubtedly an essential part of prevention, it proved overly optimistic to believe that the first prevention messages—some of which were hastily developed and quite generic—would induce widespread changes in sexual behavior. Prevention efforts clearly need to take into account both deeply rooted social mores and rapidly changing economic forces that are related in complex ways to the spread of the disease (Lurie et al., 1995a, 1995b; Feachem et al., 1995). Moreover, the level of initial response to the disease by the international community has not been sufficient to alter significantly the course of the epidemic. Additional strategies and resources are required if the spread of HIV is to be controlled.

In this connection, it may be noted that, as suggested above and confirmed by surveillance data collected to date, the HIV/AIDS epidemic has spread unevenly through sub-Saharan Africa. In fact, there is no single AIDS epidemic in Africa; rather, there are many different, interwoven epidemics (Piot et al., 1990). Initial reports of AIDS emerged in the early 1980s from Zaire and from areas surrounding Lake Victoria, particularly on the Uganda-Tanzania border. From there the epidemic quickly spread to neighboring countries as local cultural, social, economic, and biomedical conditions favored its rapid spread. Subsequently, the disease spread into the Southern African countries of Zambia and Zimbabwe and more recently into Botswana, Namibia, and parts of South Africa (U.S. Bureau of the Census, 1994; Stanecki and Way, 1994). Significantly, the epidemic has not moved westward nearly as rapidly (Caldwell, 1995). In West Africa, high levels of prevalence have been reported in Abidjan, Côte d'Ivoire, and adjacent areas of Ghana and Burkina Faso (Caldwell and Caldwell, 1993). In Nigeria the first AIDS case was detected in Lagos in 1987, but HIV sero-prevalence levels among Lagos sex workers are still under 15 percent, even though Lagos is the largest cosmopolitan city in Africa, is a major crossroads for commerce within the region, and has a highly active commercial sex industry (Caldwell, 1995). A recent study indicates that the prevalence of HIV-1 and HIV-2 among prostitutes in Lagos State may be rising rapidly (Dada et al., 1993), but a simple diffusion model clearly cannot explain adequately the set of events described above. Much more needs to be known about the role of various social, behavioral, cultural, economic, and biomedical factors that influence the nature and limits of the epidemic, and thus contribute to its differential spread.

Third, leadership of the global effort to fight AIDS is changing hands, creating an important opportunity to review what has been achieved to date and to develop a coherent global strategy for the foreseeable future. At the beginning of the epidemic, WHO assumed responsibility for the vast majority of activities related to AIDS prevention and control in Africa. In 1985, it established a Special Programme on AIDS, later renamed the Global Programme on AIDS (WHO/GPA), and began to work with ministries of health in African countries to develop their short- and medium-term plans to fight the epidemic. Furthermore, WHO/GPA offered extensive technical assistance to newly created national AIDS control programs in Africa. It provided as many as four resident expatriate advisers to some programs, all of whom were directly involved in the day-to-day implementation of HIV/AIDS-prevention efforts. Now, five additional United Nations organizations—the United Nations Children's Fund (UNICEF), the United Nations Development Program (UNDP), the United Nations Population Fund (UNFPA), the United Nations Educational, Scientific and Cultural Organization (UNESCO), and the World Bank—have made firm commitments to AIDS activities. As a result, the executive board of WHO recently recommended the creation of a joint United Nations Programme on AIDS (UNAIDS) to improve coordination among the various organizations and to boost the global response.

Fourth, for a number of reasons, current AIDS-prevention efforts may be reaching a plateau. Some donor agencies and governments in developed countries are beginning to suffer from "donor fatigue," induced partly by the realization that the epidemic is unlikely to affect the developed world as badly as was first feared, and partly by an inability to see how the money and effort expended on prevention thus far have affected the course of the epidemic. Many international donors do not want to commit themselves to providing care for the growing number of AIDS patients in countries where expenditures on health averaged less than US $15 per capita in 1990.

The most visible consequence of donor fatigue in Africa is the withdrawal of resident WHO/GPA advisers from national AIDS control programs. Because of financial constraints, WHO/GPA has been unable to sustain its initial level of support, and has been forced to reduce the number of personnel in virtually every country (see also Chapter 7). This reduction in assistance has had enormous costs, in both human and economic terms. It also increases the urgency for action by Africans and their governments. All national AIDS control programs are struggling to recover from the major withdrawal of WHO/GPA technical advisers and the concomitant reduction in funds and guidance, which have left an enormous gap in their ability to implement successful prevention programs. Instead of building on ten years of prevention experience, many programs are being forced to undergo a second infancy, and are repeating mistakes and relearning lessons (see Appendix A).

A fifth reason underscoring the need for immediate action is that AIDS is believed to be an especially costly disease, although the point has proved difficult to document. The economic consequences of AIDS stem from the direct and indirect costs to individuals, aggregated to the macro level. The direct cost of the disease is defined as the lifetime cost per patient for medical care. Estimates of this cost in Africa vary widely, from US $64 to $11,800 (see Chapter 6). The indirect cost reflects the cost to families and to society of lost potential years of productive life. AIDS tends to kill people in what should be their most productive years, and people with AIDS are often heads of households who leave behind multiple dependents. The results from one small study in Uganda, for example, suggest that the death of a household head as a result of AIDS can lead to reduced production of food crops, gradual depletion of household assets, withdrawal of children from school, and higher levels of household malnutrition (Barnett and Blaikie, 1992; see also Chapter 6). Furthermore, the disease does not affect the population uniformly. Studies in Rwanda, Uganda, Zaire, and Zambia during the late 1980s and early 1990s indicate that AIDS strikes disproportionately the wealthier, better-educated, and more skilled members of society (Ainsworth and Over, 1994a, 1994b). Consequently, the indirect cost of AIDS, which includes foregone earnings, is relatively higher among this subset of the total population. However, the absolute number of HIV cases is higher among lower socioeconomic groups. Thus there is still a great deal of uncertainty over the net impact of the epidemic on gross domestic product per capita because AIDS affects both the numerator (production) and the denominator (the size of the population).[1] Finally, the indirect cost of AIDS must include the social cost of coping with the approximately 10 million AIDS orphans expected by the year 2000.

One way to quantify the impact of AIDS in Africa is to calculate the number of "discounted healthy life years" that would be gained by averting a single new case of HIV. The benefits of averting a case—19.5 discounted healthy life years—are very high relative to other diseases; by this measure, HIV ranks lower than neonatal tetanus, but higher than other widespread illnesses such as malaria, tuberculosis, and measles. However, if one were to weigh the benefits of averting a case of HIV by an estimate of the productivity lost, HIV would rank highest among all diseases (Over and Piot, 1993).

The Need for Better Behavioral and Social Science Research

Because AIDS is an epidemic so firmly rooted in human behavior, driven by economic, cultural, and social conditions (see Chapter 2), the behavioral and social sciences have much to offer toward identifying solutions for its control. Yet to date, the vast majority of funding for HIV/AIDS research has been spent on biomedical research in an attempt to understand the nature of the virus as a logical starting point for identifying a vaccine or a cure. And the contribution of

[1]It is unclear which elements of the population will be hardest hit as the epidemic matures (see Chapter 6). For example, more highly educated African men may be first to lower their risk of infection by having fewer casual sex partners or by using condoms more often than less-educated men. In a study of HIV-1 infection in adults in rural Uganda, Nunn et al. (1994) found no statistically significant differences in HIV infection by level of occupation.

behavioral and social science research to understanding the impact of the epidemic in Africa has been minimal (Caldwell et al., 1993).

All too often it has been implicitly assumed that behavioral and social science research should take place only because there are currently no effective vaccines or treatments for the disease, as if the discovery of a vaccine or a cure would eliminate any further need for such research (Coates, 1993). As noted earlier, the assumption that availability of treatment solves all problems is simply not true. For example, the resurgence of tuberculosis has become one of the world's most serious health problems, even though a cure that is 95 percent effective has been available for almost 50 years. Moreover, historical evidence shows that mortality from tuberculosis fell sharply in England and Wales starting in the 1840s, so that a large part of the decline occurred before the introduction of an effective treatment 100 years later in 1947 (McKeown, 1979). To take another example, although treatments for other STDs, such as gonorrhea and syphilis, have existed for over 40 years, those diseases have not been eradicated, even in the United States (Turner et al., 1989), and remain a major cause of adult morbidity in Africa (Coates, 1993; Stanecki et al., 1995).

Furthermore, as noted above, even as the medical community searches for a technical solution, there is a growing realization that a vaccine or an effective treatment for HIV/AIDS will not be developed in the near future. In any event, for a vaccine or treatment to be useful in Africa, it would have to be inexpensive, easily administered, and effective against various strains of the virus (Lamptey et al., 1993). It is unlikely that the vaccines under current development would offer 100 percent protection (Coates, 1993). Millions of Africans are already infected, and it appears certain that millions more will become infected before an effective vaccine or treatment is available.

Fortunately, all African countries have implemented various forms of prevention and education campaigns to combat the spread of HIV. However, there is considerable variation in the design and execution of these programs. Good evaluations are scarce, but there are some early signs that certain prevention strategies have achieved limited success (see Chapter 5). For those programs that appear effective on a limited scale, the big questions are whether they are sustainable and whether they can be replicated successfully.

In summary, changing human behavior to slow the speed or limit the extent of transmission will always remain the first and probably the most important line of defense against HIV/AIDS. Effective prevention of the disease requires enormous and continued commitment in order to achieve lasting changes in human behavior. No one set of interventions—behavioral or medical—will be sufficient by itself to combat the HIV/AIDS epidemic. More and better behavioral, social, and medical research is needed to develop more effective and acceptable preventive strategies and to help find more effective ways of mitigating the negative impacts of the epidemic. Future efforts would benefit from a critical conceptual review of what has worked so far and why.

THE PANEL'S TASK

With the above considerations in mind, the National Research Council assembled a special panel of international experts in 1994, at the request of the U.S. Agency for International Development, to examine the nature of the HIV/AIDS epidemic in Africa from a social and behavioral viewpoint. The goal of the Panel on Data and Research Priorities for Arresting AIDS in Sub-Saharan Africa was to identify and describe the numerous behavioral and social factors that affect the spread of the HIV/AIDS epidemic in Africa, to identify or clarify strategic opportunities for donors and African governments to develop effective interventions both for preventing the spread of the epidemic and for mitigating its impacts, and to elucidate the most pressing research requirements over the next 5 to 7 years for facilitating the development of more effective prevention and control strategies in the future.

At the outset, the panel realized that this mandate was nearly impossible: the strategies and issues surrounding the HIV/AIDS epidemic are extremely complex and change constantly as the epidemic evolves. No single report could be expected to address the full range of potential issues. Therefore the panel decided to focus its efforts on identifying data and research priorities. Even so, the task is daunting. Sub-Saharan Africa is a geographically, demographically, socially, and culturally heterogeneous region (see Chapter 2). Thus, as suggested above, we do not find homogeneity in the distribution of HIV and AIDS or in the behavioral factors and social contexts that are so vital in shaping the nature and the spread of the epidemic. There are enormous differences within and among countries with regard to the rate of spread, the socioeconomic groups most severely affected, the cultural contexts of practices that place populations at risk, and the male-to-female ratio of new infections. There are also important differences among communities with regard to the level of AIDS awareness and the degree of stigmatization associated with the disease (Kaijage, 1994a, 1994b). Finally, AIDS is contracted from two different viruses—HIV-1 and HIV-2. Although the two have the same modes of transmission, HIV-2 is concentrated in West Africa, is less dangerous, and is far less common and less well understood than HIV-1 (see Chapter 3). Hence, the only way to respond effectively to the epidemic is to plan at the national, or preferably the subnational or regional, level.

A further complication facing the panel from the outset was that if AIDS research is to be successful, it must be perceived as useful and relevant by the community under study. To make the panel's efforts as participatory as possible, several members visited selected sub-Saharan African countries during the course of the panel's work and talked with many African policy makers, researchers, and planners. In addition, in January and February 1995, a subcommittee of the panel spent 3 weeks in Cameroon, Tanzania, and Zambia talking with senior African officials to solicit their views on the extent of the AIDS crisis in their countries and the appropriateness of the existing level of response (see Appendix A).

Given time and resource constraints, it was impractical to visit and talk with more than a small percentage of the large number of people working in this field. However, we attempted to survey the views of a cross-section of interested parties and tried to represent their views faithfully and accurately.

This report is the product of the panel's deliberations. We have focused on identifying research priorities that would be most useful to fund and coordinate centrally and that would have the greatest general applicability, as opposed to being useful only in a particular setting or environment. We hope this report will serve as a useful starting point for future participatory discussions among researchers from both developed and developing countries.

ORGANIZATION OF THE REPORT

This report offers recommendations in five critical areas: monitoring of the overall status and context of the HIV/AIDS epidemic in Africa, gathering of information on sexual behaviors associated with the spread of the epidemic, primary HIV-prevention strategies, strategies for mitigating the impact of the epidemic, and the need for building an indigenous capacity for AIDS-related research in Africa. Given the vast heterogeneity of the region with respect to, inter alia, the nature and severity of the epidemic and the cultural, social, economic, and political climate within which prevention and mitigation efforts are working, the relative weight given to these five areas must be judged on a country-by-country basis. Likewise, the relative priorities for recommendations offered within chapters will vary by country. Nevertheless, the panel has identified five key recommendations for immediate action.

In general, the report starts by presenting information on the societal context and basic epidemiology of the epidemic and moves to identifying strategies for preventing the further spread of the epidemic or mitigating its effects. Chapters 3 through 6 each end with a set of recommendations for future research. Chapter 7 ends with a set of recommendations for building capacity to accomplish this research. Our five key recommendations are numbered separately from our other recommendations, which are numbered by chapter in the order in which they appear.

True understanding of the HIV/AIDS epidemic in Africa cannot be achieved without an appreciation of the multiple social, behavioral, economic, and cultural obstacles to HIV/AIDS prevention in the region. The societal context within which people are born and raised, are initiated to sexuality, and lead their lives strongly influences their perceptions of risk and their sexual behavior. Social, cultural, and economic factors can act either to speed or to retard the spread of infection. Effective interventions must target not only individual perceptions and behavior, but also their larger context. Chapter 2 introduces and discusses some of the more salient features of the societal context that affect the size and shape of the epidemic.

Chapter 3 provides a comprehensive overview of what is currently known about the epidemiology of the HIV/AIDS epidemic in sub-Saharan Africa. It provides up-to-date data on the state of the epidemic and reviews what is known about the major modes of HIV transmission, including sexual, perinatal, and parenteral. A growing body of data suggests that HIV cannot be considered in isolation from other STDs because it shares with them modes of transmission and behavioral risk factors. More important, there is evidence that other STDs may increase susceptibility to and transmission of HIV, so that STD treatment and prevention may serve as an important weapon in curbing the HIV/AIDS epidemic.

Heterosexual transmission is responsible for at least 80 percent of HIV infections in sub-Saharan Africa. Information is needed on sexual behaviors, particularly numbers of partners, sexual networks and their determinants, types of safe and nonpenetrative sex, condom use, and care-seeking behavior for symptoms of STDs in order to understand barriers to the effective and rapid adoption of preventive measures; to develop more effective approaches to AIDS and STD prevention; and to provide baseline data in order to evaluate the success of an intervention. Chapter 4 focuses on social and cultural practices that may promote or inhibit the sexual spread of HIV and summarizes what we know about sexual practices and beliefs, levels of sexual activity, condom use, and levels of AIDS awareness.

Chapter 5 examines what we know about designing effective prevention programs. There are many challenges to designing effective interventions targeted to African men, women, and youth. The chapter highlights some of the strategies that have been implemented and uses case studies to illustrate both targeted strategies and comprehensive programs. Basic principles of successful intervention programs include adapting the program to local conditions, carefully targeting the audience, building local capacity, ensuring community participation, evaluating results, and using the results from evaluation studies to improve the program. Successful intervention programs should also be multidisciplinary and multifaceted and involve multiple contacts with targeted populations. As Chapter 5 explains, however, it is not easy to demonstrate the success of a particular intervention because it is difficult to define and measure outcome variables such as "better health status" and to determine whether the intervention in question was the reason for a desired change. Consequently, the need for solid evaluation research is still urgent. There is also an urgent need to design better ways to target adolescents and women for prevention messages.

Evidence from a variety of sources around Africa suggests that seroprevalence either is continuing to climb or has leveled off at discouragingly high levels. Even if the transmission of HIV were halted today, the millions of young adults and infant Africans currently infected with HIV would develop AIDS and die over the next 10 to 20 years. Increasingly, governments are obliged to spend money on mitigation assistance. Policy analysis of this problem is badly needed, both to improve the efficiency of current expenditures and to determine whether additional spending is needed. Chapter 6 reviews the evidence on the current and the inescapable future impacts of AIDS in Africa, including the social, psychological, demographic, and economic impacts on both individuals and societies. A great deal of attention has been devoted to attempting to limit the further spread of HIV. Considerably less thought has focused on identifying solutions to the problem of coping with the millions of people in sub-Saharan Africa already infected with the virus. It is obvious that the impact on infected individuals is devastating; in addition to the physical suffering and grief caused by the disease, AIDS can lead to social and economic hardship, isolation, stigmatization, and discrimination. Relatively little research has been conducted on the economic consequences of adult morbidity and mortality, which are far less obvious.

As noted above, throughout the report the panel has identified research and data priorities intended to improve our understanding of the social and behavioral factors influencing the spread of HIV/AIDS in Africa. The hope is that this understanding can in turn be used to inform the development of prevention strategies for arresting the spread of HIV/AIDS and mitigation strategies for lessening the impact of the epidemic. Undertaking effective research, however, requires that an appropriate infrastructure be in place, a prerequisite that is often lacking in Africa. As a result, virtually all research on AIDS in Africa undertaken to date has been made possible only through technical cooperation and assistance from the international community. Beyond the immediate challenge of the panel's mandate—identifying the critical research priorities—there remain enormous practical challenges surrounding the implementation of those priorities. The final chapter examines the enormous constraints to conducting research in sub-Saharan Africa and proposes means of alleviating some of these problems, including establishing a sub-Saharan Africa AIDS research institute with a strong behavioral and social science component.

At the moment there is no cure for AIDS, but prevention works, and behavioral and social science research has a critical role to play in designing more effective prevention programs. Yet access to results from studies that have been conducted throughout the region remains fragmentary; many studies have not been committed to paper, while others have not been disseminated widely, even within the country where the research was undertaken. This gap obviously hinders effective design, direction, and evaluation of programs and leads to duplication of effort. There is an urgent need to evaluate many of the strategies that have been implemented so far to determine whether they have been effective or cost-efficient and whether they warrant replication or expansion. At the same time, we note that AIDS is an extremely rapidly moving field in terms of both research and prevention.

Until new research is available, it is very important to keep trying the existing strategies, as well as designing new and innovative ones. Some interventions that did not work well one year might work well the next because the severity of the epidemic is forcing people to rethink their values and behavior and is changing the social context. Strategies and policies should be responsive to the ever-changing situation, as well as receptive to the findings of research being carried out throughout the region. An effective partnership between research and program interventions will be key to lessening the spread and impact of the HIV/AIDS epidemic in sub-Saharan Africa.

2

Societal Context

Why is it that thousands of people are still being infected every day with the HIV virus even though national AIDS control programs worldwide have conducted extensive information and education campaigns to teach people how to avoid infection? As suggested in Chapter 1, a decade of HIV/AIDS-prevention work in sub-Saharan Africa and elsewhere has demonstrated that while information and education about how to prevent transmission of HIV are necessary for inducing behavior change, such an approach by itself has been unable to induce sufficiently widespread behavioral change to alter significantly the course of the epidemic. Planners and policy makers must be cognizant of the societal context, and attempt to modify it in ways that are conducive to and supportive of change.

From this perspective emerges a distinction between proximal interventions that attempt to interrupt HIV transmission directly and contextual or indirect interventions that attempt to change the environment in which the HIV/AIDS epidemic and many other communicable and noncommunicable diseases are deeply rooted (Mann et al., 1992). Empirical evidence accumulated during more than a decade of prevention work indicates that both proximal and contextual interventions are necessary to reduce the spread of HIV, as well as to mitigate its impact (Mann et al., 1992). It is difficult to overemphasize the importance of contextual intervention as a weapon against HIV; policy makers simply must begin to consider reform of laws and policies outside the health sector as legitimate AIDS-reduction strategies. For example, discussing the merits of alternative HIV-prevention strategies for women, Heise and Elias (1995:939) conclude:

> Subsidizing the uniform and school fees of adolescent girls in Africa might actually do more to reduce HIV transmission—by eliminating the need for

Sugar Daddies—than the most sophisticated "peer education" campaign. It would also reduce unwanted pregnancy, raise the age of marriage and decrease infant mortality, not to mention promoting gender equality. One benefit of women-centered AIDS strategies is that they have positive backward links to many other development objectives.

Thus effective interventions must target not only individual perceptions and behavior, but also the larger context within which those perceptions and behaviors are shaped. In Africa, that context includes laws and policies, social and family structure, sexual debut and the construction of sexual careers, medical and program factors, and economic factors. Structural and individual factors combined produce behavior change. This chapter focuses on those contextual issues we feel may be most directly addressed through intervention.

A wide variety of social, political, and economic factors affect the societal context within which the AIDS epidemic must be viewed; similarly, these factors provide the context for the rest of this report. Among the more salient features of the societal context that affect the size and shape of the HIV/AIDS epidemic in sub-Saharan Africa are the age and gender composition of the population; the construction of sex roles and expectations within society; inequities in gender roles and power; sexual access to young girls and the acceptance of widespread differentials in the ages of sexual partners; rapid urbanization under conditions of high unemployment; considerable transactional sex fostered by limited earning opportunities for women; and lack of access to health care, particularly treatment for STDs. These factors are often exacerbated by social upheavals related to economic distress, political conflicts, and wars. Of course, sub-Saharan Africa is quite heterogeneous with regard to some, if not all, of these factors, so that there is enormous variation in the situation from country to country; particularly noteworthy are the differences between West Africa and East and Southern Africa.

SOCIAL STRUCTURE AND FAMILY ORGANIZATION

Sub-Saharan Africa is home to around one-tenth of the world's population. Its approximately 1,700 identified ethnic groups constitute over 30 percent of the world's cultures. Each group may have its own form of social organization and its own norms governing reproductive life, family formation, inheritance, and so on. Childbirth and marriage may be synonymous in some groups, or one may be expected to precede the other (in either order). Marriage may be a salient event, an extended process, or simply a convenient social label. Expectations and rules for marriage vary enormously. It may be permanent or fleeting; it may occur once in a lifetime, repeatedly over several years, or concurrently with other marriages. It may carry with it the expectation of fidelity or imply a duty of multiple partnership. Several types of unions may coexist. Some ethnographic accounts describe as many as 14 differently named transactions under the umbrella of marriage in a single society, although colonial administrations apparently attempted to narrow the field, confining amorphous unions within strictly defined legal and religious bounds (Guyer, 1994).

Clearly, the norms within a given society affect common behaviors that put people at risk of HIV infection as well as the messages that are most likely to alter those behaviors effectively. But it is vital to recognize that these norms are changing. In almost every society, sexual relations, reproduction, and marriage are governed by dynamic rules that will change in response to changes both in economic and demographic conditions and in the nature and course of the HIV/AIDS epidemic. In this age of increasing communication, researchers may well find that such changes are taking disparate cultures in a similar direction.

Studies on sexual behavior in sub-Saharan Africa share certain broad assumptions about the historical and social background of the study populations. Following is a brief description of the most common assumptions. Not all these reported findings are well substantiated, and many are probably too broad. However, they provide a review of current knowledge, demonstrate the diversity found, and reveal some of the complex structural issues that affect the epidemic.

It is widely believed that colonial urbanization fundamentally changed the terms of family life and gender relations in sub-Saharan Africa. The levers of this change were colonial administration and proselytizing, male migration to the cities, the creation of jobs—such as cash cropping—dominated by men, and the consequent economic marginalization of women. As taxation monetized the economy, women were forced to earn money where they could. In the indigenous cities of West Africa, they frequently did so through trading; as a result, West African women often have their own income and control their own budget without interference from their husbands. In colonial towns concentrated in East and Southern Africa, single women in town were often automatically associated with the exchange of sex for money or other support (Larson, 1989; Standing and Kisekka, 1989). Enforced migration and the search for support in a dislocated situation set the tone for multipartner relationships (Preston-Whyte, 1994).

Polygyny was common in nearly all sub-Saharan African societies and remains so, but to varying degrees (see Figure 2-1). Formal polygyny is more common in rural than in urban areas, probably because polygyny is well suited to agriculture. Nevertheless, various forms of multiple partnerships are also common in many urban areas, such as the taking of mistresses or "outside wives" (Larson, 1989; Standing and Kisekka, 1989; Hogsborg and Aaby, 1992; Carballo and Kenya, 1994; Rutenberg et al., 1994). Polygyny allows older men with resources to monopolize young women, leaving young men to search for sex outside stable unions (Caldwell et al., 1993). Junior wives may have limited access to family resources and need to supplement them by seeking outside support (Orubuloye et al., 1991). Some researchers have argued that the existence of polygyny may encourage a man to initiate a search for new wives during culturally prescribed periods of sexual abstinence following a birth to an existing wife (Larson, 1989; Orubuloye et al., 1993).

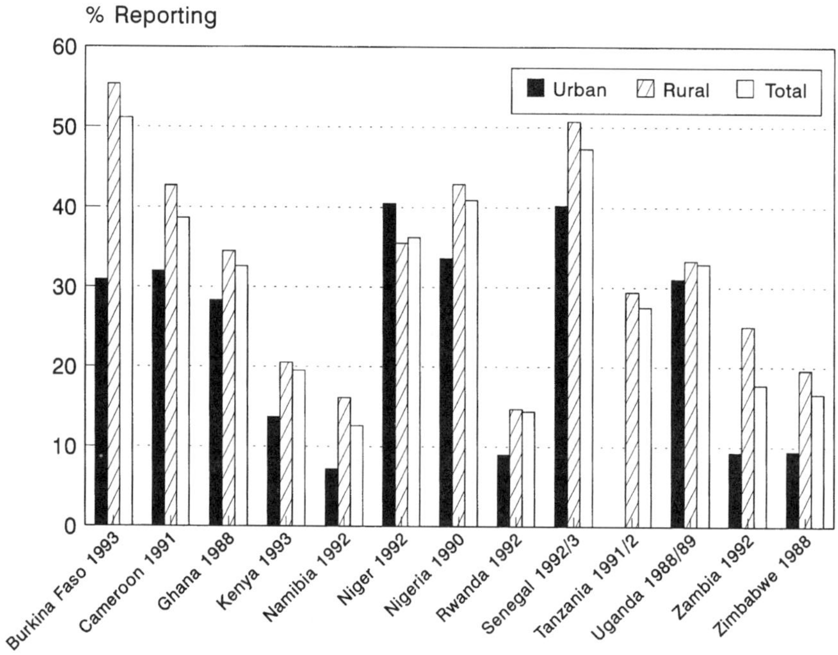

FIGURE 2-1 Percentage of Women in Polygynous Unions. SOURCES: Burkino Faso: Konaté et al. (1994); Cameroon: Balépa et al. (1992); Ghana: Ghana Statistical Service (1989); Kenya: National Council for Population and Development (1994); Namibia: Katjiuanjo et al. (1993); Niger: Kourguéni et al. (1993); Nigeria: Federal Office of Statistics [Nigeria] (1992); Rwanda: Barrère et al. (1994); Senegal: Ndiaye et al. (1994); Tanzania: Ngallaba et al. (1993); Uganda: Kaijuka et al. (1989); Zambia: Gaisie et al. (1993); Zimbabwe: Central Statistical Office [Zimbabwe] (1989).

In all sub-Saharan African societies, sexual contact forms part of an exceedingly complex network of relationships that may involve formal or informal marriage; permanent support of a woman or her children; regular or occasional gifts; or straight payment for sex, either on a repeated basis or as a single event. The same relationship may be viewed differently by different people, and the motivations of the various actors in the relationship will frequently differ as well. Both patrilineal and matrilineal kinship systems are common, and each may have different implications for sexual behavior.

Women in West Africa have traditionally enjoyed more autonomy than women in East and Southern Africa, participating in the labor force in a wide range of income-generating activities such as trading. Furthermore, it is claimed that women in West Africa who separate from their husbands can easily return to their families and usually retain their children, even in patrilineal societies

(Caldwell and Caldwell, 1993). By contrast, rural women's labor force participation in East Africa has largely been confined to subsistence farming and beer-making. In urban areas in East Africa, women are engaged mainly in the preparation and sale of food products or the production of alcoholic beverages, the latter being closely linked to the commercial sex industry (Caldwell and Caldwell, 1993). Finally, divorced or separated women in East Africa are less likely to retain their children or to be able to return to their families of origin. Therefore they are more likely, the Caldwells argue, to be forced to turn to prostitution (Caldwell and Caldwell, 1993).

SEXUAL BEHAVIOR AND HIV/AIDS

Knowledge of social and sexual networks, and of their determinants, is important in projecting the future course of the epidemic and in developing preventive strategies. Studies have begun to address how sexual and social networks channel and potentially amplify HIV transmission in sub-Saharan Africa (Dyson, 1992; Caldwell et al., 1993; Orubuloye et al., 1994; Morris et al., 1995); in addition to migration and transportation systems, such networking encompasses the role of local markets (Edmondson et al., 1993; Orubuloye et al., 1993) and local "mating networks" (Orubuloye et al., 1991; Caldwell et al., 1992; Obbo, 1993). Asymmetric age matching, whereby young women have sexual contact with older men, results in a young cohort of women being exposed to older male partners with higher HIV prevalence (Edmondson et al., 1993; Ssengonzi et al., 1995); this pattern facilitates the spread of infection from generation to generation. Perhaps even more significant, the social context of marriage and child-bearing is changing dramatically (Bledsoe and Cohen, 1993). Until recent decades, females in most African societies married at puberty, and there were strong religious sanctions against sex before circumcision or nubility or pubertal ceremonies. Now, according to some evidence, age at menarche may be declining, and formal education and other forms of training are delaying marriage. The result is an ever-rising number of postpubertal single women as a feature of society (see, for example, Antoine and Nanitelamio, 1991).

The composition of sexual networks may have strong implications for the speed or direction of viral transmission. Patterns observed in some African settings of mixing between people in high-risk core groups and others in the general population (as opposed to simple assortative mixing with strong within-group partner preference, such as pairings confined to well-defined groups) can result in substantial spread of sexually transmitted infections, including HIV, among the general population (see Anderson and May, 1992). There is also a growing realization that outside partnerships concurrent with a recognized union, including those that are stable and long term (a not uncommon phenomenon in many sub-Saharan African settings), may be frequent sources of HIV transmission—potentially as much as or more than sequential, short-term partnerships (Hudson, 1993; Morris et al., 1995).

At the same time, however, networks also serve as bases for social support and the development of new behavioral norms. When a person is well integrated into a stable social network, that network becomes a potential resource for behavioral intervention (Morris et al., 1995). Support for behavioral change, such as acceptance of condoms, can enable individuals to negotiate these matters more effectively when confronted with a resistant partner. By the same token, the absence of social networks can make behavioral change more difficult to achieve. For example, young women working in bars may have little social support for developing and negotiating safer sexual practices because they are often migrants from elsewhere and not from the local community.

Several factors lend a special character to conjugal bonds in many sub-Saharan societies: the relatively greater importance placed on lineage and intergenerational links than on marital ties; traditional separation of spousal economic activities and responsibilities; and polygyny (a common feature of married life in many sub-Saharan African populations, although its prevalence varies considerably according to region and ethnic group), which can result in substantial age differences between husbands and later wives (Caldwell et al., 1989; Goldman and Pebley, 1989; Pebley and Mbugua, 1989; Orubuloye et al., 1990). Some men choose to seek extramarital partners as a result of long periods of postpartum abstinence, particularly in West Africa (Orubuloye et al., 1991). Moreover, in certain African societies, premarital sex is an accepted practice, particularly for men. Indeed, a recent study among the Yoruba in Nigeria found that members of either sex who did not engage in such relations could be accused of being timid, sick, or afraid of disease (Orubuloye et al., 1990).[1] Although more women are attending secondary school and fewer are marrying before age 20, the proportion of young women giving birth has remained relatively constant. Because more young mothers are unmarried, premarital births as a percentage of all births to women under age 20 have risen, particularly in Botswana and Kenya, but also to a lesser degree in Uganda and Zimbabwe (Bledsoe and Cohen, 1993).

Across sub-Saharan Africa, a substantial demand for transactional sex outside marriage is met by various types of commercial sex workers. In many cities, particularly those in East and Southern Africa, a core group of prostitutes have multiple clients a week, or in some cases a day. By contrast, in other cities such a pattern is rarer, and commercial sex workers tend to have long-term, albeit sporadic, relationships with a few men over an extended period of time (Caldwell et al., 1989; Karanja, 1987). Consequently, many men surveyed in Ekiti, Nigeria,

---

[1]Again, the heterogeneity of the region makes it difficult to offer many generalizations. The description of the African family painted above may be truer of the situation in West Africa than in East or Southern Africa (see Caldwell et al., 1992).

"were reluctant to identify some of their sexual contacts as commercial, because they had known the women involved over a period of time and felt that their relationship involved more than a monetary transaction" (Orubuloye et al., 1992:344). The need for discretion in such relationships reduces condom use because use would imply that at least one of the partners has multiple outside relationships.

In the latter pattern, i.e., multiple long-term relationships, labels such as "prostitution" and "commercial sex worker"[2] are not readily applicable. Women play various roles in society; and many women who take part in what might be considered commercial sex do not view themselves, and often are not viewed by their communities, as prostitutes or commercial sex workers. Hence identifying such women for targeted interventions may be very difficult, if not impossible. In the Yoruba study, approximately one-fifth of women having premarital sex said they did so primarily for material returns (gifts in rural areas and money in town) (Orubuloye et al., 1990). Multiple partnerships, the need for discretion, and unacknowledged commercial sex all militate against the effectiveness of contact tracing or of interventions aimed primarily at "core groups" such as identifiable commercial sex workers. The economic situation of many African women results in a context where "transactions relating to sexual activity have been looked upon . . . as equally normal as those relating to work" (Caldwell et al., 1989:203).

High fertility continues to be an important survival strategy in many contexts for families in Africa, particularly for women. This imperative has at least two implications. First, females in premarital relationships tend to be under pressure to prove their fertility. The desire to have children to ensure the survival of the clan and the family in the face of AIDS reduces the probability of using condoms (Preston-Whyte, 1994). Second, to avoid jeopardizing their marital relationship, women may enter or remain in sexual unions that have the potential to place them at risk of HIV infection as a result of the extramarital activities of their husbands.

Use of modern family planning is still fairly limited in Africa. Statistics gathered from family planning programs and contraceptive surveys show low, albeit rapidly growing, acceptance and use of modern contraceptive methods. Use of modern contraceptives among women of childbearing age is below 10 percent in all but five sub-Saharan African countries; condom use is below 1 percent nationally in all sub-Saharan African countries except Botswana, Cameroon, Ghana, Malawi, and Zambia (United Nations Economic Commission for Africa, 1995). Condoms tend to be used only with an outside partner, rather than with one's spouse, and there is a tendency among both men and women to

[2]The term "commercial sex worker" is used to convey a diversity of sexual-economic exchange patterns that is not captured by the concept of full-time prostitution. For more information about the diversity in sex work and the various definitions of prostitution, see de Zalduondo et al. (1991).

regard condoms as having a stigmatizing association with promiscuity (McGinn et al., 1989; Wawer et al., 1990; Schoepf, 1992). Moreover, husbands and wives generally report little discussion of sexual matters, including family planning, with their spouses. Chapter 4 provides more detailed information on patterns of sexual behavior and HIV/AIDS in the African context.

MOBILITY

Rural-Urban Migration

One hypothesis for the emergence of the HIV/AIDS epidemic in sub-Saharan Africa is that the migration of individuals from areas of low endemicity to new, uninfected areas was instrumental in the eventual dissemination of HIV into larger, more congregated populations (Quinn, 1994). This hypothesis is supported by several findings.

First, following independence in the 1960s, many African countries experienced dramatic demographic changes, including migration from remote regions to more populous areas. For example, the number of African cities with more than 500,000 inhabitants increased rapidly from 3 in 1960 to 28 by 1980 (United Nations, 1991). By the year 2000, the projected proportion of people living in urban centers is expected to exceed one-third of the national populations in all regions except East Africa (Oucho and Gould, 1993). Demographically, migrants have tended to be young adult males. Early in the process, there was little economic or social encouragement for women to migrate; over time, however, growing numbers of women have come to the cities to work in trade and processing or in the entertainment/commercial sex work sector (Okoth-Ogendo, 1991). Ghana and Côte d'Ivoire offer paradigms of such female migration (Denis et al., 1987; Neequaye et al., 1988). Because of the large numbers of migrants to urban centers, unemployment and social disruption became common, and as a result, many individuals, mostly women, turned to commercial sex work as a means of survival. During the period of rapid urbanization, health officials noted marked increases in sexually transmitted diseases, more recently including HIV-1 infection, within the growing cities (Quinn, 1994). In addition, the economic recession may have aggravated the transmission of HIV by increasing the population at risk through increased migration, disruption of rural families, and poverty (Quinn, 1994).

Cities in East and Southern Africa have attracted a much higher proportion of male than female migrants, so that sex ratios in the cities are quite unbalanced. This pattern is also partly a legacy from the colonial period, when men were recruited for work in the mines or for blue- and white-collar jobs in urban areas, but were often prohibited from bringing their wives or families to town with them (Oucho and Gould, 1993). Sex ratios in many mining areas and cities in East and Southern Africa often exceed 110 (and sometimes 120) men to every 100 women.

Only in Abidjan, Côte d'Ivoire, is such an imbalanced sex ratio observed in West Africa. This surplus of men in urban areas has created a large demand for transactional sex that is met by prostitution (Caldwell et al., 1989, 1992; Caldwell and Caldwell, 1993).

Truck drivers, the military, and female commercial sex workers are all well recognized as high-risk populations for HIV infection, and are all highly mobile (Smallman-Raynor and Cliff, 1991; Orubuloye et al., 1993). Women involved in commercial sex work frequently move from one locality to another because of economic pressures. For example, in South Africa, the migrant labor system created a market for commercial sex in mining towns and established geographic networks of sexual relationships within and between urban and rural communities (Jochleson et al., 1991). Industrialization and the rapid growth of the mining industry led to an epidemic of STDs among migrant workers (Hunt, 1989). HIV prevalence in South Africa has been recorded as ranging from less than 1 percent among local residents to as high as 18 percent among migrants from Malawi (Quinn, 1994). Women who provide migrant mine workers with sexual services also come from socially and economically marginalized groups in rural and urban areas, many of which also have high rates of HIV infection and STDs, further enabling the spread of both (Pepin et al., 1989; Wasserheit, 1992). These data illustrate one end of the spectrum of behavior, where multiple partners and frequent partner changes are common. Thus, male labor migrants relocating to work without their spouses and commercial sex workers represent "core" populations involved in high-risk activity that act as a major engines of HIV transmission (Anderson, 1991).

Diffusion via Major Roads

Several studies have suggested that the geographic distribution of HIV and AIDS also reflects a diffusion process in which major roads act as principal corridors for the spread of the virus between urban areas and other proximal communities (Wood, 1988; Carswell et al., 1989). Such diffusion is related to contact of local populations with truck drivers, particularly between the drivers and local women, many of whom work in roadside bars or lodges but are not formally considered to be commercial sex workers. In one study of truck drivers and their assistants, one-third were found to be HIV-infected (Bwayo et al., 1991a, 1991b). Epidemiologic evidence demonstrated a wide travel history among this population involving six different countries served by the port of Mombasa, including Kenya, Tanzania, Uganda, Zaire, Burundi, and Rwanda. High seroprevalence was also documented among the female commercial sex workers and bar/hotel workers that lived along the same major highways (Serwadda et al., 1992). In a rural region of Uganda, lower community levels of HIV infection were noted to correlate with greater distance from main and secondary roads and with lower population mobility (Wawer et al., 1991; Serwadda et al., 1992). It is thus probable that the availability of adequate transportation routes to and through rural areas and the level of rural/urban migration both contribute to the speed of HIV infection. Thus, countries with well-developed transportation infrastructures and high levels of rural/urban migration may experience the rapid spread of HIV infection.

Civil Unrest and Wars

It is highly probable that the profound civil unrest and wars that many sub-Saharan African countries have experienced in the last two decades have contributed to the spread of the HIV virus. As discussed above, the military comprises predominantly single young males with high geographic mobility—factors that encourage casual sexual relationships, often with commercial sex workers. In times of war or unrest, the military are particularly aggressive and mobile, further facilitating the spread of the virus. Furthermore, in times of unrest, rape is a not uncommon tactic to intimidate a local populace and thereby force them into submission. It has been hypothesized that social and civil dislocation due to conflict has contributed to the HIV epidemic in southern Uganda and northern Tanzania (Omara-Otunnu, 1987) and to increased rates of sexually transmitted diseases in Mozambique (Gersony, 1988). In many cases, countries have undergone long periods of low-intensity warfare that have been accompanied by large-scale migrations of the local population. Between 1960 and 1980, more than 75 military coups occurred in 30 sub-Saharan Africa countries (Quinn, 1994). Civil unrest also contributes to declining infrastructure, reducing or eliminating services and slowing the extension of programs. Wars and civil unrest disrupt local authority, creating environments of lawlessness, and disrupt or destroy local economies, pushing people into cities and sex work.

MEDICAL AND PROGRAM FACTORS

Access to and use of health services (including STD treatment), HIV serological counseling, and condoms have a major bearing on HIV prevention; limitations in the availability of diagnosis and treatment for STDs may have contributed to the rapid spread of the epidemic. Many Africans do not recognize that they have an STD, and great numbers do not recognize that their partners are infected. Even when an STD is recognized, many Africans have little access to curative health services, which means that genital ulcer disease and other STDs that facilitate the spread of AIDS can remain untreated for long periods (Caldwell, 1995). Services in many health facilities in sub-Saharan Africa are woefully inadequate. Drugs are often in short supply. In some hospitals, there are far more patients than beds, and patients are forced to sleep on the floor. There is also great pressure on the families of patients to pay for care in spite of their limited means.

Problems for STD control have included ignorance of correct health-seeking behavior, a lack of inexpensive diagnostic tests for gonorrhea and chlamydia, the need for long therapeutic regimens that result in poor rates of compliance, limited treatment alternatives for pregnant women, and the need for broad-spectrum agents to treat polymicrobial STDs or multiple STDs occurring simultaneously (Stamm, 1987). A number of these problems will be alleviated once single-dose regimens of newly developed broad-spectrum antibiotics become both available and economically accessible in developing countries (Andriole, 1988; Philips et al., 1988; Steingrimsson et al., 1990; Handsfield, 1991; Handsfield et al., 1991; Plourde et al., 1991; Martin et al., 1992).

In rural Africa, poor transport and communications networks complicate STD control measures. Contact tracing is logistically difficult and potentially highly stigmatizing because household visits represent the principal means of contact. Intensive follow-up to ensure drug compliance is virtually impossible; because medications are expensive and often scarce, drugs are frequently hoarded, shared with relatives, or sold (Ministry of Health [Uganda], 1988). Such factors all contribute to the emergence of drug resistance (Pepin et al., 1989; Piot and Tezzo, 1990).

Underreporting of genital symptomatology and infection is common, further contributing to inadequate STD control. Reasons for underreporting include asymptomatic or low grade infections, particularly in women; reluctance to discuss potentially stigmatizing information; limited acceptability of genital examination; and a belief that such conditions are normal. Whereas the majority of men with gonorrhea will experience at least limited symptomatology, 50 to 80 percent of women are asymptomatic (Rothenberg and Potterat, 1990; Jones and Wasserheit, 1991).

ECONOMIC FACTORS

The AIDS crisis struck sub-Saharan Africa in the middle of its greatest economic crisis since independence. Since the 1970s, many sub-Saharan African countries have experienced declining productivity in agriculture and industry, worsening balance-of-payments positions, rising unemployment, and declining real wages. Many African countries have been forced to initiate structural adjustment programs in an effort to restore macroeconomic balance in their economies and reverse their economic declines. As government budgets have been reduced, health ministries have not been spared. Many have been forced to accept a smaller share of government expenditures (Ogbu and Gallagher, 1992).

What are the long-term implications of these economic reversals for the fight against HIV and AIDS? It is still too early to know, but certainly many individuals will be adversely affected either directly or indirectly by the crisis, and economic hardship can lead quickly to the adoption of survival mechanisms that are detrimental to health. Furthermore, the gap between the few who are affluent and the many who are left behind creates an environment conducive to exploitation and the rapid spread of the virus. For example, economic problems and structural adjustment may hinder women's access to job opportunities in urban formal-sector labor markets. With no other opportunities, women are forced to resort to commercial sex or to rely on multiple partnerships to support themselves and their children. In Zaire, for example, the economic crisis has led to an increase in the number of young rural women migrating to the towns and cities and to the proliferation of various forms of multiple-partner relationships for economic reasons (Schoepf, 1988).

In a recent review, Lurie et al. (1995) argue that the International Monetary Fund (IMF) and the World Bank's structural adjustment programs may have heightened people's risk of HIV infection by (1) reducing the sustainability of a rural subsistence economy, (2) developing a transportation infrastructure, (3) increasing migration and urbanization, and (4) reducing spending on health and social services. Although not the sole reason for the spread of HIV, such programs "may have only exaceberbated pre-existing circumstances or simply failed to reverse adverse trends" (Lurie et al., 1995:539). While one negative consequence of economic development is that it facilitates the spread of communicable disease by bringing people into closer and more frequent contact (Feachem et al., 1995), Lurie et al. (1995) argue that there is a need to develop alternative development models that strive to have a less harmful effect than current policies on the spread of HIV.

3

Epidemiology of the HIV/AIDS Epidemic

As noted in Chapter 1, the global HIV/AIDS epidemic consists of many separate, individual epidemics spread unevenly through sub Saharan Africa, each with its own distinct characteristics that depend on geography, the specific population affected, the frequencies of risk behaviors and practices, and the temporal introduction of the virus. In addition, biological factors may influence the spread of the epidemic by increasing or decreasing susceptibility to the virus, altering the infectiousness of those with HIV, and hastening the progression of infection to disease and death. Such biological factors may include the presence of classical STDs, male circumcision, and the viral characteristics of both HIV-1 and HIV-2 and their multiple genetic strains.

In sub-Saharan Africa, many of the behavioral patterns and biological conditions that can precipitate rapid HIV transmission were present at the time HIV was introduced into selected populations. Within a relatively brief period of time, massive HIV epidemics were ignited in some areas, affecting over 11 million African adults and resulting in 3 million AIDS-related deaths to date, with many more expected in the next few years (World Health Organization, 1995a). These estimates represent over two-thirds of the worldwide total of all HIV infections and AIDS cases. By the year 2000, as many as 20 million individuals on the continent of Africa will be HIV infected, and at least 8 million people will have died of AIDS (World Health Organization, 1993). It is within the African region that HIV will clearly have its greatest impact on morbidity and mortality, in addition to profound economic, demographic, and social consequences.

This chapter gives an overview of the epidemiology of the HIV/AIDS epidemic in sub-Saharan Africa, including its status and modes of transmission. The chapter ends with a discussion of remaining gaps in knowledge and a set of recommendations for future research.

STATUS OF THE EPIDEMIC

The origin of HIV continues to be an enigma, and the timing of the first human infection remains unknown. Attempts to determine the origins of the disease led to early speculation that AIDS originated in Africa. Not surprisingly, this speculation led many African leaders to resent the implication that Africans were to blame for AIDS. The controversy about the origin of AIDS resulted in a "backlash" and denial that HIV even existed within high-risk populations in sub-Saharan African countries and proved very unhelpful for designing effective prevention programs. Efforts to acknowledge that the problem existed and to initiate efforts to control its spread were delayed in some countries for several years. Because theories about where and when AIDS originated have become so entangled in politics, and because the epidemic is now too far advanced for the question to really matter, attempts to find definitive answers to these questions have been given a low priority. There are a few isolated reports in the literature in the 1970s and even earlier of people dying of opportunistic infections that have now become known as the trademarks of AIDS (Henig, 1993). However, AIDS was not recognized as a clinical entity until 1981. In Africa the first reports of AIDS-like syndromes and "slim" appeared in the literature between 1983 and 1985 (Van de Perre et al., 1984; Piot et al., 1984; Serwadda et al., 1985). Since the early 1980s, the prevalence of HIV infection among certain populations in Africa has increased dramatically, and it is expected to grow even more rapidly in the future. Factors in the spread of HIV are discussed in Chapters 2 and 4 with regard to the larger societal context and individual attitudes and behavior, respectively.

HIV/AIDS Statistics

As of December 1994, nearly 350,000 AIDS cases had been reported from the African region (World Health Organization, 1995a). As noted earlier, this sum represents one-third of the global number (1,025,073) of AIDS cases reported since the start of the epidemic. Allowing for under-diagnosis, incomplete reporting, and reporting delays, WHO estimates that more than 3 million cases of AIDS have occurred in Africa, comprising 70 percent of the global total of 4.5 million. In sub-Saharan Africa, 11 million adults are estimated to have been infected with HIV. This number represents nearly two-thirds of the estimated 18 million cumulative HIV infections that have occurred worldwide. More than half of these 11 million infected adults are women, and as many as 1 million African children are estimated to have been infected as a result of mother-to-child transmission (World Health Organization, 1994).

As discussed previously, sub-Saharan Africa is geographically, demographically, socially, and culturally heterogeneous, and the extent and spread of HIV infection and AIDS have accordingly been heterogeneous in the region. Thus, it is difficult if not impossible to generalize about the AIDS epidemic within the region. Yet some overall characteristics and trends can been seen. Wherever possible, we provide specific examples, with the proviso that the quoted rates of infection are pertinent only to the specific population and geographical area for which they are cited.

There have been only a few nationally or regionally representative seroprevalence studies conducted to date in sub-Saharan Africa, and information is available predominantly on the groups with the highest risk of HIV infection. In addition, sentinel surveillance systems have been developed to monitor changes in the levels of HIV infection among specific segments of the population, including those with high-risk behaviors, such as women engaged in commercial sex activities or patients receiving care for STDs, as well as groups more representative of the general population (i.e., at lower risk), such as blood donors and women seeking prenatal care.

HIV prevalence is not uniformly distributed even among all countries of sub-Saharan Africa. As described in Chapter 1, to date the epidemic has disproportionately affected East and Southern Africa. Among certain urban populations in the worst-afflicted parts of the region, such as those in Kigali, Rwanda, and Kampala, Uganda, up to one in every three adults is infected with HIV (Rwandan HIV Seroprevalence Study Group, 1989; Ministry of Health [Uganda], 1989). Overall HIV-1 infection patterns for lower-risk urban populations in Africa are shown in Figure 3-1. High levels of infection (in excess of 10 percent) are found among these populations in many urban areas throughout East and Southern Africa and in Abidjan, Côte d'Ivoire, in West Africa (U.S. Bureau of the Census, 1994a).

Recent data suggest that HIV seroprevalence is still low in most rural as compared with urban settings (Figure 3-2). However, HIV infection appears to be increasing in rural areas as well. In Tanzania, the Bukoba district probably always had a higher HIV seroprevalence than Dar es Salaam. However, even within the Bukoba district, urban centers exhibit higher rates of infection than do rural areas: 24 percent versus 5 percent, respectively (Mhalu et al., 1987; Schmutzhard et al., 1989).

Even within a particular geographic area, some population groups are disproportionately affected by the epidemic. The highest infection rates are usually found among men and women between 20 and 40 years old; people with STDs and tuberculosis; and, as discussed in Chapter 2, certain occupational groups, such as long-distance truck drivers, military personnel, and women employed in the commercial sex and entertainment industries (including those who work in

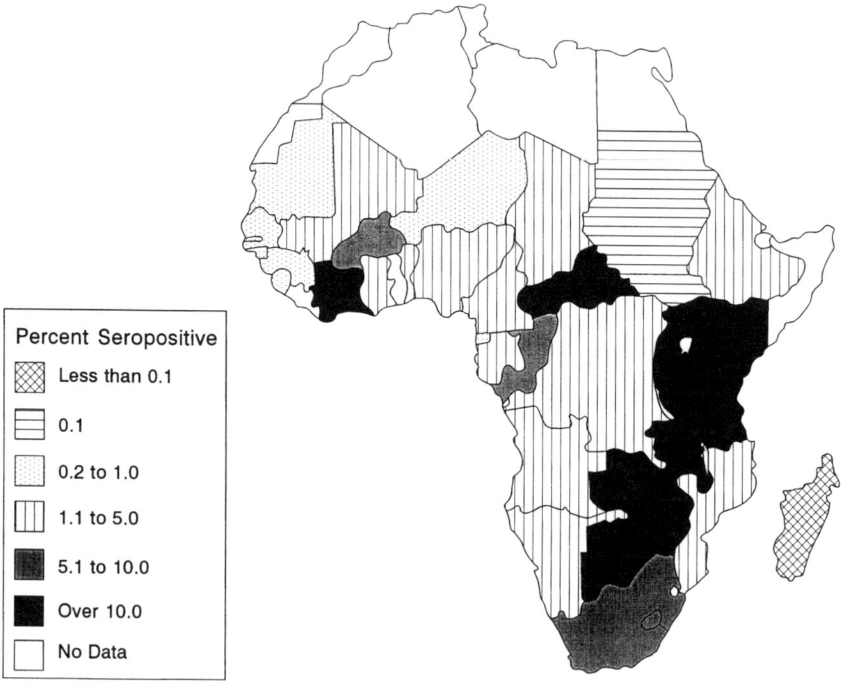

FIGURE 3-1 African HIV-1 Seroprevalence for Lower-Risk Urban Populations. SOURCE: U.S. Bureau of the Census (1994b).

bars and hotels). HIV infection rates of well over 80 percent have been reported for commercial sex workers in East and Central Africa (Piot et al., 1987, 1988; Quinn, 1991). Figure 3-3 shows the levels of HIV seroprevalence among populations of commercial sex workers in selected countries. Indeed, the AIDS epidemic in each country can be seen as a series of epidemics among subpopulations with varying levels of risk. For example, in Nairobi, Kenya, available data clearly show HIV infection spreading first and most extensively to commercial sex workers, followed by STD clinic patients—no doubt including many clients of those commercial sex workers (Piot et al., 1987). Finally, infection can be seen to be spreading among the general population, as evidenced by the initially slow but accelerating spread among pregnant women (Figure 3-4).

In serologic surveys, pregnant women are often used as surrogates for the general population. Such surveys are convenient because in many countries, pregnant women attend government clinics to receive prenatal care and may be readily tested there. To some extent, pregnant women can be considered as being at slightly higher risk than the general population because they are demonstrably sexually active. Moreover, they are drawn from a limited age range and tend to

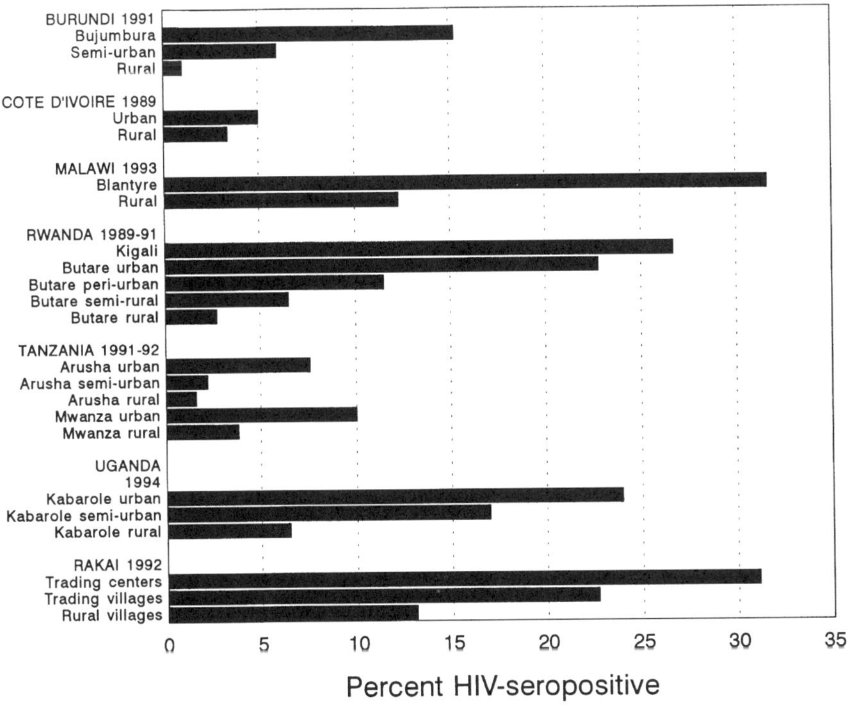

FIGURE 3-2 Urban/Rural Differentials in HIV Infection. SOURCE: U.S. Bureau of the Census (1994a).

be younger than adult women in general, given typical patterns of age-specific fertility rates. The population of pregnant women may also be biased toward those in marital (formal or informal) unions. Nevertheless, in many countries data on pregnant women provide the most representative picture of HIV infection among the general population.

Seroprevalence data from a number of studies of pregnant women conducted since the mid-1980s demonstrate the heterogeneity mentioned above (Figure 3-4) (U.S. Bureau of the Census, 1994c). There has been a consistent and rapid increase in HIV infection levels among pregnant women in Francistown, Botswana; Blantyre, Malawi; and Kampala, Uganda. By 1992, between 25 and 35 percent of pregnant women in these cities were infected. Infection rates among pregnant women rose at a much more moderate pace in Nairobi, Kenya; Bangui, the Central African Republic; and Dar es Salaam, Tanzania. However, they still reached 15 percent by 1993. Infection levels among pregnant women in Abidjan, Côte d'Ivoire, increased rapidly to about 10 percent by 1987, appeared to have reached a plateau below 15 percent through 1991, but have increased recently above 15 percent. Meanwhile, infection levels in Kinshasa, Zaire, have

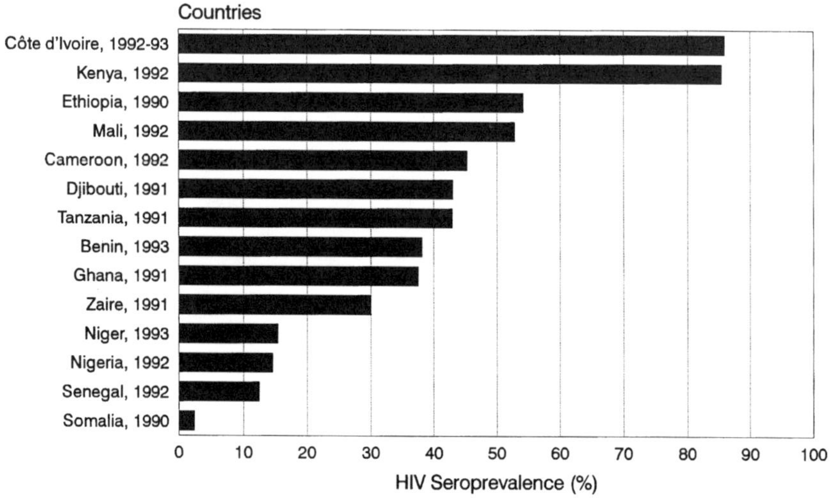

FIGURE 3-3 HIV Seroprevalence for Commercial Sex Workers in Sub-Saharan Africa: Circa 1992. NOTE: Includes infection from HIV-1 and/or HIV-2. SOURCE: U.S. Bureau of the Census (1994a).

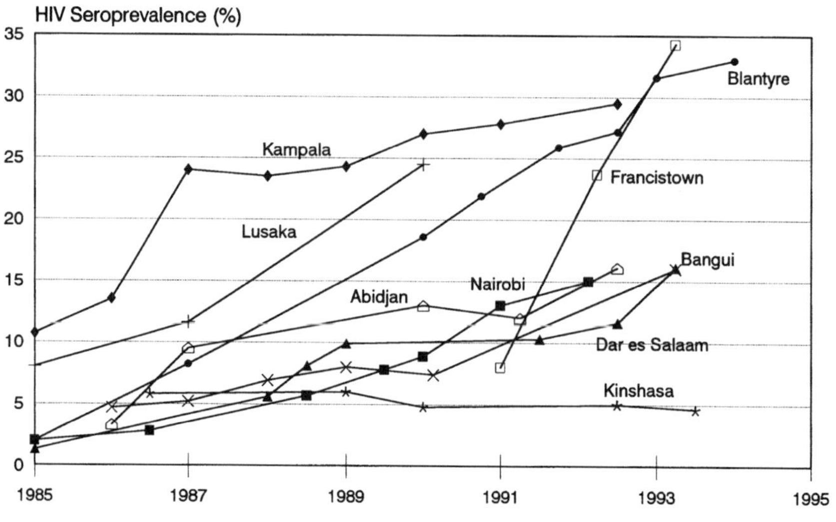

FIGURE 3-4 HIV Seroprevalence for Pregnant Women in Selected Urban Areas of Africa: 1985-1994. NOTE: Includes infection from HIV-1 and/or HIV-2. SOURCE: U.S. Bureau of the Census (1994a).

been relatively stable at 5 to 6 percent since the mid-1980s (Piot et al., 1990; Piot and Tezzo, 1990).

Although the epidemic in Africa was first recognized in Central and East Africa, and these regions continue to have the highest infection levels, there is increasing evidence that the epidemic is spreading into West and Southern Africa. In Abidjan, Côte d'Ivoire, in West Africa, HIV-1 prevalence among adults increased from 1 percent in 1986 to more than 15 percent in 1992. In Nigeria, a country with more than 105 million inhabitants, the largest population in the region, studies indicate that the prevalence of HIV-1 and HIV-2 among prostitutes in Lagos may be rising rapidly (Dada et al., 1993; Olaleye et al., 1993; see also below).

Within the last few years, investigators have noted the introduction of HIV among high-risk populations in Nigeria. Although relatively rare during the late 1980s, HIV has been increasing since 1990 throughout Nigeria, according to several surveys. This trend is of critical importance since the population of Nigeria, estimated at over 105 million, represents more than one-sixth of the total population of sub-Saharan Africa (World Bank, 1995). In one recent study, 12.3 percent and 2.1 percent of 885 female prostitutes in Lagos State were infected with HIV-1 and HIV-2, respectively, a rise from a combined prevalence of only 1.7 percent 2 years previously (Dada et al., 1993). Women in the youngest age group, ages 12 to 19, had the highest prevalence (20 percent). In addition, prostitutes residing in the port area of Lagos, which serves as a major convergence of overland and sea routes within and outside Nigeria, had the highest prevalence of HIV-1 infection. A highway region that is traversed by the overland interstate highway also had high rates. Because Lagos is the largest cosmopolitan city in Africa, the constant migratory movement of people into and out of this major trade center provides further opportunity for HIV dissemination.

The virus may be spreading even more rapidly in Southern Africa than in West Africa. For example, in Botswana, HIV prevalence among pregnant women increased from 10 percent in 1991 to 34 percent in 1993 in Francistown, and from 6 percent in 1990 to 19 percent in 1993 in Gaborone (U.S. Bureau of the Census, 1994c). Similar disturbing data are emerging from South Africa, suggesting a three-fold increase in HIV prevalence between 1990 and 1993 among women attending prenatal clinics in most regions of the country. Aggregated data collected in prenatal clinics across South Africa show a rapid increase in overall prevalence from under 1 percent in 1991 to 1.7 percent in 1992, 2.8 percent in 1993, and 6.4 percent in 1994 (U.S. Bureau of the Census, 1994a).

Thus, although HIV infection rates are high among many populations and subgroups in sub-Saharan Africa, there remains much variation in incidence and prevalence rates recorded to date, both geographically and by population subgroups. The probable causes of this heterogeneity in seroprevalence are multiple, and include behavioral, biological, and societal factors. Trying to explain the phenomenon by a single factor such as civil war, male circumcision, STDs, or rate of partner change is simplistic. Instead, it appears that the simultaneous occurrence of several risk factors for HIV transmission determines how rapidly and to what level HIV spreads among the population and who will become infected. In the absence of facilitating factors, HIV infection could remain endemic at low levels over long periods of time until a critical prevalence of infection is reached, and the spread of HIV-1 accelerates (Nzilambi et al., 1988). This epidemiologic diversity not only reflects differences in sexual and other behaviors, but also suggests that the epidemic has not reached an equilibrium in most areas.

The epidemiological evidence suggests that HIV prevalence may be stabilizing in some large urban centers (see Figure 3-4) and potentially in some rural areas (Wawer et al., 1994b; U.S. Bureau of the Census, 1994a). However, it must be recognized that a stable prevalence can conceal a significant level of new HIV infection replacing those who die (Wawer et al., 1994b). For example, in the absence of migration, a stable adult seroprevalence of 20 percent suggests that up to 2 percent of adults become newly infected each year, replacing the approximately 10 percent of the infected who are expected to die annually in African settings.

Demographics of HIV Infection

The HIV epidemic and the demographic structure of sub-Saharan populations will have complex interactions over time. The population of sub-Saharan Africa is predominantly young, in sharp contrast with the age structure in developed countries; 45 percent of the population of the region is under the age of 15, compared with one-third or less for the other major geographic regions (Decosas and Pedneault, 1992; Quinn, 1994). Among persons aged 15 and over, those in the 15-39 age group represent over two-thirds of all sub-Saharan adults; only in Latin America do young adults so predominate, whereas in Asia and the developed regions, young adults represent at most half of all adults (United Nations, 1993). In urban areas, one finds a prominent one-sided bulge caused by the migration of young males into the cities for employment (with some rural areas reporting a proportional "deficit" of young males who have migrated away) (Serwadda et al., 1992). For example, the prevalence of HIV infection among both urban and rural populations in Uganda is highest in the 25-to-44-year-old bracket among males and in the 15-to-34-year-old bracket among females (Figure 3-5) (Wagner et al., 1993; Serwadda et al., 1992).

A significant contributor to the elevated prevalence of infection in sub-Saharan Africa is the fact that behavioral factors associated with HIV transmission—including multiple partners and impermanent relationships—are generally more common among the young, this coupled with the high proportion of young adults found in sub-Saharan African countries (Anderson et al., 1991). Accordingly, the large number of young persons under age 15, who will soon enter their

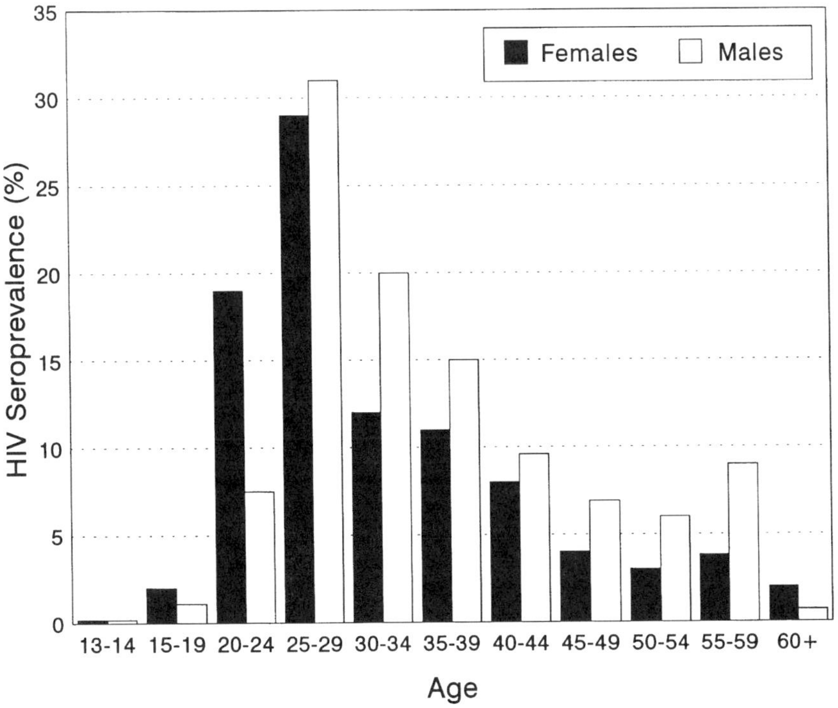

FIGURE 3-5 HIV Seroprevalence of Adult Population of Rural Rakai District, Uganda, by Age and Sex, 1992. SOURCE: Maria Wawer (personal communication, 1995).

sexual and reproductive lives, must represent a priority group for AIDS and STD prevention.

The difference in the age distribution of peak HIV prevalence between men and women occurs in the region because, on average, sexual partnerships are formed between older men and younger women (see also Chapter 2). The distortion of the urban population profile caused by male migration initially resulted in equal numbers of infected men and women (Quinn, 1994). However, male-to-female transmission of the virus is more efficient than female-to-male transmission in the absence of other cofactors (Haverkos and Quinn, 1995), so that as the epidemic has spread into the larger rural population, the absolute number of infections has become higher among women than men (Rowley et al., 1990; Anderson et al., 1991).

HIV-2 Infection

One unique feature of the AIDS epidemic in Africa is the remarkable viral heterogeneity of HIV infection. Within HIV-1 there are now nine recognized subtypes, labeled A through I, as well as the more recently identified subtype O. In addition to HIV-1, which is common predominantly in Central, Southern, and East Africa, a more distinct variant, labeled HIV-2, has been identified, predominantly in West African countries. Originally identified in 1986, HIV-2 was recognized among high-risk populations such as commercial sex workers in urban centers in West Africa. While having some genetic relationship to HIV-1, in evolution HIV-2 may be more closely related to a simian immunodeficiency virus (SIV) (Kanki, 1994). Although similar in terms of morphology, cell tropism, and overall genetic organization, HIV-1 and HIV-2 differ significantly in terms of nucleotide sequences, with only 42 percent homology (Clavel et al., 1986; Guyader et al., 1987). Genomic studies further demonstrate that HIV-2 has 70 percent or more homology with SIV. Genetic sequencing of HIV-2 isolates also shows a wide divergence among individual strains of HIV-2, similar to that observed with HIV-1. Thus, it is highly probable that the divergence of HIV-1 and HIV-2 occurred earlier than the beginning of the current epidemic (Myers, 1994). A common ancestor with similar properties and pathogenic potential may have existed a long time ago (Myers, 1994); the spread of HIV in Africa was most likely a result of simultaneous modifications of epidemiologic parameters in West and Central Africa, such as rapid urbanization and increased mobility, leading to infection of larger populations with HIV-1 and HIV-2 (Rowley et al., 1990; Anderson et al., 1991; Decosas et al., 1995) (see also Chapter 2).

Although HIV-2 can cause AIDS, it is increasingly clear that its pathogenic potential is lower than that of HIV-1. In cross-sectional studies, individuals infected with HIV-2 were found to have immunologic abnormalities similar to although less marked than those associated with HIV-1. In a prospective study among prostitutes in Senegal who were HIV-2 positive, no reduction in CD4 lymphocyte levels and no clinical abnormalities were found (Marlink, 1994). A less aggressive course of HIV-2 infection is also suggested by other observations in Dakar, Senegal; whereas HIV-2 is predominant among asymptomatic people, HIV-1 is more frequent among hospitalized patients with AIDS (Poulsen et al., 1993; Kanki et al., 1994; Marlink, 1994).

The routes of transmission and risk factors for HIV-1 and HIV-2 are similar. Like HIV-1, HIV-2 is transmitted primarily sexually (Kanki et al., 1994). However, the latency period for HIV-2 appears to be longer, and vertical transmission of HIV-2 from mother to infant is rare (Matheron et al., 1990; Poulsen et al., 1992; Adjorlolo-Johnson et al., 1994).

HIV-2 infection rates have risen steadily over the past two decades in countries of West Africa, including Côte d'Ivoire, Senegal, Guinea-Bissau, Burkina Faso, The Gambia, and Cape Verde (Kanki, 1991; Naucler et al., 1991; Markovitz, 1993; Poulsen et al., 1993). In several urban centers of West Africa, 15 to 64 percent of female prostitutes are infected. In Guinea-Bissau and The Gambia, HIV-2 is the prevalent infection, and HIV-1 is rare. In Côte d'Ivoire and Burkina

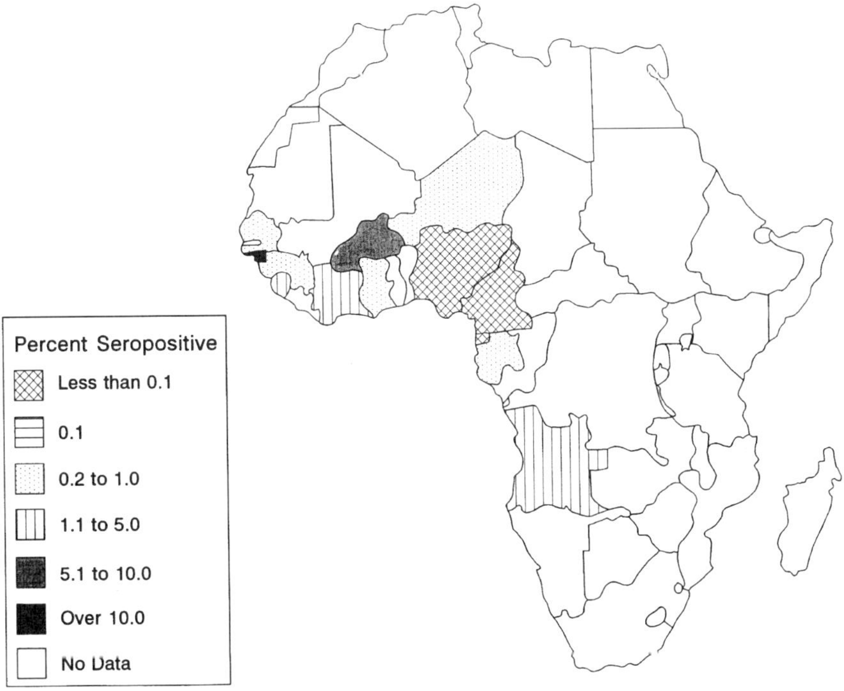

FIGURE 3-6 African HIV-2 Seroprevalence for Lower-Risk Urban Populations. SOURCE: U.S. Bureau of the Census (1994b).

Faso, HIV-2 and HIV-1 are both present among appreciable proportions of the population.

The geographic pattern of HIV-2 shows a higher prevalence in West Africa and in other African countries with a Portuguese colonial history (Kanki, 1991). Troop movements among these former Portuguese colonies and travel facilitated by cultural ties surely contributed to the spread of HIV-2 in these select countries. Conversely, several countries bordering those with substantial HIV-2 infection have as yet shown little evidence of an HIV-2 epidemic.

The highest prevalence of HIV-2 infection among high-risk urban adults is found in Côte d'Ivoire and The Gambia, where infection rates are 37 percent and 27 percent, respectively. HIV-2 seroprevalence among low-risk urban adults is far lower (see Figure 3-6); only in Guinea-Bissau does seroprevalence exceed 10 percent (U.S. Bureau of the Census, 1994b). The highest HIV-2 infection rates are found among populations with high HIV-1 prevalence, including people with tuberculosis or STDs and female prostitutes. As noted above, in contrast to HIV-1, which shows a distinct peak at ages 25 to 40, the age-specific prevalence of

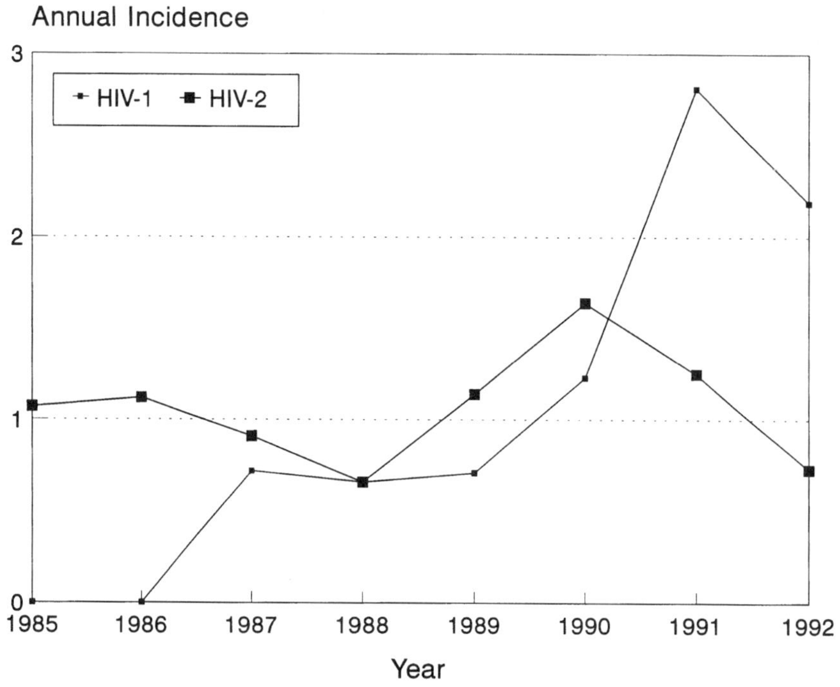

FIGURE 3-7 Incidence of HIV-1 and HIV-2 Among Female Prostitutes in Senegal. NOTE: Incidence measured as the percentage per 100 person-years of observation. SOURCE: Data from Kanki et al. (1994).

HIV-2 infection increases gradually with age. This increase may be the result of a lower case fatality rate or a longer latency period of HIV-2 infection.

It appears that with time, HIV-1 is increasing among these populations at a faster rate than HIV-2 (Kanki et al., 1994). Although HIV-2 appears to have been in West Africa longer than HIV-1, levels of HIV-1 infection have now surpassed those of HIV-2 in many West African countries. For example, in a recent study in Dakar, Senegal, 1,452 registered female prostitutes were followed prospectively between 1985 and 1993 (Kanki et al., 1994). Initially, HIV-2 was more common than HIV-1. In 1985, HIV-2 was present with a prevalence of 11.3 percent, whereas HIV-1 was present with a prevalence of 6.2 percent. The 1,277 women with a seronegative sample were evaluated over the next 8 years for evidence of seroconversion. While the incidence of HIV-2 remained stable, the annual incidence of HIV-1 increased substantially (Figure 3-7). There was a 1.4-fold increase in risk per year and a 12-fold increase in risk over the entire study period. This study suggests that the heterosexual spread of HIV-2 is significantly slower than that of HIV-1, which may reflect the differences in the viruses' infectivity potential (Kanki et al., 1994). Consistent with the idea that HIV-2 may be less virulent than HIV-1 and may have been present in West Africa for many decades, seropositivity increases with age. Among prostitutes in Dakar, Senegal, almost 100 percent of those aged 50 and over are infected with HIV-2 (Marlink, 1994).

The disparity in the speed with which HIV-1 and HIV-2 are spreading is particularly striking in Abidjan, Côte d'Ivoire, where HIV-1 has become by far the predominant virus, causing a major epidemic of AIDS. In contrast with HIV-1, HIV-2 has barely increased in Abidjan during the past 6 years (Figure 3-8). This finding suggests that under identical conditions and among populations with the same behavior, HIV-2 is less readily transmissible through sexual intercourse than HIV-1. Nevertheless, studies in Côte d'Ivoire and The Gambia have found that HIV-2 infection correlates with factors associated with HIV-1 infection, such as prostitute contact, history of past STDs, and past and current genital ulcer disease. In Côte d'Ivoire and Guinea-Bissau, 40 percent of spouses of people with HIV-2 were also infected.

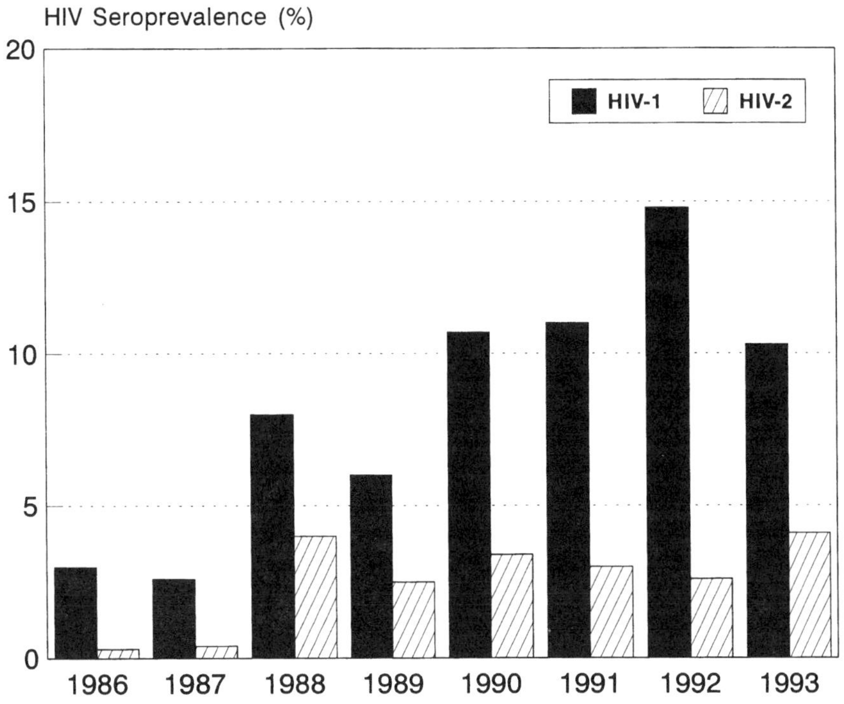

FIGURE 3-8 HIV Seroprevalence for Pregnant Women, Abidjan, Côte d'Ivoire: 1986-1993. SOURCE: U.S. Bureau of the Census (1994a).

The clinical and epidemiologic diversity between HIV-1 and HIV-2 may also have important biological and immunologic implications. Intrinsic biological properties of these viruses include infectivity and replication capacities that contribute to different epidemic curves. In addition to the higher rates of sexual and perinatal transmission and more rapid clinic course of disease associated with HIV-1, HIV-2 infection may provide some immunologic protection from HIV-1 (Travers et al., 1995). In another recent paper on commercial sex workers in Dakar, Senegal, the HIV-1 incidence was shown to be higher for seronegative commercial sex workers than for their HIV-2 infected counterparts. The lower HIV-1 seroconversion rate among those infected with HIV-2 occurred despite the same frequency of other STDs in both groups, suggesting that differences in sexual behavior between the two groups were not responsible. Further analysis indicated that HIV-2-seropositive women with CD4 cell counts of less than 800 per cubic millimeter were more likely to become infected with HIV-1 than were those women with higher CD4 counts, suggesting that with increasing immunosuppression, the protective effect of HIV-2 infection against subsequent HIV-1 may decrease (Travers et al., 1995). Further studies are needed to determine whether cross-reactive immunity can occur between different strains of HIV, and whether this information can be used in the development of more effective vaccines.

Differences in the patterns of infection are likely to be the result of different types of interrelations and contacts within West Africa, where HIV-2 predominates, and between West Africa and Central Africa, where HIV-1 predominates. In general, it seems likely that the migration of sexually active, high-risk populations played a major role in the observed spread of these sexually transmitted viruses. One example is seasonal migration of young men and women in Senegal and The Gambia. In one study of 3,230 persons residing in rural Senegal, 0.8 percent were HIV-2 seropositive, and 0.1 percent were HIV-1 seropositive. Seropositivity was directly associated with seasonal migration and a history of blood transfusion, injections, or STDs (Pison et al., 1993). In another study of 278 female prostitutes from Ziguinchor, Senegal, HIV-2 seroprevalence was associated with women from Guinea-Bissau and with increased years of sexual activity. Women from Ghana and Guinea-Bissau also constituted a significant portion of study participants (commercial sex workers) in other sites in Senegal (Kanki et al., 1992). Both of these nationalities were associated with higher HIV-2 prevalence.

These findings suggest that even in rural areas, with the exception of a few cases of transmission by blood transfusion or injection, HIV-2 is transmitted mainly sexually from migrant female prostitutes to adult men, and secondarily to their wives or regular partners upon return home. Ghanaian and Gambian prostitutes report that they migrate and work in a number of other West African countries, such as Burkina Faso, Côte d'Ivoire, and Mali, all having significant HIV-

2 rates (Pepin et al., 1991; Pickering et al., 1992; Dada et al., 1993; Olaleye et al., 1993).

Several cases of mother-to-child transmission of HIV-2 have been reported from The Gambia. However, the risk of perinatal transmission of HIV-2 is much lower than that of HIV-1 (Adjorlolo-Johnson et al., 1994). In a community-based survey in Guinea-Bissau, all HIV-2-seropositive infants lost HIV-2 antibodies before the age of 9 months, and no evidence of mother-to-child transmission of HIV-2 was found in prospective studies in Burkina Faso or Côte d'Ivoire. Additional data from prospective studies are needed before the risk of HIV-2 transmission from mother to child can be more accurately assessed.

HIV-2 infection can also be acquired by blood transfusion. This is illustrated by studies among hospitalized patients in Guinea-Bissau, where previous blood transfusions were found to be a risk factor for HIV-2, and in Côte d'Ivoire among children with multiple transfusions, who had an increased prevalence of infection with HIV-2 (Horsburgh and Holmberg, 1988; De Cock and Brun-Vezinet, 1989).

MODES OF TRANSMISSION

The primary mode of HIV transmission is sexual, with heterosexual transmission accounting for at least 80 percent of adult HIV infections in sub-Saharan Africa (Piot et al., 1988). HIV is also acquired through perinatal and parenteral transmission.

Sexual Transmission

Risk Factors in Sexual Transmission

Behavioral risk factors for HIV transmission among heterosexuals include number of sex partners, frequency of unprotected intercourse, commercial sex, a history of or concurrent infection with an STD, lack of male circumcision, and anal intercourse; many women are at risk only because they have unprotected intercourse with a regular partner or spouse who is infected. Of these factors, the importance of STDs as a cofactor for HIV transmission among heterosexuals has been emphasized in a number of studies (Wasserheit, 1992). The increase in seroprevalence in recent years among STD clinic patients in comparison with the increase among the overall population was 2-fold in Tanzania, 3-fold in Zambia, 4-fold in Burundi, and 20-fold in rural Rwanda (Plummer et al., 1991; Laga et al., 1993). Even among commercial sex workers, the transmission of HIV is associated with the presence of STDs.

The statistical risk of HIV transmission appears to be small for any single episode of penile-vaginal intercourse, regardless of which partner is infected (Haverkos and Quinn, 1995). Studies of male-to-female transmission suggest that the risk may be as low as 0.1 percent per episode of intercourse. Female-to-male transmission by intercourse is less efficient than male-to-female spread (Mastro et al., 1994; Haverkos and Quinn, 1995). Reasons for the greater susceptibility of women may include greater trauma to the genitalia and the vaginal epithelium in women during intercourse and longer exposure to HIV when infected ejaculate is retained in the vagina. Similar mechanisms may account for greater female susceptibility to non-ulcerative STDs, such as gonorrhea, chlamydia, and trichomoniasis (Wasserheit, 1992). Studies of HIV transmission among heterosexual couples have demonstrated a seroprevalence of 20 to 50 percent among originally discordant couples; in two African studies, annual seroconversion rates among discordant couples were on the order of 4 to 9 percent per year (Allen et al., 1992; Serwadda et al., 1995). From European data, factors that appear to increase heterosexual transmission include anal-receptive intercourse, more advanced illness in the male partner, and history or presence of STDs (de Vincenzi, for the European Study Group on Heterosexual Transmission of HIV, 1994).

It is generally accepted that homosexual contact between men is a minor route of HIV transmission in sub-Saharan Africa, given that such behavior is reported only rarely in the region (see Chapter 4). Although homosexual transmission may be rare, underreporting of such behavior may be common because homosexuality is highly stigmatized in most African societies. However, when homosexual sex does occur, male-to-male transmission may play a part in sustaining the epidemic; there is little reason to think that the risk factors would not be similar to those in Western countries, where anal-receptive intercourse appears to be a primary risk factor for homosexual transmission of HIV. Similarly, other studies among male homosexual populations have demonstrated an association between HIV-1 and other STDs, such as syphilis and herpes.

HIV and STDs

A growing body of data suggests that HIV transmission cannot be considered in isolation from the classical STDs, principally syphilis, gonorrhea, chlamydia, chancroid, trichomoniasis, and herpes simplex virus type 2 (HSV-2). HIV shares modes of transmission and behavioral risk factors with these other STDs. More important, there is evidence that classical STDs may increase susceptibility to and transmission of HIV; their control may thus serve as an important element in curbing the HIV epidemic. Thus, the following sections on sexual transmission, as well as some subsequent sections on behavior and care seeking, refer to both HIV and the classical STDs.

Prevalence of STDs in Africa Although accurate determination of the prevalence of STDs in Africa is hindered by a lack of population-based data and adequate surveillance, existing information suggests that infection rates are very high in many African settings. Serological evidence of a prevalence of syphilis ranging from 11 to 21 percent has been documented among women attending prenatal clinics in a number of sub-Saharan countries (Ratman et al., 1982; Watson, 1985; Cooper-Poole, 1986). Between 7 and 15 percent of pregnant women have been found to have *Neisseria gonorrhoeae* (*N. gonorrhoeae*) infection in similar settings (Nasah et al., 1980; Mabey et al., 1984; Laga et al., 1986; Mason et al., 1989; Welgemoed et al., 1986; Widy-Wirsky and D'Costa, 1989). In a recent study of pregnant Ugandan women, Nsubuga et al. (1994) found a prevalence of 42.5 percent for trichomoniasis, 10.4 percent for active syphilis, and 7.5 percent for chlamydia. *Hemophilus ducreyi* (chancroid) is a frequent etiologic agent of genital ulcers (World Health Organization Expert Committee on Venereal Diseases and Treponematoses, 1986; Mabey et al., 1987). Of 293 male STD clinic clients in Nairobi, 149 had acquired genital ulcer disease following contact with a prostitute; chancroid was clinically diagnosed in 89 percent of the cases (followed by genital herpes in 5 percent) (Cameron et al., 1989). Nonulcerative *Chlamydia trachomatis* (*C. trachomatis*) infection is another common genital tract pathogen, isolated in over 13 percent of male and female patients with urethritis or discharge in several studies (Bowie et al., 1977; Mabey and Whittle, 1982; Ballard et al., 1986; Leclerc et al., 1988).

Data from community-based cohort studies suggest that high STD rates are not confined to self selected, urban clinic populations. High rates of positive syphilis serology, indicative of active syphilis in over 10 percent of the adult population, have been reported from population-based studies in rural Uganda (Mulder, 1993; Hudson, 1993). Preliminary data from another predominantly rural district of Uganda indicate that up to half of the rural women in Rakai residing in small towns on secondary roads have *Trichomonas vaginalis* infection (Wawer et al., 1995a).

In contrast with HIV, whose prevalence has been found to vary widely within countries or districts in relation to the degree of urbanization and proximity to roads, the classical STDs may be more uniformly distributed among the general population within a given region. In Uganda, adult HIV rates ranged from 11 percent in the stratum of relatively isolated agrarian villages to over 30 percent in communities along main roads (Wawer et al., 1991). In contrast, the rates of active syphilis varied far less, from 9 percent in the most rural stratum to 13 percent in the main-road towns (Nelson K. Sewankambo, personal communication, 1995). The older infections may have become established more uniformly over time in any one particular region; given that STDs may enhance HIV transmission, the data also suggest that STDs represent an important risk factor in a very wide segment of the African urban and rural populations. Given the data described above, however, it is obvious that the rates of classical STDs may vary substantially across regions, and such underlying rates may have contributed to the unequal pace at with which HIV infection has spread in different parts of Africa.

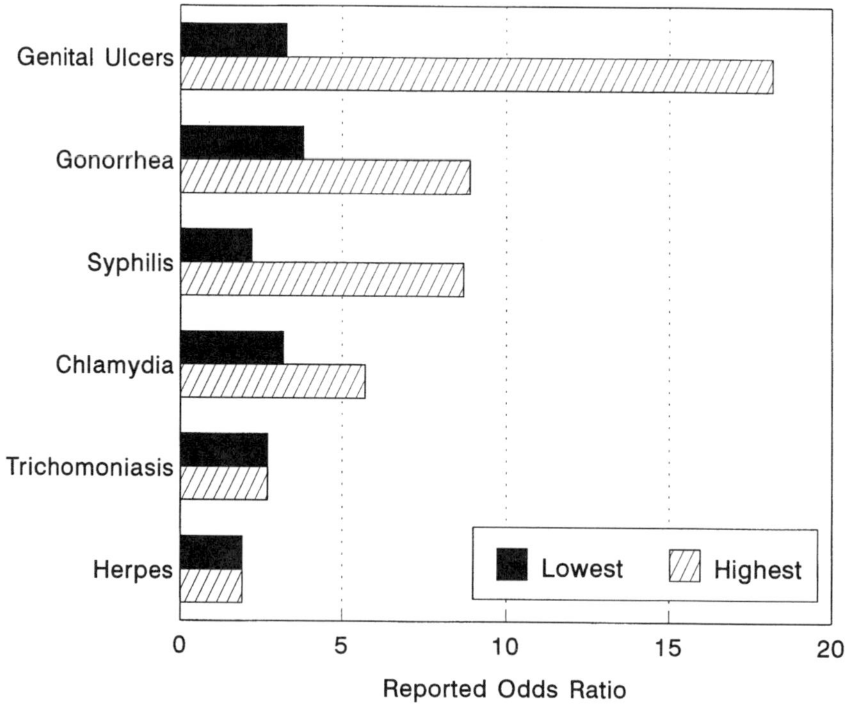

FIGURE 3-9 Relative Risk of HIV Infection by Type of STD. NOTE: Summary of risk estimates of STDs and HIV infection, drawn from prospective cross-sectional or case control studies. All reported studies included physical examinations and/or laboratory confirmation of the STD and multivariate adjustment for behavioral risk factors. Data reported are for heterosexual men or women. All risks are expressed as odds ratios and indicate the highest and lowest reported risk (odds ratio) of HIV infection in the presence of the STD, as compared with subjects without the STD. SOURCE: Wasserheit (1992).

Synergy of HIV and STDs A number of studies conducted in sub-Saharan Africa have demonstrated that both genital ulcers—mainly chancroid, syphilis, and herpes—and non-ulcerative STDs—such as gonorrhea, chlamydial infection, and trichomoniasis—are associated with increased risk of sexual transmission and acquisition of HIV (Figure 3-9).

That HIV-1 can be isolated directly from genital ulcers strongly suggests the potential for increased transmission associated with genital ulcers (Kreiss et al., 1989); the reduced epithelial integrity of the ulcers may render uninfected sexual partners more susceptible to HIV infection. In a prospective study in Kenya, Cameron et al. (1989) demonstrated a high incidence of HIV infection among men who developed genital ulcer disease after contact with a commercial sex worker. Among the same population of seropositive female commercial sex workers, HIV was detected by culture from 4 of 36 ulcers (11 percent).

The case for non-ulcerative STDs as risk factors for HIV transmission/acquisition is less well documented. Cervical inflammation has been shown to be associated with cervical shedding of HIV DNA (Kreiss et al., 1994). In a prospective study among female prostitutes in Kinshasa, Zaire, gonorrhea, chlamydia, and trichomoniasis during the presumed period of exposure were all significantly associated with HIV seroconversion, even after controlling for sexual exposure in terms of the number of sexual contacts and frequency of condom use (Laga et al., 1993).

Based on data from this observational cohort study, Laga et al. (1994) reported lower HIV incidence among those sex workers who regularly attended clinical services for STD diagnosis and treatment as compared with workers who received STD services irregularly, after adjustment for condom use. Among prostitutes in Nairobi, Kenya, genital ulcer disease was independently associated with HIV infection (Simonsen et al., 1990). It should also be noted that although the association with HIV infection is generally stronger for ulcerative than non-ulcerative STDs, the latter are more prevalent. It is thus possible that in many settings, the increase in attributable risk to the whole community of HIV infection due to the presence of other STDs may be greater as a result of non-ulcerative STDs than genital ulcer disease (Piot and Laga, 1989; Wasserheit, 1992). In addition, as suggested above, although the high prevalence of untreated STDs found in many African settings may have contributed to the generally rapid spread of HIV in the region, underlying differences in STD rates may play a role in the unequal spread of HIV on the continent.

It has been argued that the consistency of the findings and the strength of the associations between HIV infection and STDs lend strong support to a causal association: that STDs facilitate HIV transmission. However, interpretation of the findings is difficult because of potential confounding variables. Classical STDs may be markers of sexual activity and not causal risk factors, and accurately controlling for the sexual activity of the patient and of his/her partner(s) is frequently not possible (Pepin et al., 1989; Wasserheit, 1992). Even longitudinal observational studies do not provide conclusive evidence because of potential misreporting of partner information, problems in determining the time sequence of the infections (the latter being dependent on the frequency of HIV testing and the accuracy of the information regarding the time the STD was acquired), the variable delay in HIV seroconversion following infection, and the inability to assess accurately the STD status of the partner(s) of the index case (Pepin et al., 1989; Piot and Laga, 1989; Mertens et al., 1990). It has thus been proposed that "a more direct approach to establish a causative association would be through the conduct of randomized controlled trials, which seek to determine whether intervening against STDs reduces the transmission of HIV" (Mertens et al., 1990:63).

The attributable risk of STDs for the transmission of HIV remains to be determined, as does the impact of STD control on the spread of HIV-1.

Data from a recent randomized community-based intervention trial conducted in Mwanza, Tanzania, indicate significantly lower HIV incidence among adults residing in communities that received improved STD case management at the primary health care level, as compared with control communities (Grosskurth et al., 1995). HIV incidence was lower for both males and females, and for all age groups between 15 and 54, in the treatment communities as compared with the controls; the data further suggest that the observed differences were not due to factors such as condom use or numbers of partners. However, the study had only limited information on STD end points, and no significant reductions in STD rates were observed. The authors hypothesize that "the most plausible explanation for our results is that the STD treatment programme reduced HIV incidence by shortening the average duration of STDs . . ." (Grosskurth et al., 1995:535).

A number of other randomized controlled community-based trials of STD prevention and treatment are under way currently in Africa (Wawer et al., 1995b; Mulder et al., 1994a). Data from these trials should elucidate further the effects of STD reduction on HIV transmission among the general population and should add to our understanding of the role of individual STDs, and of symptomatic and asymptomatic infections, in HIV transmission in the community setting.

HIV may also have a reciprocal effect on other STDs; that is, HIV infection may alter the natural history, diagnosis, and response to therapy of other STDs (Johnson et al., 1991; Wasserheit and Holmes, 1992; Aral and Wasserheit, forthcoming). For example, although data are as yet limited, there is some evidence that the incidence of pelvic inflammatory disease may be greater among HIV-positive women with gonorrhea than among HIV-negative women with gonorrhea (Plummer et al., 1989). Increased rates of chancroid treatment failure have been reported among HIV-infected persons in Zimbabwe and Kenya (Latif, 1989; MacDonald et al., 1989). More research is needed to determine whether HIV infection results in atypical STD presentations, including more resistant lesions or more frequent recurrence (Aral and Wasserheit, forthcoming), which could presumably result in greater STD transmission.

Aral and Wasserheit (forthcoming) conclude that the multiple potential interactions between STDs and HIV, coupled with their joint modes of transmission, result in epidemics that are "inextricably intertwined, particularly in heterosexual populations. . . . These interrelationships mean that HIV infection and other STDs may amplify one another by establishing a mutually reinforcing spiral of infection. . . . Clearly, this suggests that in communities with high rates of STDs, augmented STD prevention and control efforts should be a central HIV prevention strategy."

Other Health Consequences of STDs Regardless of the STD/HIV synergy, STD control is highly desirable in itself. STDs result in substantial acute adult morbidity; male and female infertility; maternal postpartum complications; fetal loss; and other negative reproductive outcomes, including congenital sequelae.

High incidence of pelvic inflammatory disease has been reported in several African countries (Muir and Belsey, 1980), with *C. trachomatis* and *N. gonorrhoeae* being the two most frequently recognized pathogens (Mabey et al., 1985; Frost et al., 1987). In a prospective Kenyan study, the incidence of postpartum upper genital tract infections was 20 percent, nearly one-third of these being infections caused by *N. gonorrhoeae*, *C. trachomatis*, or both (Plummer et al., 1987).

Pelvic inflammatory disease is thought to have contributed substantially to the historical "infertility belt" of Central Africa, a region that includes Cameroon, the Central African Republic, northern Zaire, the Congo, Gabon, and parts of Uganda (Arya et al., 1973; Arya and Taber, 1975; World Health Organization Scientific Group on the Epidemiology of Infertility, 1975; Frank, 1983). Based on World Fertility Survey and Demographic Health Survey data from 17 sub-Saharan African countries, Larsen (1994) estimates that at the age of 34, the proportion of sterile women ranges from between 33 and 41 percent in Cameroon to between 10 and 15 percent in Burundi, Kenya, Ondo State, Nigeria, and Togo. These data, as well as those from a WHO-sponsored multicenter collaborative investigation of infertility, are strongly suggestive of previous genital infection (World Health Organization Scientific Group on the Epidemiology of Infertility, 1975). Indeed, it has been estimated that between 50 and 80 percent of cases of female infertility in Africa may be due to reproductive tract infections; in industrialized countries, the proportion is from 10 to 35 percent (Cates et al., 1985; Wasserheit and Holmes, 1992). Brunham et al. (1991) have estimated that a 20 percent prevalence of gonorrhea among sexually active adults may produce up to a 50 percent reduction in net population growth, an estimate consistent with fertility rates observed in parts of Uganda. Male fertility is also affected by STDs: sexually transmitted organisms, in particular *N. gonorrhoeae* and *C. trachomatis,* are the most common cause of epididymitis among heterosexual men under the age of 35. Epididymitis and occlusion of the vas deferens are associated with reduced male fertility (Berger, 1990). Such conditions arise more frequently in Africa than in other regions because of inadequate treatment (Mputo et al., 1986; Arya and Taber, 1975).

STDs can also result in adult mortality, particularly among women, through a number of major complications, including ectopic pregnancy and postpartum infection. It should be noted further that in addition to the reproductive effects of STDs in adults, the cardiovascular and neurological sequelae of syphilis represent important public health concerns.

Pregnancy and birth outcomes are also affected by STDs. A Zambian study determined that 57 percent of pregnancies among women with untreated syphilis ended in abortion, stillbirth, preterm birth, or low birth weight, as compared with 10 percent among women without syphilis (Hira et al., 1990). Shulz et al. (1987)

have estimated that with a 10 percent prevalence of syphilis among pregnant women—not uncommon in Africa—5 percent or more of all pregnancies surviving past the twelfth week of gestation will have congenital syphilis or one of the other serious adverse syphilitic outcomes of the type cited above.

The incidence of many other STD-related birth sequelae is poorly documented, but data suggest that *Trichomonas vaginalis* and *C. trachomatis* can also be associated with negative pregnancy outcomes (Berman et al., 1987; Sweet et al., 1987; Cotch and Pastorek, 1991). Approximately 30 to 45 percent of infants exposed to gonorrhea in utero acquire gonococcal eye infection (gonococcal ophthalmia neonatorum or GON) in the absence of prophylaxis; GON rates of 4 to 6 percent have been documented in African centers (Laga et al., 1986; Shulz et al., 1987; De Schryver and Meheus, 1990; Hammerschlag, 1991). Bacterial vaginosis is characterized by a marked (20- to 1,000-fold) increase in vaginal *Gardnerella vaginalis, Mycobacteria hominis, Ureaplasma urealyticum,* and various anaerobic bacteria and reduced numbers of peroxide-producing Lactobacillus species (Hillier et al., 1992; Eschenbach, 1993; Hillier, 1993; Hillier et al., 1993). Bacterial vaginosis, particularly in early pregnancy, has been associated with chorioamnionitis and intramniotic infection; such infections may lead to premature rupture of the membranes and premature delivery (McDonald et al., 1991; Gibbs, 1993; McGregor et al., 1993; Read and Klebanoff, 1993; Riduan et al., 1993).

In another example of STD and HIV interactions, it has been hypothesized that STDs that compromise the integrity of the placental membranes and result in placental barrier defects may increase the rate of vertical (mother-to-child) HIV transmission (St. Louis et al., 1993). There is some evidence that active genital ulcer disease in the mother at the time of delivery also increases maternal-to-infant transmission (Wabwire-Mangen, 1995).

In addition to the substantial, direct effects of STDs on adult and infant health, STDs have major social and economic implications. Although male infecundity may be responsible for up to one-third of all "couple" infecundity, the woman is more likely to be identified as the responsible partner and to suffer the social consequences (de Bruyn, 1992). To avoid rejection and divorce, the woman in an infertile couple may seek an outside partner to make her pregnant, feeding a vicious cycle of STD-HIV transmission. Economically, STDs place substantial demands on the health systems of sub-Saharan Africa, representing one of the top five reasons for clinic attendance in many settings (Meheus et al., 1990). STDs have been found to account for up to 10 percent of adult outpatient visits in Zambia (Hira and Sunkutu, 1993). The substantial negative effects of congenital syphilis, gonorrhea, and chlamydia on child growth, development, and survival, described earlier, also affect the provision of health and social services.

More intensive STD control is thus critically needed, in particular since evidence from countries such as Burkina Faso and Kenya suggests that the prevalence and incidence of STDs are rising (Damiba et al., 1990; Hammerschlag,

1991; Cates and Hinman, 1991). Although some of the reported increase may be due to improved diagnosis, the trends appear to be real, presumably driven by the same social factors (mobility, urbanization, changing mores) that are fueling the HIV/AIDS epidemic.

Transmission Models of STDs and HIV The basic biological and behavioral factors that determine the transmission dynamics of STDs, including HIV, are reflected in the formula $R_0 = \beta Dc$ (Anderson and May, 1988). R_0 represents the reproductive rate of infection of a particular pathogen, i.e., the number of new infections transmitted by one infected person in the susceptible population. There are three direct determinants of R_0, or the rate of spread:

β, which represents the mean probability of sexual transmission per partnership
D, the mean number of years an infected person remains infectious
c, the average rate of new sexual partner selection per year

Each of these variables can be viewed as a category that encompasses certain classes of risk factors. If R_0 exceeds 1.0, the disease will grow, whereas if R_0 is less than 1.0, the disease will die out since each new infection will fail to replace itself. Added complexity is introduced since the duration of the infectious period, the probability of transmission, and the rate of new partner acquisition will certainly vary among individuals.

Each STD, including HIV, has unique biological characteristics that affect its transmissibility or β. The number of infectious particles necessary to establish infection, or the infectious dose, is an example. A factor associated with HIV infectiousness is increased viremia, seen in acute primary infection or advanced clinical disease. Moreover, as indicated above, conditions that compromise the vaginal mucosal or penile epithelial barriers, such as genital ulcers or inflammatory conditions provoked by non-ulcerative STDs, may increase susceptibility to HIV infection. It has also been postulated that HIV infection, by compromising immunocompetence, may lead to longer duration of infection by classical STDs. Theoretically, cervical ectopy (a condition in which part of the cervical surface becomes covered by the delicate mucus-secreting columnar cells that normally line the cervical canal), such as that arising during pregnancy or use of some contraceptives (Moss et al., 1991; Daly et al., 1994), may increase β by increased viral shedding or susceptibility to infection. Adolescent females may be at higher risk of HIV infection because of a larger zone of cervical ectopy that is associated with puberty; the effect could be direct, or indirect through increased susceptibility to gonococcal or chlamydial cervicitis (Bulterys et al., 1994). It has also been suggested that the immunosuppression of pregnancy may have similar effects (Biggar et al., 1989). Some of the broad number of biological and behavioral

TABLE 3-1 Factors That Affect Infectiousness of or Susceptibility to HIV

Infectiousness	Susceptibility
Acute primary HIV infection	Genital ulcerations
Advanced clinical stage of HIV	Other STDs
Genital ulcerations (chancroid, syphilis, herpes)	Cervical ectopy
Other STDs (gonorrhea, chlamydia, trichomoniasis)	Lack of male circumcision
Cervical ectopy	Traumatic sex
Antiretroviral therapy (decreased infectiousness)	Lack of condom use
Consistent condom use (decreased infectiousness)	Anal intercourse
	Sex during menses

factors that may influence either the infectiousness of or susceptibility to HIV are listed in Table 3-1.

Areas with the highest HIV prevalence correspond roughly to geographic areas where most men are not circumcised (Bongaarts et al., 1989; Caldwell and Caldwell, 1993; Caldwell, 1995a, 1995b; Piot et al., 1994). Lack of circumcision in men has been associated with an increased prevalence and incidence of HIV in several studies in Nairobi (Cameron et al., 1989), although not in studies in Rwanda or Tanzania (Borgdorff et al., 1991, cited in Piot et al., 1994; see also Chapter 4). Vaginal trauma or abrasions caused by traumatic sex or vaginal application of plant extracts or desiccating products have been associated with an increased risk of HIV acquisition among women in several countries (see Chapter 4).

Since β is defined as the probability of transmission per partnership, it depends in part on sexual behaviors, such as coital frequency, anal intercourse, and dry sex. The most important measure of sexual behavior is c, the rate of sexual partner change within a population (which through its effect on STDs also affects β). Note that c is not the average annual number of new sexual partners per person, μ, but instead is $\mu + \sigma^2/\mu$, where σ^2 is the variance of the number of new sexual partners per year. It is the number of partners associated with the average new partnership, which exceeds the average number of new partners per person, just as the size of the city in which the average person resides exceeds the average size of cities. The lesson is that both mean and variance matter. Those few individuals with many new partners ensure that infections will spread more rapidly.

The structure of the sexual mixing environment—sexual interactions among individuals—has a major influence on the shape of the HIV/AIDS epidemic (Anderson and May, 1992). A high number of sexual partners within a relatively circumscribed group partially explains the very rapid rise of HIV infection among homosexual men in the early phase of the epidemic in the United States. In Africa, sexual contact with commercial sex workers, who represent a group of high-frequency transmitters, may have been partially responsible for escalating and sustaining the epidemic in urban settings. The activities of such a core group sustain the hyperendemic levels of STDs and HIV within the core; because the core is not a closed population, the epidemic is spread and sustained beyond the core. As discussed earlier, in sub-Saharan Africa, female commercial sex workers, their male clients, truck drivers, migrant workers, and the military form the core groups of heterosexual HIV transmission, resulting in the high HIV seroprevalence and seroincidence described earlier.

It should also be noted, however, that once HIV infection has achieved high levels among the general population, the role of multiple sexual partnerships and core groups in sustaining the epidemic becomes less important (Wawer et al., 1994a). Serwadda et al. (1992) report that in rural Uganda, having one sexual partner in communities with high underlying HIV prevalence was associated with as much risk of HIV infection as having multiple partners in areas of lower prevalence. Thus, where prevalence is already high, programs targeted at high-risk groups may have limited impact. In addition, concurrency—a pattern of long-term overlapping relationships—provides the basis for stable connected networks that can amplify HIV spread through populations (Morris and Kretzschmar, forthcoming; Kretzschmar and Morris, forthcoming). Such concurrent relationships are not uncommon in African settings (Pison, 1989; Parkin and Nyamwaya, 1987).

In Africa, the high prevalence of STDs, low rates of male circumcision, substantial incidence of commercial sex, heterogeneous sexual mixing, low rates of condom use, and long duration of the HIV/AIDS epidemic may explain the current high levels of heterosexual transmission of HIV as compared with the levels in other regions of the world. Nevertheless, the recent explosion of HIV infection among heterosexuals in Asia demonstrates how quickly HIV can spread within core groups, in this case commercial sex workers, their clients, and injecting drug users, and from these groups to the general population.

Underlying ecological and behavioral factors that operate through one or more of these direct determinants of the spread of the epidemic lie on a continuum. Some of the factors are more remote and cannot be readily modified, such as cultural, economic, and social history. Factors that are more proximate on the continuum, and more modifiable, include a number of behaviors influenced by recent technological and commercial product development, such as use of condoms and spermicides for family planning and STD/HIV prevention, care seeking for STDs, and patterns of alcohol and illicit drug use (which influence sexual behaviors).

Of particular interest is the potential effect of a vaccine against HIV on the course of the epidemic. The efficacy of a vaccine can be expressed as the product of three factors (Blower and McLean, 1994): the vaccine take (the fraction of recipients in whom the vaccine induces any immunological effect), the degree of the vaccine (the reduction in susceptibility per sexual partnership among those in whom the vaccine takes), and the fraction of those ceasing sexual activity before the vaccine-induced protection wanes. Whether a vaccine could ultimately lead to eradication of HIV and if so, the extent of coverage necessary to achieve eradication depend on R_0, the reproductive rate of HIV. Modeling results show that vaccines with moderate efficacy or those administered to a population with a severe HIV epidemic (as measured by R_0) could not achieve eradication; for example, 100 percent of the population at risk would need to be vaccinated if R_0 were 2.0 and the efficacy of the vaccine were 50 percent (Blower and McLean, 1994). These calculations assume no change in risk behavior.

Perinatal Transmission

The second major mode of HIV transmission in Africa is perinatal, which accounts for approximately 15 to 20 percent of all AIDS cases in sub-Saharan Africa, in contrast with 5 to 10 percent worldwide (Quinn et al., 1994). The large numbers of infected children in Africa are explained by the high proportion of women infected with the HIV virus and the large number of children each women bears. Serologic surveys of pregnant women in Africa find that between 6 and 30 percent are HIV-positive (U.S. Bureau of the Census, 1994c). Sub-Saharan Africa accounts for three of every four women who have been infected with HIV worldwide (World Health Organization, 1995b).

Perinatal transmission may occur in utero through transplacental infection, at the time of delivery, or through breastfeeding or other routes. The probability of mother-to-child transmission varies according to different studies: 27 percent in Kampala, Uganda; 30 percent in Kigali, Rwanda; 39 percent in Lusaka, Zambia; 39 percent in Nairobi, Kenya; 39 percent in Kinshasa, Zaire; and 42 percent in Brazzaville, Congo (Ryder et al., 1989; Hira et al., 1989; Lallemant et al., 1989; Miotti et al., 1990). In comparison, transmission rates have been lower in North America and Europe, ranging from 7 to 30 percent (Blanche et al., 1989; Rogers et al., 1989; Oxtoby, 1990; European Collaborative Study, 1991). Unfortunately, the results of various studies published to date are not strictly comparable because of differences in recruiting strategies for prospective studies and the criteria used to determine HIV infection among children. Nevertheless, risks of perinatal transmission reported in African studies appear to be generally higher than those reported in North American and European studies, probably because of large differences between the duration and intensity of breastfeeding by seropositive women in Europe and North America compared with women in sub-Saharan Africa. To resolve the issue of lack of standardization of study protocols, a consensus meeting was held in Ghent, Belgium, in 1992. It resulted in a definition of HIV infection in children and a clinical classification of HIV-infected mothers.

Factors that affect the probability of perinatal transmission include the disease stage and immune status during pregnancy, as measured by CD4 and CD8 cell counts; the conditions of pregnancy and delivery; the particular viral strain involved; the infectious, parasitic, and nutritional environment in which the mother and child live; the presence of chorioamnionitis and funisitis; and whether the infant is breastfed (Ryder et al., 1989; St. Louis et al., 1993; Semba et al., 1994). Of these factors, the rate of transmission associated with breastfeeding is most difficult to evaluate because infants are often exposed to HIV infection during pregnancy and at birth, as well as postnatally. Although the majority of transmission occurs pre- or intrapartum, there have been several documented cases of postnatal transmission to the infant in which the mothers were infected after delivery (Van de Perre et al., 1991; Lepage et al., 1987). Transmission in these cases occurred from mother to infant during the first year of life while the infant was being breastfed. Postnatal transmission in these instances was probably facilitated because the mothers were seroconverting and therefore had a high level of viremia, and because no immunity was passively transferred to the infants transplacentally or through breast milk. The rate of postnatal transmission estimated from these studies might be higher than that estimated for asymptomatic seropositive mothers who breastfed their infants, but is still likely to be low. The majority of infants who are infected with HIV-1 acquire the infection in utero or during childbirth. When the mother is infected prenatally, the additional risk of HIV-1 transmission via breastfeeding is estimated to be 14 percent (Dunn et al., 1992); when the mother is infected postnatally, the risk of HIV-1 transmission is 29 percent (Dunn et al., 1992). As noted earlier, the risk of perinatal transmission is much higher for HIV-1 than for HIV-2.

All babies born to an HIV-infected mother carry passively acquired maternal antibodies to HIV. Those infants who are not infected will gradually lose those antibodies, which may nevertheless persist in some cases beyond a year. Since standard tests for HIV can detect only HIV antibodies and not the virus itself, they cannot be used reliably to determine which infants born to HIV-positive mothers have been infected until the maternal antibodies have been lost (Hardy, 1991). The problem, therefore, is that the HIV status of infants born to HIV-infected mothers cannot be ascertained until well after birth. It is possible that a new inexpensive HIV test will be developed that can reliably yield positive results only if the infant is HIV-positive when cord blood is tested, although a negative result would not mean conclusively that the infant was HIV-negative (Miles et al., 1993). If such a test were developed, HIV-positive mothers might be advised that an infant who tested positive could be breastfed.

There has been much discussion concerning whether breastfeeding should be discouraged in areas where HIV is very prevalent. In 1992, a special group representing WHO/UNICEF concluded that breastfeeding should be promoted in all developing countries, regardless of HIV infection rates (World Health Organization, 1992). Breastfeeding provides a mechanism for increased spacing of births, as well as better nutrition and protection against diarrheal diseases, pneumonia, and other infections. Where the primary causes of infant deaths are infectious diseases and malnutrition, the benefits of breastfeeding outweigh the risk of HIV transmission via breastfeeding, even for women known to be infected with HIV. However, in areas with low infant mortality rates from infectious diseases, women known to be infected with HIV should be advised to use a safe feeding alternative to breastfeeding; women whose HIV status is unknown should be advised to breastfeed (World Health Organization, 1992). Several studies support the WHO/UNICEF recommendations (Choto, 1990; Kennedy et al., 1990; Nicoll et al., 1990; Ryder et al., 1991; Dunn et al., 1992; Hu et al., 1992).

Mortality among HIV-infected infants is much higher in Africa than in North America or Europe. In examining mortality rates, it is necessary to distinguish between African studies, in which survival is reported globally for infants born to seropositive mothers because of difficulty in diagnosing HIV infection during the first year, and American studies, in which mortality is often reported among infected infants only (Quinn et al., 1994). In Africa, the ultimate cause of death is not easily determined because the diagnostic tools are lacking, and because infants whose clinical deterioration is rapid do not always reach the hospital before they die. In Kinshasa, Zaire, and Brazzaville, Congo, mortality at 12 months was found to be 21 and 37 percent, respectively, for children born to HIV-seropositive mothers and 4 percent for controls (Ryder and Hassig, 1988). In a study in Malawi, mortality rates were 32 percent for the first 24 months for infants born to seropositive mothers and 11 percent for controls (Taha et al., forthcoming). In rural Rakai, Uganda, infant mortality rates were 210 per 1,000 live births for children born to HIV-seropositive mothers and 111 per 1,000 for those born to HIV-seronegative mothers (Sewankambo et al., 1994).

High mortality rates among HIV-infected children are due not only to the direct effects of HIV, but also to the profound disruption of the family unit associated with the infection (Preble, 1990). In many cases, the parents themselves are incapacitated by HIV infection, becoming progressively less capable of caring for their families. Parental loss and worsening socioeconomic status affect the survival of children in the family regardless of HIV serologic status.

In countries with large numbers of HIV-seropositive women, the impact of AIDS on overall childhood survival is already being felt. In Zimbabwe, approximately half of pediatric hospital admissions were from HIV-associated illness. However, the extent of illness among hospitalized children that is due to HIV infection and AIDS is unknown because of the difficulty involved in making a diagnosis in young children. Using available HIV seroprevalence data for women living in several African countries, Valleroy et al. (1990) estimated the percentage increase in infant-child mortality rates that is due to HIV-attributable mortality. They estimated that infant mortality rates would increase by 6 to 38 percent in Kampala and by 1 to 6 percent in Nairobi as a result of HIV infection (Valleroy et al., 1990). WHO also estimated that within the previous 10 years, nearly 500,000 infants in Africa had been born with HIV infection (Chin, 1990). By the year 2000, there will be an additional 10 million HIV-infected children in Africa. In addition, 5 to 10 million children under age 10 are expected to become orphans during the 1990s because of the death of one or both parents from AIDS. During the decade, it is estimated that infant and child mortality rates in some African countries will increase by 50 percent as a result of AIDS.

Parenteral Transmission

The third mode of HIV infection is parenteral transmission, which includes blood transfusions, injections, and scarification. This mode represents less than 10 percent of all HIV cases in sub-Saharan Africa (Piot et al., 1988).

Blood transfusion with HIV-infected blood is known to be a very efficient means of transmission, with over 90 percent of recipients becoming infected. Unfortunately, blood screening, which is universal in industrialized countries, is not widely available in many developing areas of the world. The impact of not screening is substantial. In Central Africa, HIV seroprevalence is between 2 and 18 percent among blood donors (Mhalu and Ryder, 1988). The public health impact of exposing African populations to unscreened blood units has been documented in several countries. In one survey of 2,384 health care workers in Kinshasa, 9 percent of HIV-seropositive individuals had received blood transfusions as compared with 5 percent of HIV-seronegative individuals (Mann et al., 1986c). In a study of children who were admitted to general pediatrics or measles wards and whose mothers were HIV-seronegative, 31 percent of seropositive children had received blood transfusions, as compared with only 7 percent of seronegative children (Mann et al., 1986a). In another study of older children admitted to a pediatrics ward but not diagnosed with AIDS, 60 percent of children infected with HIV had received blood transfusions, whereas only 33 percent of the HIV-seronegative children had received transfusions (Mann et al., 1986b).

HIV transmission via blood transfusion is often associated with preventable endemic tropical diseases. In pediatric populations, malaria-associated anemia is highly prevalent, and patients are often given multiple transfusions for treatment. In one study in Kinshasa, 87 percent of blood transfusions at one hospital had been given to children for malaria-induced anemia. In that study, it was estimated that as many as 561 new pediatric cases of HIV infection would occur each year in one hospital if donated blood were not screened for HIV (Greenberg et al., 1988).

With increasing awareness of the transmission of HIV through blood transfusion, transmission through infected blood and blood products is being reduced as appropriate screening of donated blood is introduced. Other measures being taken to protect the blood supply include recruiting donors from among low-risk population groups on a voluntary and unpaid basis. Health-care workers are also being encouraged to revise their guidelines on transfusion to ensure that the procedure is carried out only when absolutely necessary, and that saline solutions are used as blood substitutes whenever possible.

Needles and other sharp instruments used by traditional African healers are an unproved but possibly important mode of HIV transmission (N'Galy et al., 1988; Berkley et al., 1989). Traditional healers normally establish patient practices in a village, or have a mobile practice in which they visit a circuit of different towns and villages. Many practitioners give their patients injectable antibiotics; injection equipment used is sterilized poorly or not at all. Ironically, the practice of giving prophylactic antibiotics may facilitate HIV transmission because the patient receives an additional injection with blood-contaminated needles and syringes. Because needle use is so ubiquitous in Africa, it is difficult to determine a true causal relationship between needle use and needle transmission. Cosmetic scarification, with its custom of using communally shared cutting utensils, is another possible mode of HIV transmission, as is tattooing with unsterilized needles.

HIV transmission through the use of unsterilized paraphernalia by injecting drug users has not been documented as a major mode of HIV transmission in Africa. In contrast with the situation in developed countries, injectable drugs such as heroin or cocaine are not commonly found or used in Africa, although they are becoming more popular in certain port areas and among the more affluent population (World Health Organization, 1994). The low incidence of injectable drug use in Africa has been attributed to the expense of the drugs and associated paraphernalia.

REMAINING GAPS IN KNOWLEDGE

Limitations of Existing African Behavioral Data

With a more complex set of data, it would be possible to understand better the social and behavioral processes that underlie the HIV/AIDS epidemic. To develop more effective AIDS- and STD-prevention strategies, additional information is needed on sexual behaviors (including sexual networking), particularly their determinants (as discussed in Chapter 4), and on barriers to the effective and rapid adoption of preventive measures, including reduced numbers of partners, safe and nonpenetrative sex, condom use, and care seeking for symptoms of STDs (as discussed in Chapter 5). Specifically, data on timing of entrance into a sexual network, dominant sexual practices, and timing of permanent or transitory exit from and re-entry into sexual networks would provide a better understanding of the social and behavioral aspects of HIV transmission. More complex data would also provide information on the conditional probability of infection and its association with particular practices, the presence of other diseases, and possible duration dependencies.

Unfortunately, social science research related to sexuality, AIDS, and STDs in Africa has most frequently been conducted in urban areas and among groups that fit the Western concept of high-risk behavior, such as commercial sex workers and the military; other groups in the general population that may also be at high risk because of elevated underlying HIV prevalence are less likely to be contacted (Udvardy, 1990). Logistical problems associated with community-based research have further resulted in a preponderance of urban clinic, hospital, and high-risk group studies, and more recently, community-based urban and rural serosurveys involving little or no behavioral research (Kaheru, 1989; Rwandan HIV Seroprevalence Study Group, 1989). The number of studies combining HIV serologic and behavioral research among representative community-based populations, particularly among rural dwellers, remains small (Konde-Lule et al., 1989; Killewo et al., 1990; Serwadda et al., 1992; Mulder et al., 1994b). The need for such research is underlined by the fact that the vast majority of Africans reside in rural areas, and may account for the bulk of the region's HIV infection.

Only recently have researchers started to collect data on actual African sexual practices and patterns. It has been noted that "anthropologists have devoted relatively little attention to the systematic study of sexual behavior. There are many studies of marriage and divorce, of the social, economic and ritual roles of women, of changes in male-female relationships and in other institutionalized forms of gender behavior. Where sexual practices are mentioned, however, they are often of a generalized nature" (Brokensha, 1988:167-168). Similarly, data on sexual networks and the determinants of partner selection remain limited in quantity and scope (Orubuloye et al., 1990; Obbo, 1993), so that empirical findings are incomplete at best.

We still have much to learn about the acceptance of and barriers to other aspects of HIV/AIDS prevention, including condom use. As yet, there are inadequate data on care seeking for STDs and AIDS, and on the determinants of acceptance of HIV serological testing.

When considering available data, as well as data that will become available in the next decade, we must be careful not to overgeneralize findings from one African setting to another (Ntozi and Lubega, 1990). As emphasized throughout this report, Africa is culturally diverse, and neighboring groups of closely related peoples can have very different cultural expectations. Given evidence of variability in sexual beliefs and practices, the utility of overarching models of African sexuality has been questioned (Schoepf, 1990).

To summarize, available social and behavioral data have limitations from the viewpoint of supporting the development of more effective AIDS-prevention strategies or projecting future transmission. Little is known about the range of sexual options open to individuals; the types of sexual practices conducted with different partners; and changes brought about by migration, various degrees of urbanization, and AIDS itself. The next chapter surveys the available knowledge on these issues. Chapter 7 examines means of building an indigenous capacity for HIV/AIDS-related research in Africa.

The Need to Combine Epidemiological and Social/Behavioral Research

To date, the interpretation and utility of much epidemiological and social/behavioral research have been limited by the lack of a multidisciplinary approach. Data on reported behavior change may be difficult to assess in the absence of biological validation that such change is sufficient to reduce STD/HIV acquisition. Efforts to model the demographic effects of the HIV/AIDS epidemic are hindered by a paucity of data sets that combine fertility, mortality, migration, and other sociodemographic information with HIV serology. Conversely, serological studies that fail to collect adequate behavioral data miss an important opportunity to assess the effects of factors such as sexual practices, sexual networks, and injecting drug use practices within given populations. There is also a growing realization that the design, execution, and analysis of clinical trials for HIV vaccines, STD control, antiretroviral drugs, and genital barrier methods/viricides all depend on appropriate behavioral research to guide enrollment, ensure adherence to trial protocols, and permit adequate interpretation of epidemiological results (including the very basic need to control for potential differential behavioral change among study groups).

The disjunction between epidemiological and social/behavioral research has been due in part to a perception by behavioral scientists that biological specimen collection is difficult, intrusive, and unacceptable to subjects and to caution among clinical/epidemiological researchers in posing questions about potentially intimate behaviors within the context of studies that collect substantial biological samples. However, such reluctance to implement multidisciplinary research is rapidly losing its rationale as the STD/HIV epidemic continues to intensify and as techniques for and experience in the application of combined epidemiological/social science studies improve.

On the biological front, assessment of HIV prevalence/incidence has been greatly facilitated by the development of serological collection methods that do not call for venous blood collection. Finger prick/filter paper and saliva tests are now well established as tools in HIV epidemiology (Behets et al., 1992; Belec et al., 1994; Nyambi et al., 1994; Pappaioanou et al., 1993; Frerichs et al., 1994), and HIV assessment from urine samples is under development (Cao et al., 1988; Berrios et al., 1995). Such samples can be collected by lay personnel in nonclinic settings. Urine samples can also be used to quantify gonorrhea and chlamydia prevalence (Chernesky et al., 1994; Lee et al., 1995; Smith et al., 1995), and there is positive experience with home-based collection of self-administered vaginal swabs for trichomonas culture (Wawer et al., 1995a) and the determination of bacterial vaginosis (Nugent et al., 1991; Speigel et al., 1983). From the behavioral viewpoint, detailed data on sexual networks and practices have been collected on subjects in diverse cultural settings (Dyson, 1992; Caldwell et al., 1993; Orubuloye et al., 1994).

A few studies have integrated biological specimen and detailed behavioral information collection in community surveys and have achieved high participation rates (Mulder et al., 1994a; Wawer et al., 1995a). The Demographic and Health Surveys (DHS) project is currently planning a pilot survey that would combine biological sample collection with standard DHS sociodemographic and contraceptive information (Cynthia Stanton, personal communication, 1995). Although experience is still limited, data suggest that a combined epidemiological/social science research approach will prove acceptable in many clinic and population-based settings.

Ethical Issues in STD/HIV Research

According to guidelines for research involving human subjects developed jointly by the Council for International Organizations of Medical Sciences (CIOMS) and WHO, when research is conducted by investigators of one country on subjects of another, the ethical standards applied should be no less exacting than if the research were carried out in the initiating country (Council for International Organizations of Medical Sciences and World Health Organization, 1992). It has also been noted, however, that "the great complexity, varied presentation, and wide distribution of HIV infection challenge this stance" (Christakis, 1988:31) and that the stated purpose of the CIOMS/WHO guidelines is, in part, to anticipate such issues and suggest they can be applied to the special circumstances of developing countries (Christakis, 1988).

Ethical standards related to biological and behavioral data collection, and to intervention trials of medical and behavioral prevention modalities, include voluntary informed consent, confidentiality, randomization, avoidance of physical/psychological risk, and provision of STD/HIV counseling and preventive services (Christakis, 1988; Barry, 1988). The concept of justice is also relevant, particularly in the case of international research: the burdens of research should be justly distributed, and disadvantaged communities should be assured of reaping an equal share of potential benefits—such as access to effective vaccines that have been tested in part in developing countries (Beauchamp and Childress, 1983; Christakis, 1988; Garner et al., 1994). Each of these issues is complex, and only a few salient points can be summarized here.

Voluntary informed consent represents an ethical imperative in behavioral and medical research. In studies conducted in Africa (or other regions, for that matter), informed consent procedures must take cultural practices into consideration. Thus, community-based research may require the consent of the head of the household prior to the enrollment of other household members, in addition to confidential individual consent. It is obvious that consent forms require careful translation into the local language (or prevalent European language or dialect, if appropriate). In addition, the legalistic language required by U.S.-based institutional committees is frequently incomprehensible and inappropriate for African contexts. Some flexibility is required to develop appropriate formulations, while safeguarding the inviolate principal of voluntary and informed participation in research activities.

A recent review of HIV/AIDS intervention research concludes that the majority of behavioral intervention studies reported in the literature were methodologically inadequate for assessing intervention effectiveness (Oakley et al., 1995). The authors consider randomized controlled trials most appropriate for evaluating the effectiveness of behavioral interventions, but note that "it is commonly argued by behavioral researchers that random allocation to experimental groups is ethically more dubious than the uncontrolled experimentation resulting from less robust designs or from the implementation of unevaluated programs." The authors conclude that the resulting methodological weaknesses have led to a situation in which there is "a troubling lack of . . . soundly based preventive interventions," and they call for more randomized controlled trials to provide adequate guidance for investment in HIV/AIDS behavioral interventions (Oakley et al., 1995:484). A similar call for controlled trials has been sounded by Aral and Peterman (1993). Involving subjects in inadequately controlled trials is itself ethically questionable, as it requires commitment (and potentially some inconvenience and risk) on the part of study subjects with no assurance that this commitment will result in useful data or effective programs.

Assessment of reasonable research risk must take into consideration existing services, prevention strategies, and medical care in a given setting. It is obvious that regardless of where it is conducted, research must never take advantage of a lack of alternative services to test strategies that are of dubious benefit or are associated with inappropriate risk. However, in places where diagnostic and service delivery alternatives are very limited, testing of STD/HIV prevention, diagnostic, and treatment strategies that would not be applicable in the North American or European context may be appropriate, provided such research offers distinct potential for the development of locally appropriate and sustainable approaches that would otherwise not exist. Examples include innovative STD interventions based on limited diagnostics. In any case, the involvement of host country researchers, care givers, and policy makers in ethical decision making is essential in weighing the local risks and benefits of particular research efforts.

A potential barrier to the integration of behavioral and epidemiological research has been the perception that serological testing for HIV must always include mandatory HIV counseling (i.e., that for ethical reasons and in keeping with U.S. domestic federal regulations, subjects cannot be enrolled unless they agree, a priori, to receive their HIV results). Researchers (both behavioral and other) have thus shied away from collecting blood specimens or at best have collected unlinked, anonymous specimens, thus severely constraining the analysis and interpretation of results. In reality, the desirability of voluntary HIV counseling may be dictated by both the value of enrolling truly representative population samples in some intervention trials (and not only those persons who agree to receive their results) and host country regulations and standards. Indeed, large population-based HIV studies in countries such as Uganda and Tanzania have adopted voluntary testing strategies, with the proviso that HIV results be made readily available and that the programs provide information and motivation for subjects to receive their results. In Nairobi, Kenya, women were tested in perinatal HIV transmission studies after giving voluntary informed consent and were given an appointment one week later to collect their results. Among the 243 women who were told that they were infected, three-quarters did not report their HIV-positive status to their partner, 1 committed suicide, 7 were beaten, and 11 were replaced by another wife or expelled from their home. The investigators subsequently adopted a policy respecting women's right not to know their HIV test results (Temmerman et al., 1995).

Finally, although it is ethically important to provide an appropriate level of HIV education and prevention services to all study participants, in a randomized trial it is also important to ensure sufficient difference between treatment and control groups to allow interpretation of data. Studies that "overtreat" control group subjects and thus do not meet this basic criterion are themselves of questionable ethical standing, as they may lead to false conclusions and subsequent ineffective programs or the dismissal of a useful approach to HIV prevention. Services provided to control-group subjects must at a minimum meet local standards of care; it is not necessarily appropriate for them to meet U.S. standards of care. To borrow an example from medical interventions, WHO recently concluded that comparing simplified intrapartum Zidovudine (AZT) regimens with untreated controls can be ethically appropriate in settings where AZT is not otherwise available, even if such a control group would no longer be appropriate in the United States (World Health Organization, forthcoming).

RECOMMENDATIONS

KEY RECOMMENDATION 1. Basic surveillance systems for monitoring the prevalence and incidence of STDs and HIV must be strengthened and expanded.

Good social science research is as dependent as public health and medical research on reliable and valid HIV/AIDS surveillance data. With the implementation of various interventions aimed at controlling HIV transmission, periodic monitoring of STD and HIV prevalence and incidence among selected populations is essential both for assessment of the impact of these programs and for decision making on program design and implementation.

Recommendation 3-1. More emphasis must be placed on HIV incidence studies for monitoring trends in HIV infection rates.

Although seroprevalence provides important information regarding currently infected individuals in an area, measuring incidence is also critically important for estimating the rate of change in the spread of HIV infection in a given population. In particular, data on current incidence provide the most direct and immediate information regarding the potential effects of a given intervention. Together, prevalence and incidence studies can provide information regarding the current status of the epidemic in terms of numbers of infected individuals and the rate of spread within a given population on an annual basis.

Recommendation 3-2. STD and HIV prevalence and incidence data should be combined with behavioral and demographic information.

Current surveillance systems are often limited, incomplete, and inconsistent, and they rarely measure behavioral or demographic variables. Given new, noninvasive techniques for the collection and analysis of biological specimens (including blood, urine, vaginal secretions, and saliva), accurate assessment of STD and HIV prevalence and incidence can readily be combined with behavioral and demographic information.

In conjunction with periodic serosurveys, demographic information is needed to elucidate the differential spread of STD and HIV infection in rural and urban settings and variations in seroprevalence and incidence by gender, educational level, profession, income level, age, and other demographic factors. This type of information is critical for targeting prevention messages to selected groups at risk of acquiring and transmitting HIV and for projecting the effects of HIV and other STDs on a population over time.

4

Sexual Behavior and HIV/AIDS

This chapter discusses what we know about sexual behavior and HIV/AIDS in Africa. Given that the epidemic is being sustained by heterosexual transmission (see Chapter 3), information on sexual behavior is needed to help project the future course of the HIV/AIDS epidemic, to develop more effective prevention strategies, and to provide baseline data for evaluating the effectiveness of alternative prevention strategies. Consequently, this chapter provides important background information for the next chapter, which deals with prevention.

Published papers on sexual behavior and HIV/AIDS in sub-Saharan Africa show a remarkable uniformity in their point of departure and their destination. They tend to begin with the observation that in the absence of a vaccine or cure, changing sexual behavior is the only way to halt the spread of the HIV/AIDS epidemic in the region, and they end with a call for more research. What lies between diverges widely in methodology, focus, presentation of results, and conclusions. This chapter reviews some of this literature, attempting to identify common threads and define the boundaries of what we know. It concentrates on work dealing with general populations, although reference is made to some of the larger body of work on high-risk groups, such as commercial sex workers. The sections that follow address sources of information on sexual behavior in Africa, patterns of sexual activity, sex-related risk factors for HIV/AIDS, sexual practices and beliefs, AIDS awareness, the role of condoms, and behavior change. The chapter ends with conclusions and a set of recommendations for future research.

SOURCES OF INFORMATION

Researchers have often noted the dearth of studies on sexual behavior in sub-Saharan Africa. According to Larson (1989:9), "data on actual practice [of extramarital sex] are extremely rare and probably worthless." What little was known about sexual behavior in Africa at the time was exhaustively reviewed by Standing and Kisekka (1989). Accordingly, while some mention is made here of the early ethnographic work they reviewed, this chapter focuses on work published subsequently.

This chapter relies heavily on the results of a series of nine surveys coordinated by the World Health Organization/Global Programme on AIDS (WHO/GPA) that were carried out in 1989 and 1990. Eight of the surveys were national in coverage, while the ninth was conducted in Lusaka, Zambia. These surveys provide information on age at sexual initiation; broad patterns of sexual activity within and outside of stable unions; levels of commercial sex; and many other issues, such as perceived risk.[1]

QUESTIONS OF METHODOLOGY

The two principal sources of information about sexual behavior are ethnographic accounts and survey methods. Ethnographic accounts typically focus on sexual behavior only insofar as it relates to family, marriage, and kinship. Anthropological research uses primarily qualitative methods and participant observation for data collection. The goal usually is not to quantify the behaviors, but to understand their intent and meanings. This research is important to the design of interventions, but says little about the number of times an event occurs, its duration, or other factors of concern to disease transmission models. Large-scale surveys are designed to provide information that is comparable across cultures, but are forced to use sweeping, standardized definitions for complex and highly varied concepts such as marriage. Increasingly, researchers are designing studies that aim to bridge the gap between detailed observation of particular societies and broad characterizations of patterns and trends, for instance by combining survey data with diaries and in-depth interviews.

The principal danger with using survey methodology to collect data on sexual behavior is that respondents may simply say what they think researchers want to hear and that without elaborate probing, such methods may lead to a serious undercount of the true situation (Bleek, 1987). Women are believed to be particularly prone to giving normative answers. Indeed, women are sometimes excluded from surveys altogether for fear that their responses will be worthless

---

[1]See Ferry (1995a) for more details regarding the characteristics of the WHO/GPA surveys and a detailed assessment of the data quality.

(Hogsborg and Aaby, 1992; Orubuloye et al., 1992). Nevertheless, there is also evidence that people are not entirely swayed by social norms when reporting their own behavior. For instance, several studies report a large gap between proportions expressing disapproval of premarital sex (typically high) and those reporting virginity at marriage (frequently low) (see, for example, Anarfi, 1993).

Public health researchers, independent of discipline, use both qualitative and quantitative methods to improve our understanding of behaviors. In an effort to verify independently the WHO/GPA estimates of sexual behavior, the WHO/GPA survey material is therefore supplemented here, as the authors of those studies urge, with less-generalizable surveys and information derived from ethnography, observational studies, serosurveys, and focus group interviews. Study designs differ substantially; those of the principal papers used in this chapter are summarized in Table 4-1. The following subsection makes some general observations about difficulties common to several studies.

Concerns about large-scale comparative survey research include the selection, operationalization, and validation of responses to items in the questionnaire. For example, researchers frequently need to use broad and sometimes arbitrary categories for comparability across research sites (e.g., partner categories such as regular and casual). Many of the difficulties that arise in conducting survey research are compounded when one is conducting research about intimate topics such as sexuality (Bleek, 1987). In the quest for comparability, large-scale surveys sacrifice information that may help explain local differences in sexual networking. Nor are international surveys likely to contribute much to our understanding of motivations for behavioral change. However, such surveys can be useful in highlighting patterns that link sociodemographic variables and personal behavior. As the editors of the WHO/GPA volume observe, single-round surveys are also good at describing the climate of public opinion and measuring the incidence of certain behaviors (Cleland and Ferry, 1995). Moreover, repeated over time, nationally representative surveys can help track behavior change.

Sampling proved problematic in many of the WHO/GPA studies reviewed. Although the WHO/GPA surveys covering the Central African Republic, Côte d'Ivoire, Guinea-Bissau, Togo, Burundi, Kenya, Lesotho, and Tanzania sought to be nationally representative, sampling difficulties appear to have led to an overrepresentation of women and urban residents in some cases. The remaining WHO/GPA survey in mainland sub-Saharan Africa, that in Lusaka, Zambia, leaned heavily toward the more educated.

Family formation norms vary widely throughout the African continent, and marriage in many African societies has often been described as being more akin to a process than a discrete event. It has proved difficult to develop easily understood definitions for sexual partners, and many of the subtleties of various forms of marriage are lost when all forms of unions are coded using a small number of standardized categories. For example, the WHO/GPA surveys make no distinction between regular partnerships and marriages, "regular" partnership

TABLE 4-1 Details of Some Studies of Sexual Behavior Cited in This Chapter

Reference	Study Population	Sample Size	Main Methodology	Limitations
Anarfi (1993)	Ghana, rural, urban	1,360	Cross-sectional survey	Unclear reference periods
Anarfi and Awusabo-Asare (1993)	Ghana, various lineal groups	360	Cross-sectional survey	Interviewers known to respondents; no clear definitions of marriage
Hogsborg and Aaby (1992)	Guinea-Bissau, urban (both sexes, but diary respondents all male)	422 25	Cross-sectional survey Diaries	Diary men purposively chosen
Hunter et al. (1994)	Nairobi, Kenya, prenatal clinic attenders	4,401	Serosurvey	
Irwin et al. (1991)	Kinshasa, Zaire, male factory workers	1,796	Serosurvey, focus groups	
Kisekka (no date)	Hausa groups, Nigeria; Baganda, Uganda	n.a.	Focus groups	
Konde-Lule (1993)	Rakai, Uganda	35 groups of 8-12 respondents	Focus groups	
Lindan et al. (1991)	Kigali, Rwanda prenatal clinic attenders	1,458	Serosurvey	
Meekers (1994)	DHS data, 7 African nations	n.a.	Survey data analysis	
Messersmith et al. (1994)	Ile-Ife, Nigeria (men aged 18-59, women aged 18-49)	1,149	Cross-sectional survey	Excludes adolescents

Meursing et al. (forthcoming)	Bulawayo, Zimbabwe, sexually abused children	54	Clinical examination, record review, focus groups	
O'Toole Erwin (1993)	Ado-Ekiti, Nigeria, prenatal clinic attenders	113 455	Clinical examination Cross-sectional survey	
Ogbuagu and Charles (1993)	Calabar, Nigeria	500	Cross-sectional survey	High nonresponse rate; partnerships not clearly defined
Orubuloye et al. (1991)	Ekiti, Nigeria, urban and rural	400	Cross-sectional survey	Unclear reference periods, denominators, and partner definitions; no cross-checking of spousal replies possible
Orubuloye et al. (1992)	Ekiti, Nigeria	488	"The lawyer's cross-examination method of investigation by exhaustion"	
Pickering et al. (1992)	The Gambia, prostitutes (p) and clients (c)	248p 795c	Prospective survey, diaries	
Preston-Whyte (1994)	Kwazulu/Natal, adolescents	n.a.	Focus groups, intervention	All mixed-sex focus groups
Schopper et al. (1993)	Moyo, Uganda	1,486	Cross-sectional survey	
Serwadda et al. (1992)	Rakai, Uganda, trading towns, rural	1,292	Serosurvey	

n.a. = not available
DHS = Demographic and Health Surveys

being any union that continues or is expected to continue, however sporadically, for at least a year. "Casual" is anything outside that, and any partnership that lasts under a year and involves the exchange of money, gifts, or favors in exchange for sex is classified as "commercial." In the standard partner relations questionnaire,[2] it is frequently difficult to distinguish one category from another, and secondary regular partners may be double-counted as casual, unless the interviewers were very skillful. In a study designed to test the validity of the WHO/GPA survey instrument, Schopper et al. (1993) showed that among 392 women whose answers could be cross-checked with those of their partner, 12 percent reported they had co-wives when their husbands declared themselves monogamously married, thus illustrating the difficulty of watertight categorization. Other surveys use entirely different definitions, so that even comparing data on premarital sex becomes fraught with difficulty.

Discrepant reference periods do little to clear the confusion. Without defining the term "current," several West African studies make a distinction between current partners and partners within the previous week (e.g., Orubuloye et al., 1991; Anarfi, 1993). As documented by Orubuloye et al. (1991), consistently more men and women in both urban and rural areas reported abstinence in the last month (and, except for rural males, in the last 12 months) than reported abstinence currently, which leaves us with a puzzle for interpretation. That respondents are confused by definitions emerges also from a study by Ogbuagu and Charles (1993). In that study, 55 percent of women reported more than one current partner. However, when asked directly if they kept other partners outside their regular partnership, 66 percent answered no.

Sources of bias are sometimes incompletely documented. Often studies state or imply significant levels of nonresponse, but give no information on possible refusal bias (Ogbuagu and Charles, 1993; Omorodion, 1993; Oyeneye and Kawonise, 1993). Bias can also arise from the injudicious or unclear use of denominators; for instance, excluding virgins from the denominator will bias downward the mean age of onset of sexual activity in the youngest cohorts (Konings et al., 1994).

The question of age cut-offs is relevant to almost every study. Although overwhelming evidence of early sexual activity is provided in existing sources such as the Demographic and Health Surveys (DHS) series, the successor to the World Fertility Surveys (WFS), very few studies include people under age 15. Indeed, some investigate only the behavior of people over age 18 (e.g., Messersmith et al., 1994), and many exclude women after they reach age 50.

[2]The WHO/GPA surveys used one of three questionnaire types: (a) a knowledge, attitudes, beliefs, and practice (KABP) questionnaire that investigated general attitudes and behaviors related to HIV/AIDS; (b) a partner relations (PR) questionnaire that focused more narrowly on sexual behavior; and (c) a combination of (a) and (b). In Tanzania, surveys of both types (a) and (b) were conducted.

Other shortcomings common across studies are a lack of information about economic status (education is often the only proxy for socioeconomic status) and a failure to include information about the content of public education campaigns, data that might help us understand local knowledge and attitudes.

The Issue of Validity

Self-reported data on sexual activity are of course more or less impossible to verify absolutely. But other checks can be made. For example, are study results consistent with what we know from other sources? The answer would appear to depend on the context. The age at first intercourse reported in the WHO/GPA surveys does not differ strikingly from the available DHS data (Schopper et al., 1993; Meekers, 1994). On occasion, however, reported condom use differs greatly, appearing much higher for a given country in the WHO/GPA surveys than in subsequent DHS surveys (Cleland and Ferry, 1995). This discrepancy may occur because people's answers differ according to the intent of the survey.

Are data mutually consistent? In the WHO/GPA surveys, consistency is difficult to check because there is no device for linking two halves of a couple when each individual has been randomly selected. Since questions are not repeated within the same interview, internal consistency checks are difficult as well. There is, however, broad aggregate agreement between the sexes on coital frequency and number of regular partners. In Schopper et al. (1993), a study using the WHO/GPA survey instrument, 392 couples were identified among the 1,486 individuals randomly selected for interview. Although it was confirmed that results were good on an aggregate basis, there were significant disparities on the individual couple level in reports of coital frequency between monogamous couples reporting no outside partners.[3] Similar results are cited by Rutenberg et al. (1994) using Tanzanian DHS data for 1991/1992; men reported on average 35 percent more sexual contacts than women. That study shows further that women are just as likely as men to report higher frequency than their partner.

Studies on sexual behavior consistently find that men report more partners than women. For instance, Konings et al. (1994) show men reporting around 10 times as many partners as women. This discrepancy may occur because men overreport their partners, because women underreport theirs, or because a large number of men network with a small number of women who have a high turnover of partners. Many researchers point out that their study populations are unlikely to capture sex workers; few indicate whether they include men likely to be clients

[3]This discrepancy is perhaps to be expected; recalling coital frequency is not easy. Differences in coital frequency, though apparently small, can add up to quite large differences in overall sexual activity (because a larger proportion of men is sexually active at any given time).

of sex workers, such as truck drivers or the military—highly mobile groups that might escape the sampler's net.

One way of teasing bias out of a single-round survey is to supplement it with other methods. Repeated interviews at short intervals and respondent diaries have been shown to be effective in this regard. Using this method, studies in Guinea-Bissau and Senegal suggest overreporting of coital frequency in surveys, but underreporting of numbers of partners (Hogsborg and Aaby, 1992; Enel et al., 1994). Similarly, Pickering et al. (1992) used diaries to show that prostitutes in The Gambia consistently gave higher totals of client contacts in surveys than when reporting daily; comparison with questionnaires administered to clients emerging from their rooms showed that the women also overreported condom use in surveys.

More cross-referencing of questions might help identify bias in normative responses. In focus group interviews of schoolgirls in Zimbabwe, most denied they had sugar daddies, that is, older men as boyfriends who gave them presents or money for sex; however, in answer to a later question, half volunteered ways of keeping presents from sugar daddies hidden from parents, indicating that their earlier responses may have been less than wholly honest (Vos, 1994). Individual interviews might have avoided this discrepancy. Ethnographic models may also be applied to resolve discrepancies in single-round survey results (Stone and Campbell, 1984).

It is clearly premature to reach any firm conclusions about the reliability or validity of survey data on sexual behavior in developing countries. However, after a review of the evidence, Dare and Cleland (1994) are guardedly optimistic that the information gathered in most surveys is solid enough to allow broad conclusions to be drawn.

PATTERNS OF SEXUAL ACTIVITY

This section examines patterns of sexual activity in sub-Saharan cultures, including sexual initiation and premarital intercourse, sex within marriage or a stable union, extramarital and casual sex, and commercial sex.

Sexual Initiation and Premarital Intercourse

Marriage has long been considered a proxy for the onset of sexual activity. In cultures where female sexuality is strongly proscribed, an increase in premarital sex is often believed to be synonymous with the amoralizing influence of modernization. In premodern times, marriage for most sub-Saharan African women took place around puberty. Now, in some African societies, changes associated with modernization, such as increasing urbanization and greater emphasis on formal education for women, have led to an increase in the age at first marriage for women.

In some sub-Saharan African civilizations (although by no means universally), marriage has been an unfolding process rather than a salient event (Meekers, 1992). As Bledsoe (1990:118) writes:

> The first problem is that of defining when marriage begins and ends. African marriage is often a long, ambiguous process rather than a unitary event. It may extend over a period of months or even years, as partners and their families work cautiously toward more stable conjugal relationships. A girl, sometimes with her family's implicit permission, may test out potential relationships with several young men before establishing a more permanent one.

This ambiguity presents researchers with an additional problem of interpretation, since the answer to the question "Were you a virgin at marriage?" clearly depends on how the respondent dates marriage. If a union turned out to be successful, the respondent may in retrospect date the marriage from the start of that union, even though it was at the time a tenuous and potentially transitory liaison (van de Walle, 1993).

A substantial body of work addresses the question of premarital sex. Inevitably, definitions vary widely. In the WHO/GPA surveys, for instance, the term refers to any sex before first regular partnership. Other surveys define the term as any sexual activity before legally or traditionally sanctioned marriage, thus including early sex between people who subsequently go on to marry. Table 4-2 gives some of the findings reported by the various studies.

As mentioned earlier, several studies show a discrepancy between a persistent ideal of virginity at marriage and actual levels of premarital activity, both now and in the past. In Anarfi (1993), three-quarters of both men and women said they believed women should be virgins at marriage, but barely 1 in 10 of either sex maintained that he or she was. Further, two-thirds of ever-married men and half of ever-married women reported having had two or more premarital partners. Some 40 percent of respondents in Ogbuagu and Charles' (1993) study in Calabar, Nigeria, said they hold virginity at marriage as an ideal, but fewer than half that proportion could report no sex before marriage. While Botswana and Kenya display strong evidence of a rise in premarital sex, Meekers (1994), using data from a variety of DHS studies, shows that there is generally a substantial fall in the proportions of single women currently reporting sexual activity as compared with the proportions of married women saying they experienced sex before marriage. While the figures are distorted by the fact that many single women who are still virgins may go on to have premarital sex, this observation also hints that it may be easier to report socially dubious behavior after the fact than at the time of its occurrence.

Several researchers note that women sometimes feel under pressure to prove they are fertile by getting pregnant in order to increase their chances of marriage (e.g., Standing and Kisekka, 1989). Because of a ubiquitous age difference at marriage between men and women, any decline in polygyny—as long as popula-

TABLE 4-2 Percentage of Respondents Reporting Premarital Sex in Various Studies

Reference	Country	Population	Study Period	Percent Reporting Premarital Sex	
				Women	Men
Cleland and Ferry (1995)	Burundi	singles (15-19)	12 months	3	10
Meekers (1994)	Burundi	all single	ever	5	n.a.
Meekers (1994)	Burundi	all ever-married	ever	20	n.a.
Balépa et al. (1992)	Cameroon	all single	ever	57	n.a.
Cleland and Ferry (1995)	CAR	singles (15-19)	12 months	56	69
Cleland and Ferry (1995)	Côte d'Ivoire	singles (15-19)	12 months	28	43
Anarfi & Awusabo-Asare (1993)	Ghana	all respondents	ever	75	90
Anarfi (1993)	Ghana	all respondents	ever	87	n.a.
Meekers (1994)	Ghana	all single	ever	47	n.a.
Meekers (1994)	Ghana	all ever-married	ever	60	n.a.
Cleland and Ferry (1995)	Guinea-Bissau	singles (15-19)	12 months	30	51
Cleland and Ferry (1995)	Kenya	singles (15-19)	12 months	44	54
Meekers (1994)	Kenya	all single	ever	50	n.a.
Meekers (1994)	Kenya	all ever-married	ever	61	n.a.
Cleland and Ferry (1995)	Lesotho	singles (15-19)	12 months	16	33

Meekers (1994)	Liberia	all single	ever	81	n.a.
Meekers (1994)	Liberia	all ever-married	ever	59	n.a.
Meekers (1994)	Mali	all single	ever	6	n.a.
Meekers (1994)	Mali	all ever-married	ever	13	n.a.
Kourguéni et al. (1993)	Niger	all single	ever	10	n.a.
Messersmith (1994)	Nigeria	all respondents	ever	53	85
Ogbuagu and Charles (1993)	Nigeria	all respondents	ever	82	83
Federal Office of Statistics (1992)	Nigeria	all single	ever	41	n.a.
Barrère et al. (1994)	Rwanda	all single	ever	12	n.a.
Cleland and Ferry (1995)	Tanzania	singles (15-19)	12 months	24	37
Rutenberg (1994)	Tanzania	all single	ever	44	72
Cleland and Ferry (1995)	Togo	singles (15-19)	12 months	3	18
Meekers (1994)	Togo	all single	ever	61	n.a.
Meekers (1994)	Togo	all ever-married	ever	65	n.a.
Cleland and Ferry (1995)	Lusaka, Zambia	singles (15-19)	12 months	10	16
Meekers (1994)	Zimbabwe	all single	ever	26	n.a.
Meekers (1994)	Zimbabwe	all ever-married	ever	48	n.a.

n.a. = not available
CAR = Central African Republic

tions are growing—would increase the pool of available women of marriageable age relative to potential husbands in older cohorts. This increase would be likely to intensify competition for husbands, reinforce pressures to prove fertility, and erode lingering disapproval of premarital sex.[4] Already, 1 in 10 urban respondents in Ado-Ekiti, Nigeria thinks that no one is a virgin at marriage these days, and some men and women report that virginity is considered antisocial (Orubuloye et al., 1991). Qualitative work with teenagers in Kwazulu/Natal, South Africa, led Preston-Whyte (1994) to observe that whatever parents preach, they will usually help care for offspring of their unmarried teenage daughters. Social sanctions on premarital pregnancy do not run deep, although perhaps deep enough to make sexual education and services targeted at young teens politically difficult.

WHO/GPA survey data show that education is associated with an increase in premarital sex in the teen years, particularly in societies with generally low levels of sexual activity. However, in data analyzed by Meekers (1994), the association more or less disappears when age is held constant. The implication is that since extra years of schooling are likely to delay marriage, they increase exposure to premarital sex. Any observed increase in premarital sexual activity may thus be a function more of later marriage (or changing definitions of marriage) than of earlier first sexual experience.

If we look at sexual initiation regardless of marital status, rates of sexual activity recorded in the WHO/GPA surveys for men and women converge dramatically. In West Africa, sexual initiation tends to occur relatively early: in Côte d'Ivoire and the Central African Republic, 45 to 60 percent of both sexes are sexually active by the age of 15 (see Table 4-3). In Calabar, Nigeria, Ogbuagu and Charles (1993) report lower figures: over one-third of men and 17 percent of women have had sex by the time they are 15. In East and Southern Africa, WHO/GPA surveys show that sexual activity starts slightly later, with a wider gap between the sexes. In some studies (e.g., Anarfi and Awusabo-Asare, 1993, Ghana), people recall that they first had sex when as young as 8 or 10. This young age at sexual debut is important when targeting populations for intervention, particularly in light of the work by Konings et al. (1994) showing a correlation between the early onset of sexual activity and large numbers of partners.

Sex Within Marriage or a Stable Union

It appears that marriage may have been a relatively informal concept in many African societies throughout much of history, becoming more narrowly defined only in response to the dictates of colonial administrators and missionaries. Some

---

[4]It would also tend to give men greater opportunity to marry at an earlier age, which could cut the extent of sexual networking for young men.

TABLE 4-3 Approximate Percentage of Those Currently Aged 15 Already Sexually Active

Study Area	Male	Female
Burundi	27	7
Central African Republic	46	43
Côte d'Ivoire	47	60
Kenya	24	29
Lesotho	36	6
Tanzania	29	29
Togo	19	15
Lusaka, Zambia	43	24

SOURCE: Cleland and Ferry (1995).

suggest that formalization is currently being reversed, although, as Guyer (1994) points out, there are no clear data to support this conclusion that many anthropologists have reached by observation.

Certainly, informal unions are very common. In some cities in the developing world, nearly half of all adults are living in unions not formally legitimized (Caraël, 1995), so distinguishing between marital and extramarital relations can be problematic. What emerges clearly from the WHO/GPA data is that multiple concurrent partnerships are frequent in Africa. In Lesotho, with low organized polygyny but high rates of migrant labor, over half of men and two in five women report more than one current regular partner. In Côte d'Ivoire, over one-third of men are in two or more unions simultaneously, but no women report more than one regular partner, while in Lusaka, Zambia, twice as many men as women have two stable relationships. In general, women are aware of their partners' other partners; the surveys show a very high correlation between men reporting more than one partner and women reporting the same of their husbands.

The WHO/GPA surveys report high levels of abstinence within marriage or regular partnership (Table 4-4), in part the consequence of either long periods of abstinence following the birth of a child or terminal abstinence following the birth of a grandchild. One-quarter of married women in Togo reported no sex with their regular partner in the 12 months preceding the study. (Figure 4-1 shows that women in Togo also average more months of postpartum abstinence than most other women in Africa.) In most countries, 4 to 8 percent of currently

TABLE 4-4 Percentage of Currently "Married" Men and Women (15-49) Reporting Sex with Their Regular Partner and Mean Coital Frequency in the Last Month

	Burundi		Côte d'Ivoire		Lesotho		Tanzania		Togo		Lusaka, Zambia	
Percent Reporting	M	F	M	F	M	F	M	F	M	F	M	F
No sex this year	6	8	4	8	4	6	6	8	11	24	2	2
Sex this year but not this month	27	26	38	42	46	54	28	28	31	34	42	43
Sex this month	68	66	58	50	50	41	66	64	58	42	56	55
Mean coital frequency	5.5	5.7	2.9	2.0	3.0	1.9	4.9	4.4	2.9	1.5	3.4	3.7
Sample size	735	826	865	1,136	356	805	1,119	1,642	811	961	594	738

SOURCE: Cleland and Ferry (1995).

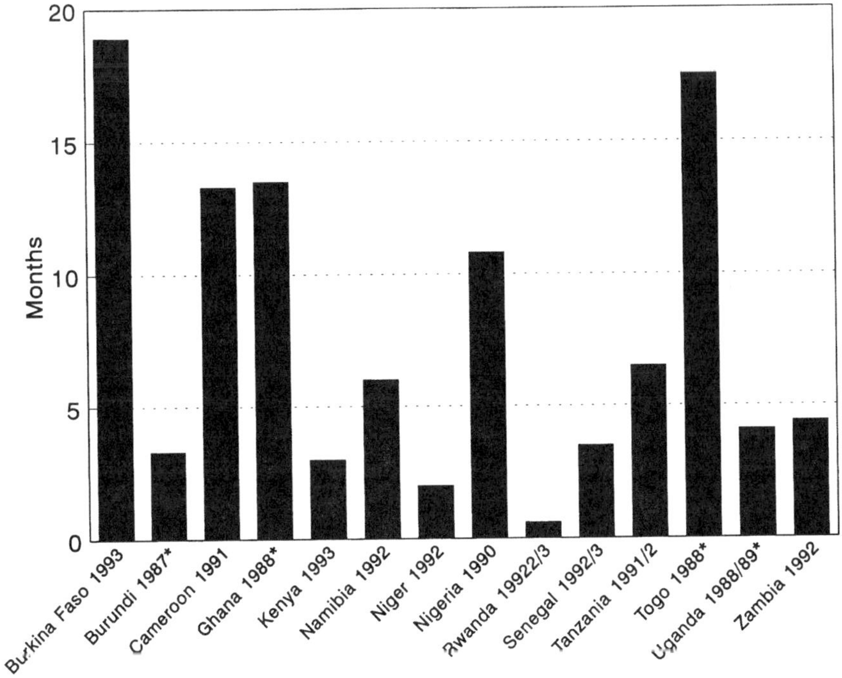

FIGURE 4-1 Average Number of Months of Postpartum Abstinence. NOTE: Asterisk indicates mean number of months of postpartum abstinence. All other figures are median number of months. SOURCES: Burkino Faso: Konaté et al. (1994); Burundi: Segamba et al. (1988); Cameroon: Balépa et al. (1992); Ghana: Ghana Statistical Service (1989); Kenya: National Council for Population and Development (1994); Namibia: Katjiuanjo et al. (1993); Niger: Kourguéni et al. (1993); Nigeria: Federal Office of Statistics (1992); Rwanda: Barrère et al. (1994); Senegal: Ndiaye et al. (1994); Tanzania: Ngallaba et al. (1993); Togo: Agounké et al. (1989); Uganda: Kaijuka et al. (1989); Zambia: Gaisie et al. (1993); Zimbabwe: Central Statistical Office [Zimbabwe] (1989).

married respondents reported not having sex with their regular partners for a year or more. In a single month, 35 to 45 percent typically had no sexual contact with their spouse or regular partner.

Extramarital and Casual Sex

Given that marriage is difficult to define, defining what constitutes extramarital sex is also problematic. A woman may consider her husband's relationship with another woman to be an extramarital affair, while the man may see it as a stable union of some emotional significance. What a researcher considers it to be will vary from study to study.

Much of the nonquantitative literature assumes that extramarital sex must have a primarily economic underpinning, with women accepting material support, gifts, or money from their lovers. "African women do not trust their boyfriends and believe that several are needed as a financial insurance," declare Awusabo-Asare et al. (1993:71). Indeed, two out of three rural women in a Nigerian study justified their extramarital affairs on the basis of economic security, although half of all extramaritally active urban women said they had sex outside marriage just for fun (Orubuloye et al., 1991). Even among market traders, a group often thought highly likely to supplement their income through sexual relations (e.g., Orubuloye et al., 1992), nearly one-quarter said they had affairs for pleasure (Omorodion, 1993). In-depth interviews in Uganda suggest that the most common reaction by men to their wives having extramarital affairs was to try to avenge oneself by sleeping with the wife of the offending man—a powerful push toward extramarital sex (Obbo, 1993a).

An interesting variation on the theme of extramarital sex as a survival strategy is proposed by Guyer (1994). She maintains that easily dissolved marriages and increasingly common informal unions may be insufficient to ensure support for women, who are instead turning to childbearing as a survival strategy. Because men in most of sub-Saharan Africa are happy to claim paternity, and extended families are happy to absorb additional members, bearing a child may give a woman a stake in a man's family resources, regardless of whether she has married into the family or not. Bearing several children to different men will potentially allow the woman a claim to the resources of several families. Where conception and childbirth are the prime goal of a union, the prognosis for condom use as an AIDS-prevention strategy cannot be good.

It appears that a woman's postpartum abstinence may well be a strong motivation for men to seek sex outside marriage. Messersmith et al. (1994) show strong aggregate agreement between the sexes when reporting their own or their partner's pregnancy and lactation; but while only 12 percent of breastfeeding women reported having sex in the last 4 weeks, the proportion was three times as high among men who declared that their main partner was lactating.[5] Hogsborg and Aaby (1992) report that 68 percent of women observing postpartum abstinence or their male principal partners said the male partner had sex with others during that time.

Levels of extramarital sex with nonregular partners vary, though once again comparisons are difficult because of differences in definition.[6] WHO/GPA sur-

[5]Men in this situation may have been having sex with other regular partners during this time. The study does not distinguish regular from casual partners in this context.

[6]Nevertheless, levels are generally much higher than in non-African countries for which representative data are available (the United States, the United Kingdom, France, Belgium, Singapore, Sri Lanka, and Mauritius) (see Cleland and Ferry, 1995). The only country shown thus far to have levels of nonmarital sex comparable to those of Africa is Thailand.

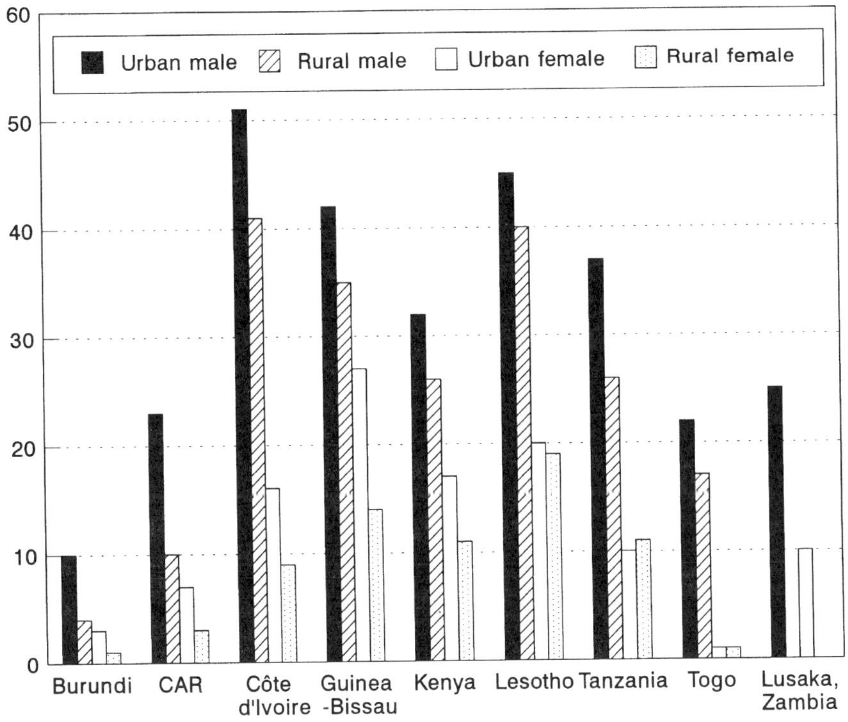

FIGURE 4-2 Percentage of All Men and Women Reporting Nonregular Sex in the Last Year, by Residence. SOURCE: Cleland and Ferry (1995).

veys show proportions of men reporting nonregular sex ranging from 51 percent in urban Côte d'Ivoire to 4 percent in rural Burundi (a figure the researchers regard as surprisingly low in view of the area's high HIV seroprevalence). Women tend to report less than half of male levels of nonregular sexual activity (Figure 4-2). In a study that looked only at most recent sexual partners in Ghana, around two-fifths of women, and a slightly higher proportion of men, reported that their most recent partner was not their spouse, although only a fraction of those relations would be defined as extramarital by the WHO/GPA surveys (Anarfi, 1993). Beliefs about partners can be revealing: in high-HIV-prevalence Rwanda, nearly 9 women in 10 said they believed most married men are unfaithful, and 44 percent said they believed most married women are, too (Lindan et al.,

1991). It may also be noted that women are far more likely to have extramarital lovers if they are the younger wives in a polygynous marriage than if they are the only wife (Orubuloye et al., 1991).

With whom are the men having sex? In Ekiti, Nigeria, Orubuloye et al. (1992) report that two-thirds of men's extramarital partners are single, and, perhaps disturbingly, one-third are described as schoolgirls.[7] This pattern is confirmed by Hogsborg and Aaby (1992), who conclude that in Guinea-Bissau, single women under age 26 appear to constitute the pool of nonmarital partners for men of all ages.

And who are the men? The WHO/GPA surveys show a strong aggregate correlation between men reporting casual sex in the last year and men reporting more than one regular partner. This finding would suggest that where overall levels of sexual activity are high, women who have no sex outside regular partnerships will still be at increased risk for HIV. Stronger still is the correlation between men reporting casual sex and men not cohabiting with their regular partner (a figure that reaches 43 percent in Côte d'Ivoire and is lowest in Tanzania at 11 percent). Not surprisingly, men reporting more than five casual partners in the last month are disproportionately likely to live in countries with generally high levels of sex outside regular partnerships. Interestingly, there is no apparent correlation between levels of commercial sex reported and the proportion of men with five or more casual partners, though this surprising result may perhaps be explained by the imprecise definition of "commercial" sex in the surveys.

Commercial Sex

The WHO/GPA survey instruments defined "commercial" sex as any sex in which money, gifts, or favors are exchanged in partnerships lasting under a year. Interviewers were told that the term did not include relationships in which the exchange was not the prime motive or reason for sex. Use of this definition once again led to the possibility that the same sexual experience would be classified differently by the man and woman involved. In terms of overall proportions reporting commercial sex, men dominated everywhere, though the gender gap was narrower in Côte d'Ivoire than elsewhere. However, in most sites, a higher proportion of all nonregular sex was classified as commercial by women than by men. The incidence of commercial sex during the past year ranged from 3 percent of all men in Burundi to 25 percent of all men in Tanzania (Figure 4-3A)

[7] Kisekka and Otesanya (1988, quoted in Standing and Kisekka, 1989), report that commercial sex workers in Uganda impersonate schoolgirls to appear to have "low HIV risk."

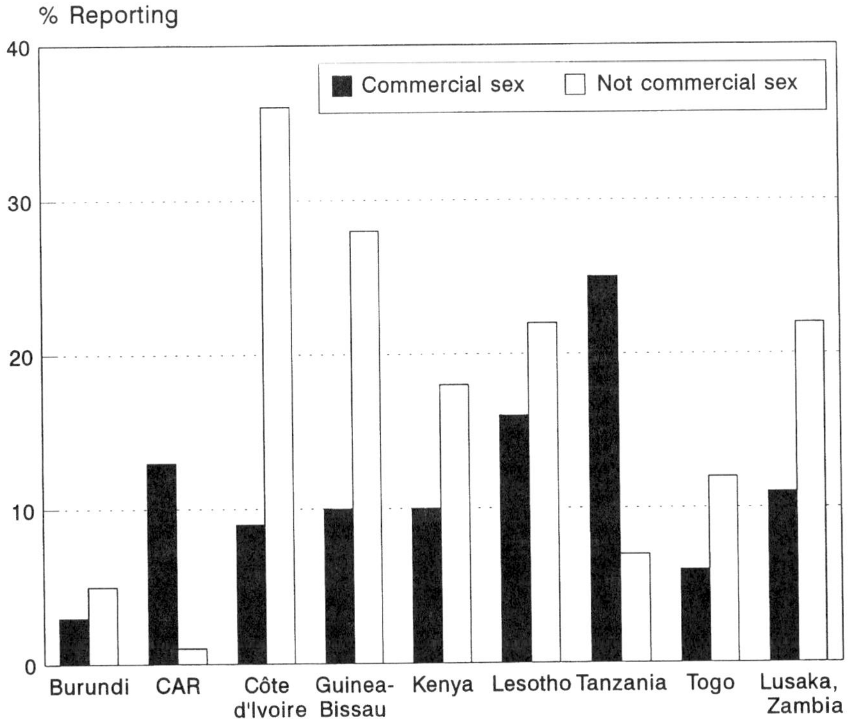

FIGURE 4-3A Percentage of Men who Reported in the Last Year (1) Commercial Sex and (2) Nonregular but Not Commercial Sex. SOURCE: Cleland and Ferry (1995).

and from 0.2 percent of all women in Burundi and Togo to 11 percent of all women in Tanzania (Figure 4-3B).

The confusion surrounding transactional sex is apparent elsewhere. In Ekiti, Nigeria, Orubuloye et al. (1992) note a profusion of sex workers incompatible with the low levels of commercial sex reported by men. Only 1 percent of extramarital partners of men surveyed were reported to be sex workers, but 38 percent were classified as street traders, whom the authors describe as an important source of commercial sex. Further, the authors note that when a man visits a sex worker regularly, the relationship may cease, in his mind, to be one of commercial sex. Indeed, such sex would not have been classified as commercial in the WHO/GPA surveys if the relationship lasted more than one year. In another Nigerian study, a far higher proportion of men (14 percent) reported having paid for sex with a sex worker (Messersmith et al., 1994). Relatively high proportions (16 percent) of schoolboys in Zimbabwe surveyed by Wilson et al. (1989) reported sex with a prostitute.

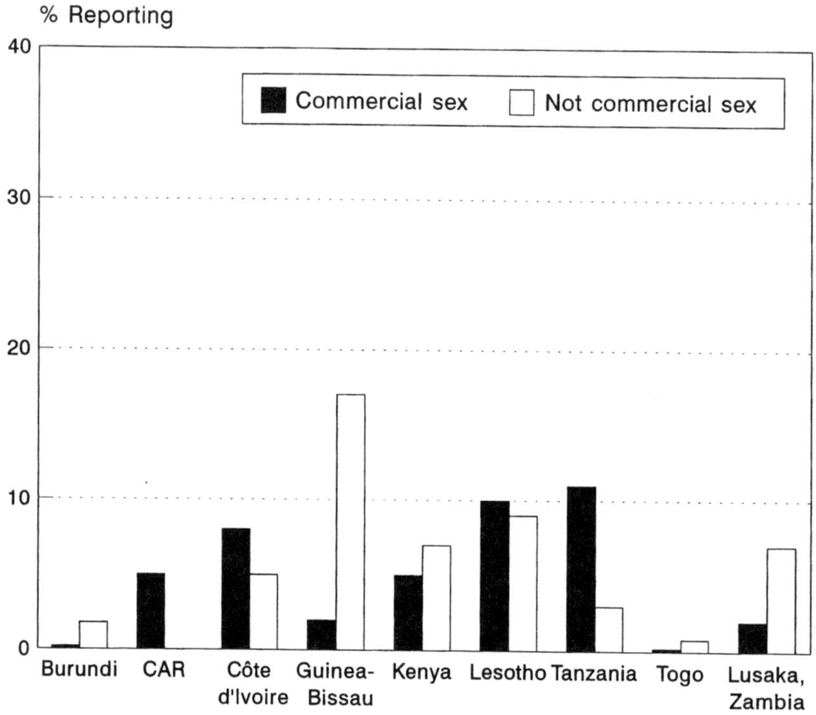

FIGURE 4-3B Percentage of Women who Reported in the Last Year (1) Commercial Sex and (2) Nonregular but Not Commercial Sex. SOURCE: Cleland and Ferry (1995).

Many authors comment that economic hardship, particularly that caused by structural adjustment programs, has increased the need for and incidence of transactional sex (e.g., Larson, 1989; Caldwell et al., 1993). Although the spectrum of women engaging in transactional sex is broad, commercial sex workers are often portrayed as hapless victims of extreme poverty and family breakdown in surveys and focus group interviews (Pickering et al., 1992). However, in an extremely thorough prospective study of prostitutes and their clients in The Gambia that led to invitations to the commercial sex workers' family homes, the researchers reported that many of the women were from well-off families; their work appeared to be a life-style choice. A concurrent study (Pickering and Wilkins, 1993) calls into question the common assumption that many widowed, divorced, or separated women, shorn of their partner's support, are obliged to turn to sex as a means of generating income. Through income/expenditure diaries, formerly married women were shown to generate two-thirds of their income by providing services, such as laundry and cooking, that require few skills, but are commonly required in cities in which men greatly outnumber women. That these women had discovered viable alternatives to casual transactional sex was supported by the fact that levels of syphilis among formerly married women were found to be nearly identical to those among currently married women, and one-third those among a well-defined group of professional prostitutes.

SEX-RELATED RISK FACTORS

In examining which sociodemographic, behavioral, or attitudinal characteristics might be linked to an elevated risk of contracting HIV/AIDS, studies fall into two categories. In the first, the HIV status of study participants is known, usually only after information on explanatory variables has been collected. In the second, analysts must rely on proxy markers of risk that have been determined by clinical studies of the first kind; these markers include high numbers of partners, unprotected sex with commercial sex workers, and the presence of STDs.

This section examines sex-related risk factors associated with HIV/AIDS, including a high number of partners/commercial sex, perceived risk, age, education, marital status, residence, migration, STDs, circumcision and traditional medical practices, and alcohol.[8]

High Number of Partners/Commercial Sex

In analyzing the WHO/GPA survey data, researchers define "risk behavior" as having one or more nonregular partners in the last 12 months, while "high-risk behavior" is having "commercial" sex in that time period. Although the definitions may appear to capture a wide range of behavior, they are lent credence by serostudies. Lindan et al. (1991) show that in Kigali, Rwanda, while one-quarter of the women reporting only a single lifetime partner were seropositive, the proportion rose to 47 percent for women reporting more than one lifetime partner. In Nairobi, Kenya, where overall prevalence is much lower, Hunter et al. (1994) found a strong positive association between the number of lifetime partners and seropositivity, even at low number of partners. Lindan et al. (1991) also found that 42 percent of Rwandan women reporting that their partner had visited commercial sex workers tested HIV-positive, as compared with 30 percent of those who answered negatively or did not know.

The risk inherent in the rate of partner exchange is of course affected by the background prevalence of HIV infection. While the odds of being HIV-positive increase with the number of sexual partners in various urban and rural locations,

---

[8]Some observers have suggested that religion may play a significant role in shaping social and behavioral responses to the epidemic, but the role of religion has not been the subject of significant research. Because there would be significant policy implications if religion were found to be an important factor, research into the role of religion may well be a fruitful topic for future work.

the danger at any given level of sexual activity is greater where HIV is more prevalent (Serwadda et al., 1992).

Perceived Risk

Surprisingly, there does not seem to be a strong correlation between perceived risk and risk behavior. People who report risk behavior do not seem to feel more threatened by HIV than people who do not, and in the WHO/GPA data, no relationship between the two appears when the effects of other factors are simultaneously controlled. Conversely, Lindan et al. (1991) report that those who perceive themselves to be at risk of AIDS (62 percent of them through their partner's sexual behavior rather than their own) are actually no more likely to be seropositive than those who feel less threatened. It does, however, emerge from that study that women who feel powerless to prevent HIV/AIDS are more likely to be infected.

The WHO/GPA data suggest that risk behavior is itself positively correlated with AIDS awareness and knowledge of its lethality and sexual transmission routes. While this finding may dim hopes that knowledge will lead to behavior change, the relationship may be spuriously caused by the fact that formal schooling leads simultaneously to better AIDS awareness and a socioeconomic status that makes it easier to acquire more partners.

Age

In the WHO/GPA surveys, risk behavior is associated with age. In some African societies, for example, Central African Republic, Guinea-Bissau, and Kenya, over half of all those aged 15 to 19 are already sexually experienced (Caraël, 1995). In contrast, in other societies such as Burundi, around 90 percent of those aged 15 to 19 are still virgins (Caraël, 1995). However, by age 20, the level of sexual experience is close to 90 percent among most of the populations studied in the WHO/GPA surveys. Never-married men aged 15 to 19 reported that in the last 12 months they had had between 1.6 and 2.5 partners; women in the same age range reported between 1.0 and 1.9 partners.

Condom use for sexually experienced men aged 20 to 24 varies from under 20 percent in Lesotho, Tanzania, and Togo to over 50 percent in Guinea-Bissau and Lusaka, Zambia (Mehryar, 1995). Reported condom use for women in this age range was significantly lower. Only in Lusaka, Zambia, did more than 20 percent of sexually experienced women in this age range report ever using a condom, and in Central African Republic, Togo, and Lesotho, fewer than 10 percent of women in this age range reported ever having used a condom (Mehryar, 1995).

Education

In the comparable national WHO/GPA studies, more education is associated with more casual sex everywhere except Lesotho. The effect, which is most powerful when secondary education and primary or no schooling are compared, remains when the effects of other variables are controlled.[9] However, the WHO/GPA analyses do not include economic status. It is likely that the effect of education is confounded by the fact that for men, education opens the door to resources, and resources can make it easier to acquire access to commercial or casual sex. In Rakai, Uganda, seropositivity shows a linear rise with education and with occupational status for both sexes, with the exception of female bar and hotel workers (Kivumbi, 1993).

Marital Status

Lindan et al. (1991) report that among women, the unmarried were found to be far more likely to be seropositive than the married, with the monogamously married safest of all. In Rakai, Uganda, and Nairobi, Kenya, the same pattern was found (Serwadda et al., 1992; Hunter et al., 1994). In Nairobi, single sexually active women were found twice as likely and formerly married women three times as likely as married women to be HIV-positive. The high rates among the formerly married are not altogether unexpected. In high-prevalence areas, the formerly married may well be AIDS widows and therefore at extremely high risk of exposure. Alternatively, some women may have been divorced because they were suspected to be HIV-positive.

In terms of risk behavior, Rutenberg et al. (1994) used DHS data to show that in Tanzania, single women have the highest rate of partner change, with the formerly married just behind, while for men the two groups are roughly the same. In the WHO/GPA surveys, formerly married women were typically more likely to report casual sex than married women, with single women being intermediate. Among the three surveys for which multivariate analyses were performed, however, a significant effect of marital status was found only in Côte d'Ivoire. Among men, marital status in these three countries appears to be a less important influence on risk behavior.

Residence

The WHO/GPA surveys in every case reported more casual sex in urban than in rural areas, though the data show an extremely strong correlation between

[9]It should be noted that at the time of this writing, multivariate analysis of the WHO/GPA surveys was available only for Côte d'Ivoire, Burundi, and Lusaka, Zambia.

urban and rural rates of casual sex within each country. There was little difference across place of residence in the percentage of men who reported having commercial sex in the last 12 months, although among men reporting commercial sex, the mean number of partners was higher in urban areas (Caraël et al., 1994). In a result that surprised researchers, however, the effect of residence evaporated in multivariate analysis, suggesting that it is greatly confounded by other variables, such as education, marital status, and age (Cleland and Ferry, 1995). Thus there is little support for the hypothesis that sexual life-styles are divided merely across urban-rural lines. Instead, sexual behavior in towns and cities appears culturally linked to sexual behavior in rural areas, and risky behavior is present in both urban and rural areas (Caraël et al., 1994).

Orubuloye et al. (1991) report astonishingly similar levels of multiple partners in rural and urban areas of southwest Nigeria. Rutenberg et al. (1994) report that in Tanzania, single men who were not virgins were far more likely to have multiple partners if they lived in rural areas, but, perhaps because of lower levels of polygyny, married men were more likely to have extramarital partners in town. Anarfi (1993) reports earlier sex in urban than in rural areas of Ghana. In multivariate analysis of DHS data for several sub-Saharan African countries, Meekers (1994) shows little effect of urban/rural residence on age at first intercourse, although when asking retrospective questions in cross-sectional surveys, it is difficult to determine where first sex took place, or if onset of sexual activity might be linked in some way to migration.

Migration

A widening rural-urban gap in income and availability of social services and a subregional variability in development have generated large movements of people in Africa. Increasing urbanization is associated with a lower proportion of customary marriages relative to consensual unions (Caldwell et al., 1989; Orubuloye et al., 1990). Such conjugal situations often weaken the financial security of women and their children. Because migrants are most often young adult men, one outcome of migration is a very high ratio of men to women at the points of destination. Most West and Central African cities (except Abidjan, Côte d'Ivoire) have sex ratios close to parity, in contrast to the situation in East and Southern Africa (see above). In such settings, high sex ratios in favor of men have generated growing demand for commercial sex, which is often satisfied by widowed, divorced, and single women because of their bleak economic situation (Anarfi, 1993). Mining or industrial centers often have particularly high concentrations of young men who have migrated to seek employment; these sites are highly vulnerable to the spread of HIV infection. Lesotho, Swaziland, and several other countries in Southern Africa face the dual challenge of sustaining economies that are largely dependent on their export of labor to South Africa and reducing the consequent vulnerability of migrant workers and their families to HIV/AIDS (Phits'ane, 1994).

Migration in Africa commonly takes the form of people leaving their villages on a seasonal or temporary basis in search of work, hoping to move back eventually to their place of origin. In this pattern of migration, an infected individual may spread HIV/AIDS to others at both the sending and the receiving ends of the cycle. In Ghana, the risk is heightened in rural areas by a tendency among returning migrants to flaunt wealth and acquire partners (Anarfi, 1993). The same study showed that international migrants are more likely than internal migrants to report high numbers of partners (Anarfi, 1993). Rutenberg et al. (1994) show that migration in the last 3 years (presumably largely within Tanzania, although this implication is not stated) makes no substantial difference in levels of sexual activity.[10] The issue of migration as a factor in the spread of HIV/AIDS is discussed in further detail in Chapter 2.

Sexually Transmitted Diseases

As discussed in Chapter 3, there is a strong relationship between STDs and HIV. Lindan et al. (1991) report that HIV infection among women with a history of STDs in the previous 5 years is twice as high as among women with no STD history.

Responses about symptoms of STDs over the last 12 months in the WHO/GPA surveys show a strong correlation between reported risk behavior and venereal infections. In many nations, those reporting STD symptoms are two or three times as likely to report casual sex as those apparently unaffected. The correlation grows stronger as partner numbers increase, and stronger yet with a history of contact with commercial sex workers. Messersmith et al. (1994) report a 12-fold increase in STD history for respondents with five or more lifetime partners and previous contact with a prostitute as compared with those having a single lifetime noncommercial partner.

Treatment (often of both partners) can be crucial in limiting the importance of STDs as a cofactor for HIV transmission. Although high proportions of those reporting STD symptoms in the WHO/GPA survey said they obtained treatment, only half reported telling their regular partner. In Cameroon, one-quarter of STD patients in one study continued sexual relations during their illness, and of those nearly two-thirds stated that they used condoms on every occasion (IRESCO, 1994). Caldwell et al. (1993) assert that much sex in sub-Saharan Africa takes place in the dark without hand-to-genital contact, making it difficult for people to ascertain whether their partner is infected with an STD.

---

[10]Doubtless other large-scale movements of refugees, such as those associated with famine, civil unrest, and military coups, also contributed to the rapid spread of the epidemic, but such situations rarely lend themselves to careful study (see Chapter 2).

In a Nigerian study, a sizeable majority of STD sufferers said they had sought treatment in hospitals or with private doctors, though turning to traditional healers and self-medication was not uncommon. In Nigeria, abstention and effective treatment were much more common among women who knew their illness to be sexually transmitted than among those who thought it "natural" (O'Toole Erwin, 1993).

Where levels of STD-induced sterility are high and the connection between the two is well known, single women may refrain from seeking treatment for fear of being stigmatized and jeopardizing their chances of marriage. The high cost of treatment, lack of available services, and the attitude of the staff toward the client may also be further reasons to deter women from attending STD clinics. In a society where fertility is an all-important key to family support and resources, barrenness may drive women to towns and to commercial sex work (Southall, 1961, cited in Standing and Kisekka, 1989). Where barrenness is the product of chronic or untreated STDs, the implications for HIV transmission are clear.

Circumcision and Traditional Medical Practices

Generally, male circumcision is thought to be protective against HIV transmission and female circumcision a risk factor, although some dispute these claims. Female circumcision continues to be widely practiced among some groups throughout Africa (Kouba and Muasher, 1985). In the most recent DHS in northern Sudan, 86 percent of women aged 15 to 19 were circumcised and/or had experienced infibulation (Ahmed and Kheir, 1992). There have been no studies that have actually attempted to examine the relationship between female circumcision and HIV transmission, although the practice may put women at risk if unsterile instruments are used; it is also likely to increase the risk of bleeding during intercourse and therefore of HIV transmission.

Lack of male circumcision has been associated with some sexually transmitted diseases, including chancroid, syphilis, and gonorrhea (Cook et al., 1994), but there has been a good deal of debate in the recent literature on the link between lack of male circumcision and the risk of HIV infection. On one side, Bongaarts et al. (1989), Moses et al. (1990, 1995), and Caldwell and Caldwell (1993) have argued that there is a statistically significant positive association between estimates of the extent to which ethnic groups in various regions traditionally do not practice circumcision and the prevalence of HIV, so that absence of male circumcision may be a crucial factor in the spread of HIV in Africa. Using micro-level data, Hunter et al. (1994) show in a multivariate analysis that having an uncircumcised partner is a risk factor for seropositivity for women even when other factors, including number of partners, are held constant. Adopting a more cautious tone, others argue that the causal relation is far from proven, and that confounding factors such as behavioral differences may account for these findings (de Vincenzi and Mertens, 1994; Conant, 1995). For instance, a study of rural Uganda revealed that circumcised men tend to be Moslem traders concentrated in high-prevalence trading towns (Serwadda et al., 1992). Although circumcision is found to be protective, the authors do not investigate whether there are behavioral factors associated with being Moslem that might also be protective. Further research is required to illuminate not only the association between male circumcision status and acquisition of HIV, but also the causal factors and specific mechanisms involved (Mertens and Caraël, 1995).

Alcohol

Drinking is often thought to be associated with lower self-control and greater risk-taking behavior with regard to sex. However, few studies have examined the effects of alcohol consumption on sexual behavior in sub-Saharan Africa, although some income expenditure studies show that a significant portion of disposable income is spent on the consumption of various forms of alcoholic beverages. Bars and nightclubs that sell alcohol are often popular meeting places and are frequented by people looking for commercial or casual sex. Six of the nine WHO/GPA surveys in sub-Saharan Africa included a module on drinking habits (Central African Republic, Côte d'Ivoire, Guinea-Bissau, Lesotho, Tanzania, and Lusaka, Zambia). Analysis of these data established that alcohol consumption is common in these countries and that it is positively associated with risk behavior, even when other factors are held constant (Ferry, 1995b).

In Uganda, alcohol and sexual activity are linked in both commercial and social spheres (Olowo-Freers and Barton, 1992). The brewing of various forms of alcoholic beverages is a major source of cash income for many women, particularly in urban slum areas. The alcohol trade is closely intertwined with commercial sex activity. Many women who make and sell beer are also known as prostitutes (Olowo-Freers and Barton, 1992). In Kampala, beer gardens are popular places for finding casual sexual partners. Drinking is particularly heavy among students and urban slum dwellers. In one study of urban slum dwellers in Kampala, over 60 percent of heads of households drink daily (Kayobosi, 1988, cited in Olowo-Freers and Barton, 1992).

SEXUAL PRACTICES AND BELIEFS

While quantitative studies are useful in defining the incidence of common practices, they will never identify all of the beliefs and practices that, albeit far from universal—indeed sometimes apparently at odds with survey data—may help indicate acceptable interventions with the potential for having some impact on behavior. This section reviews some of the beliefs and practices examined by the literature on sexual behavior in sub-Saharan Africa, particularly qualitative studies.

The Notion That Men Need Sex

It is widely held in sub-Saharan Africa that men have an all-but-insatiable need to copulate (what Anarfi [1993:47] calls "the repetitive and overpowering nature of the sexual appetite in males") and that this need must be satisfied if they are to remain in good health. The idea that retained semen is somehow poisonous and dangerous to health is frequently expressed. Caldwell et al. (1993) state that African cultures hold frequent sex to be healthy and strengthening, and some researchers contend that men measure their health status by their ability to achieve multiple orgasms. Poewe's 1981 study in Zambia (quoted in Standing and Kisekka, 1989) reports the belief that sexual deprivation may cause emaciation and madness.[11] In focus groups in Zimbabwe, men and women agreed that men must find a way to release their sexual tensions, and may even be "forced by nature" to rape (Meursing et al., forthcoming), and women immodestly dressed are considered by both sexes to be provoking just such a situation and to deserve what they get (Vos, 1994).

Coercive Sex

Coercive sex or rape is a behavior that no quantitative survey will ever adequately describe. But there is no shortage of evidence that it is present in all societies and even common in some, particularly during periods of intense ethnic conflict. As documented by Orubuloye et al. (1992), 4 percent of Nigerian men reported themselves guilty of rape or coercion at first intercourse, while 3 percent of women in a Ghanaian study reported that they were forced into first sex and a further 8 percent that they were lured or deceived (Anarfi, 1993). Standing and Kisekka (1989) quote many anthropological papers giving accounts of ritual or commonplace violence in marital and sexual relations. The authors also detail rape cases, often involving very young victims.

In a study of the rape of children in Bulawayo, Zimbabwe, Meursing et al. (forthcoming) show a linear rise in reported rape cases in recent years. Over half of the 54 child victims of rape (the youngest 2 years old) referred to central hospitals in the city in the final 6 months of 1992 contracted STDs. Although this high proportion may partly reflect the increased likelihood that a rape resulting in an STD will be reported, the risk for a young girl to be subjected to violent sex must be high in a population where STDs are common. Since STDs are a cofactor for HIV transmission, HIV, too, is a potential consequence of rape.

[11]These are two common outcomes of opportunistic infections associated with AIDS. The implication that they can be cured through a more vigorous sex life should be viewed with concern.

Health Beliefs

Some women who report knowingly having sex with an STD-infected partner say they did so because of a belief that sex could cure venereal diseases (Awusabo-Asare et al., 1993). This belief apparently extends to AIDS. Blue-collar respondents in Ugandan focus groups reported a belief that frequent sex could diminish the viral load of the HIV-infected. Focus groups in Uganda reported a belief that young girls were "safe"; adolescents reported that infected men bribed young girls for sex or raped them (Konde-Lule, 1993; Obbo, 1993b). In Zimbabwe, female traditional healers reported that their male counterparts sometimes encourage men to have sex with young women (especially family members) to "cleanse" themselves of HIV (Meursing et al., forthcoming).

Dry Sex

There are a number of reasons "dry sex" practices intended to decrease vaginal secretions might be associated with an increased probability of HIV transmission. The insertion of crushed leaves, powders, or mineral infusions into the vagina can lead to tearing, lesions, or inflammation in the vagina, increasing the likelihood of transmission of STDs and HIV. Lesions or inflammation may also mask symptoms of ulcerative or non-ulcerative STDs (Sandala et al., 1995). Dryness alone may lead to abrasive sex and lesions, with the same effect. Finally, strong preferences for dry sex may interfere with condom effectiveness or acceptability of vaginal microbicides (Kisekka, no date; Dallabetta et al., 1995).

Dry sex practices have been reported in many countries in sub-Saharan Africa, including Nigeria, Zaire, Zambia, Malawi, Zimbabwe, and South Africa (see Sandala et al., 1995 and references therein). In one study in Ghana, schoolchildren of both sexes said that they preferred the vagina dry and tight, and most could describe drying agents (Bleek, 1976, quoted in Standing and Kisekka, 1989). The same was also true for older women (but not schoolgirls) in focus groups in Zimbabwe (Vos, 1994). Among some teenagers in Natal, South Africa, wetness is thought to indicate promiscuity (Preston-Whyte, 1994).

In a thorough study in Zaire, men and women alike expressed a preference for a dry, tight vagina during intercourse (Brown et al., 1993). All men and women studied could contribute at least 1 of a total of 30 drying methods spontaneously mentioned, and over two-thirds of the women said that they had used such a method themselves. Although most of the women said that the procedure increased their sexual pleasure, some complained of inflammation and itching. Clinical examination showed that many of the methods had led to lesions or swellings in the vagina.

In Blantyre, Malawi, a study of women attending an antenatal clinic, designed to assess the prevalence of dry sex practices and its association with HIV infection, found that 34 percent of the women had used an intravaginal agent for treatment of discharge and itching, while 13 percent had used traditional drying agents exclusively for tightening the vagina. The study found that a significantly higher proportion of HIV-infected than uninfected women had used intravaginal agents for treatment purposes, but no difference was found in HIV status among women who used these agents for tightening (Dallabetta et al., 1995). In Lusaka, Zambia, 50 percent of women attending an STD clinic reported having ever engaged in dry sex behavior (Sandala et al., 1995). A variety of practices was reported, including drinking an elixir or "porridge" before having sex. There was no evidence of a strong relationship between these practices and HIV infection (Sandala et al., 1995).

Oral/Anal Sex

Conventional wisdom holds that oral and anal sex are uncommon among most sub-Saharan African groups. However, this belief may reflect the fact that studies rarely investigate levels of nonvaginal sex. IRESCO (1992), studying sexual practices among commercial sex workers and their clients in Cameroon, found that 26 percent of commercial sex workers and 28 percent of their clients reported experience with anal intercourse, while over one-third of men and one-quarter of women in the group reported having experienced oral sex. In focus group studies in Uganda, some heterosexuals said they engaged in anal sex while women were menstruating (Standing and Kisekka, 1989). In a study of 329 women attending an STD clinic in Lusaka, Zambia, 8 percent of women reported ever engaging in anal intercourse (Sandala et al., 1995).

Homosexuality

Although very little sound research appears to have been done on homosexuality in sub-Saharan Africa, its existence is overwhelmingly denied in academic publications. This claim may result because "homosexuality" as a lifelong sexual identity is rare or unknown, rather than because men never have sex with men.

Ahmed and Kheir (1992) report homosexual behavior to be common though clandestine in northern Sudan. The authors express a concern that a recent government crackdown on female commercial sex workers may increase the incidence of homosexual sex, thus perhaps increasing the spread of HIV. Male-with-male sex featured prominently in focus group discussions among the Hausa in Nigeria (Kisekka, no date). Other studies give evidence of homosexual behavior among the Kikuyu in Kenya, the Hausa in Nigeria, and mine-workers in South Africa (Standing and Kisekka, 1989). According to D. Moodie et al. (1988, quoted in Standing and Kisekka, 1989), the mine-workers most likely to have boys acting as "mine-wives," that is, performing domestic and sexual services for them, were Mozambican migrants who also had the highest HIV prevalence.

Postpartum and Other Abstinence

Postpartum abstinence probably evolved simply as a means of birth spacing, but became ritually sanctioned so that it would be maintained. In Bamako and Bobo-Dioulasso, two cities of the Sahel region, the prevailing belief among women interviewed in 1983 was that women must not have sex while they are breastfeeding because the ingestion of semen will spoil the mother's milk (van de Walle and van de Walle, 1991). As was pointed out earlier, it is common for men to seek other partners during the postpartum period; indeed, many researchers believe postpartum abstinence is a principal prop of high levels of sexual networking, and call for the promotion of condoms to breastfeeding women as a means of eliminating the danger of "dirty milk" (e.g., Hogsborg and Aaby, 1992). Anarfi (1993) suggests that a possibly related dynamic is under way in Ghana: women are limiting their postpartum abstinence in an attempt to keep husbands from seeking other sexual partners. He reports an average of 12.4 months of abstinence in Ghana, where, he says, the taboo period was much longer in the past.[12] Half of the women in his sample reported contraceptive use, versus a national average of 13 percent among currently married women (Ghana Statistical Office and IRD/Macro Systems, 1989). However, repeated surveys sometimes contradict the conventional wisdom that postpartum abstinence is everywhere on the wane. In Cameroon, the average length of postpartum abstinence remained at 13.9 months between 1978 and 1991 according to WFS and DHS data, while in Kenya the mean number of months rose from 2.9 in 1977/78 to 5.9 in 1989. The median length of postpartum abstinence measured by the 1993 DHS in Kenya was 3.0 months (Figure 4-1).

Couples may abstain from sex for other reasons, such as during a woman's menstrual period or in times of mourning. Researchers report that in some contexts, the definition of "abstinence" may be flexible, extending to situations that include sleeping with a person only on a single occasion. Such misconceptions, if common, would diminish health educators' recommendation of "abstinence" as a protection against HIV/AIDS.

Levirate Marriage

Standing and Kisekka (1989) report that passing on wives to the brothers or family members of dead husbands remains common in some societies, particu-

[12]No evidence for this claim can be found in the trends from the 1979-1980 WFS, the 1988 DHS, or the 1993 DHS in Ghana. Anarfi's measure is higher than the 1979-1980 WFS mean of 10 months (Central Bureau of Statistics [Ghana], 1983), but lower than the 1988 DHS mean of 14 months (Ghana Statistical Service and IRD/Macro Systems, 1989) and the 1993 DHS mean of 14 months (Ghana Statistical Service and IRD/Macro Systems, 1994).

larly in Uganda (see also Olowo-Freers and Barton, 1992). The practice also remains quite common in parts of West Africa. In East African patrilineal societies, such as the Masai, Nandi, Kikuyu, Kisii, and Meru in Kenya, widow-inheritance used to be the rule, and widows had limited rights of appeal (Lesthaeghe, 1989). Nowadays, widows often have more choice in the matter (Lesthaeghe, 1989; Olowo-Freers and Barton, 1992). They may choose among the potential heirs or even choose not to remarry at all (Olowo-Freers and Barton, 1992).

AIDS AWARENESS

Almost all studies report a very high awareness of the existence of HIV/AIDS, with the WHO/GPA surveys recording that over 9 out of 10 people know of the disease everywhere except Francophone West Africa (Table 4-5). The lowest awareness recorded in any study was in Togo, where just under two-thirds of respondents had heard of AIDS, and where the sex differential in knowledge was also greatest. In multivariate analysis, media exposure and education appeared as major predictors of AIDS awareness. Controlling for education diminished the independent effect of age. This section reviews levels of AIDS awareness with respect to the specific issues of modes of transmission, asymptomatic transmission, severity and perceived threat, attitudes toward sufferers, and testing.

Modes of Transmission

Most studies concur that among those aware of AIDS, the overwhelming majority are aware of actual modes of transmission and genuine risk behaviors (Irwin et al., 1991; Lindan et al., 1991; Hogsborg and Aaby, 1992; Messersmith et al., 1994). In most sub-Saharan Africa WHO/GPA surveys, sex with prostitutes was recognized as risky by over 90 percent of those respondents who were aware of AIDS, although in Guinea-Bissau, nearly 3 in 10 respondents did not think of the practice as dangerous (Ingham, 1995). However, in a Nigerian study reporting very high awareness of sexual transmission, just 29 percent of women and 17 percent of men mentioned the route of sex with prostitutes spontaneously (Messersmith et al., 1994). The suggestion here of deliberate denial—especially in this case by men who were broadly more educated and aware than women—was reinforced in the same study by the sex differentials in answers to questions about prevention. Of those who knew of AIDS, women were nearly twice as likely as men to mention condom use and avoidance of sex workers, and were also slightly more likely to mention partner reduction. Men who had a history of contact with sex workers were less likely than those who did not to regard sex workers as a source of danger, and the proportion of men saying fewer partners could reduce the risk of HIV infection fell as their number of partners over the

TABLE 4-5 Awareness of AIDS and Accuracy of Knowledge of Suggested Routes of Transmission

	Percent Aware of AIDS		Among Those Aware of AIDS, Percent Responding Accurately on Routes of Transmission				
Study area	Male	Female	Prostitute (Yes)	Touch (No)	Mosquito (No)	Vertical (Yes)	Curable (No)
Burundi[a]	96		94	77	38	89	97
CAR	87	78	93	60	26	78	95
Côte d'Ivoire	94	86	n.a.	51	23	n.a.	n.a.
Guinea-Bissau	77	72	69	45	71	86	84
Kenya	90	89	78	75	51	68	95
Lesotho[a]	98		93	67	n.a.	86	83
Tanzania[a]	96		92	66	41	81	97
Togo	73	56	92	40	11	80	71
Lusaka, Zambia[a]	98		77	88	n.a.	88	93

[a]Both sexes.

Prostitute = having sex with a prostitute
Touch = touching someone with AIDS
Vertical = mother-to-child transmission
Mosquito = transmitted by mosquito bite
Curable = AIDS is curable

CAR = Central African Republic
n.a. = not available

SOURCE: Cleland and Ferry (1995).

last years rose. Moreover, in every survey, respondents demonstrated a high propensity to respond positively to questions on biomedically erroneous modes of transmission, and even to report spontaneously that HIV could be transmitted, for example, by the wind or by eating chicken (Messersmith et al., 1994).

In a regression analysis of WHO/GPA survey data, education was the strongest predictor of accuracy about ways of contracting HIV, both correct and incorrect. Despite fears that a belief in casual transmission will act as a disincentive to protect oneself from contracting HIV sexually, such erroneous beliefs do not seem to be independently associated with a lack of behavior change.

Asymptomatic Transmission

Some investigators report that local concepts of disease may not encompass the idea of a healthy carrier (Irwin et al., 1991; Hogsborg and Aaby, 1992). Among women questioned by Lindan et al. (1991), 70 percent believed that everyone infected with HIV was clinically ill, and one in five thought one could tell if someone was seropositive by looking at him or her. A study of AIDS-related knowledge in Zimbabwe, undertaken in 1994, revealed that while virtually all Zimbabwean men and women have heard of AIDS, 15 percent of men and 26 percent of women do not believe that a healthy-looking person can carry the AIDS virus (Central Statistical Office [Zimbabwe] and Macro International Inc., 1995). It is surprising, then, to find such high levels of awareness of asymptomatic transmission among respondents to the WHO/GPA surveys. This awareness, however, may be more apparent than real as a result of bias in the question.[13]

Severity and Perceived Threat

Although most people who know of AIDS consider it a dangerous disease, a substantial proportion believe it is curable. This is the case even in countries such as Lesotho, where there is broad access to AIDS information. In Kigali, Rwanda, one of the highest HIV-prevalence areas in the world, over one-third of women said they thought AIDS was curable or possibly curable (Lindan et al., 1991), while in Zaire, the vast majority of subjects in a study of factory workers said they thought a cure was available (Irwin et al., 1991). The WHO/GPA surveys show that high proportions of those who think most people infected with AIDS will die of it also think that a cure is available, presumably because most people will not be able to get access to it.

A large proportion of respondents in most WHO/GPA survey countries spontaneously mentioned AIDS as a major health threat to both the world and their nation. Some respondents thought the problem less pressing in their own regions. High proportions in Guinea-Bissau and Burundi said AIDS was a national threat, but only around 1 person in 10 in those countries thought it an immediate threat to his or her community, although more thought the danger would grow over the next few years. Respondents in some heavily afflicted areas (e.g., Tanzania and Lusaka, Zambia), though very much aware of the immediate threat AIDS poses to their community, appeared not to fully understand the implications of the epidemic; lower proportions saw it as a medium-term rather than a current con-

[13]In the standard protocol, the surveys asked people "whether someone who has the AIDS virus but looks healthy can transmit the virus to others" (response options: yes/no/don't know), wording that assumes the person's infection. For discovering the determinants of behavior, a more accurate picture might be given by a question such as "Can you get AIDS from someone who looks healthy?"

cern. Such optimism is unlikely to be warranted. People's perceptions may change rapidly once vaccine trials begin. It is possible that a mass vaccination campaign would induce negative changes in risk behavior. In particular, there is concern that those vaccinated would believe themselves to be at reduced risk of acquiring HIV, and consequently increase their rate of acquisition of new partners or decrease their use of condoms (Lurie et al., 1994; Chesney et al., 1995).

What emerges from these responses is that ordinary people are genuinely concerned about AIDS as a public health problem. Those governments concerned with the opinions of their citizens would appear to have nothing to lose and much to gain by putting the epidemic high on their national agendas.

Beyond the public threat, to what extent do individuals feel they themselves are at risk? Here expected relationships fail to emerge. To return to a point made earlier, we might expect, assuming an understanding of HIV transmission and accurate reporting, to find that people with several partners feel themselves most at risk. The WHO/GPA data show that this expectation often does not hold. In Francophone countries, for example, many people who reported no intercourse for 12 months still felt themselves to be at risk. Only in Lusaka, Zambia, did a clear majority of respondents say they did not consider themselves to be at risk of contracting HIV. This majority included half of the men who reported five or more casual sex partners. Nonusers of condoms with "commercial" sex partners also frequently reported that they felt in no danger of infection.

These discrepancies cannot be neatly reconciled by pointing to erroneous beliefs about modes of transmission. In multivariate analysis, belief in casual transmission was associated with higher perceived risk only among men in Lusaka, Zambia, and women in Côte d'Ivoire. That finding might explain why women in Côte d'Ivoire who were apparently not at risk perceived that they were, but it does not explain why men in Lusaka who did report high-risk behavior felt safe.

In sites surveyed under the auspices of WHO/GPA, there were few differences between men and women in perceived personal vulnerability to HIV infection. Multivariate analysis of a subset of these surveys showed that marital status was related to perceived personal risk for women, but not for men. In two surveys, married women reported significantly higher risk than unmarried women, and in the third the difference was in the same direction, though not significant. However, in a study of sexually active women in Kigali, Rwanda, 84 percent of women who lived alone felt at risk of HIV infection, as compared with just one-quarter of monogamously married women (Lindan et al., 1991). In fact, this was exactly the fraction of monogamously married women that turned out to be seropositive, a potent reminder that women are probably more at risk from their partner's behavior than from their own. That awareness is evident from the responses of women living with men who had other wives: 9 in 10 felt at risk of infection.

Even in high-prevalence Kigali, Rwanda, 56 percent of women reporting at least one factor shown in the HIV-seropositivity study to be an HIV/AIDS risk still thought themselves to be in no danger of contracting the disease. Astonishingly, the WHO/GPA surveys showed that proportions feeling themselves vulnerable to the disease were generally much lower in the higher-prevalence areas of East and central Southern Africa than in lower-prevalence West Africa.

Perhaps the explanation for the weak links between behavior and risk perception can be found in Hogsborg and Aaby (1992). Respondents reporting feelings of vulnerability in that study were also liable to report that "it depends on God." This fatalism was taken one step further by focus group participants who were aware of modes of transmission and risk reduction. Kisekka (no date) and Obbo (1993a) report that the sentiment "after all, you have to die of something" has become a common justification for continued high-risk behavior.[14]

Attitudes Toward Sufferers

In heavily affected Rakai district, Uganda, Konde-Lule (1993) found that AIDS patients were little stigmatized except by adolescents, who thought that since the means of transmission were known, people had only themselves to blame if they fell ill. This feeling was among the most sympathetic attitudes expressed elsewhere, however. Factory workers in Kinshasa, Zaire, stated that anyone known to be HIV-positive would be shunned by his or her neighbors (Irwin et al., 1991), while many respondents in the WHO/GPA survey in the Central African Republic thought AIDS patients deserved no care, and nearly one in five stated flatly that they should be killed. Anarfi (1993) found similar sentiments in Ghana: "The general opinion is that sufferers of the disease must be killed or at best confined" (Anarfi, 1993:65).

The extent of variation even within countries is illustrated in two reports on AIDS from different regions of Tanzania. Kaijage (1994a:15) states that in Kagera, AIDS stigmatization is declining:

> Although the problems raised above are still fairly widespread, denial and stigma are less prevalent now than they used to be in the earlier days of the epidemic. . . . [A]lmost every family, especially in Bukoba, Muleba, and to some extend Karagwe, has been affected by AIDS. People are therefore generally more sympathetic to persons with AIDS (PWAs) than used to be the case. And, for a PWA in Kagera, having AIDS is no longer such a peculiar experience. AIDS is less a disease of shame than it used to be. It is now euphemistically referred to as "this disease," which suggests familiarity with it.

However, Kaijage (1994b:14) comments as follows about Arusha:

---

[14]See also Chapter 5 for further discussion of the underreaction to the AIDS epidemic.

> Stigmatization of AIDS patients in Arusha is far worse than it is in Kagera. The reason is that the disease is not so prevalent in Arusha, and lots of myths still surround it.

Testing

If some of the attitudes described above are indeed common, there is a real risk that HIV/AIDS will be driven underground, and its spread will become yet more difficult to control. One might expect the above rather harsh views on HIV/AIDS-infected individuals to translate into a reluctance to be tested, or at any rate a desire not to have test results known. Surprisingly, the WHO/GPA surveys indicate no such fear of testing. Around 90 percent of respondents in all areas except Lusaka, Zambia, said they would undergo testing and would want to know the results, and the vast majority also said they would want their families to know the results.

Similar responses were found in another survey in Guinea-Bissau (Hogsborg and Aaby, 1992), but the authors observe that the professed willingness to share information with partners was at odds with actual behavior. In a serosurvey in the same area, all people testing positive were invited to bring their partners back for free counseling. Not one did. The likelihood that survey results reflect what respondents feel to be the "correct" answer rather than the truth is supported by focus group discussions. While participants in Zaire said they would want to know test results, many men said they would not want their wives or partners to be told (Irwin et al., 1991). In Uganda, the majority of those discussing the issue said flatly that they did not want to know their HIV status (Konde-Lule, 1993). And in a recent study of female partners of AIDS patients in a hospital in Kampala, Uganda, only 12 percent of women correctly identified their husbands' diagnosis as "slim" or AIDS (Baingana et al., 1995). Most women (54 percent) thought that the disease was tuberculosis. Others thought that it was some other disease or simply did not know. Furthermore, although just over half of the women felt that they needed to be tested for HIV, only 5 percent had actually done so at the time of the survey (Baingana et al., 1995).

THE ROLE OF CONDOMS

Knowledge of condoms varies widely both across countries and, in many surveys, between the sexes.[15] More men than women knew of condoms in every country surveyed by WHO/GPA, a disparity that remains even after holding

---

[15]An exception to generally low awareness is the study by Ogbuagu and Charles (1993), which reports that 87.1 percent of women and 89.9 percent of men surveyed in Calabar, Nigeria, knew of condoms. This result compares with a national figure reported in the DHS of 24 percent for all women.

media exposure, education, and residence constant. Of those who said they knew of condoms (including answering affirmatively to prompting), a high proportion could not say where they might be obtained. In the WHO/GPA surveys, a maximum of 38 percent (males, Côte d'Ivoire) knew of a source and lived or worked within 30 minutes of it.

Some surveys have found that people's declared knowledge of condoms depends on the context of the questioning. Messersmith et al. (1994) report that in their study of sexual behavior and condom use in Ile-Ife, Nigeria, condoms were known as a means of family planning by more people of both sexes than as a means of protecting against STD transmission, although more actually used condoms for the latter purpose.

Condom Use

Perhaps the same dynamic is at work with reports of condom use: people asked in the context of STD prevention whether they have ever used condoms may underreport their use as contraceptives. Condom social marketing projects in many African countries have been remarkably successful in the recent past, and the number of condoms sold has increased dramatically (see Chapter 5). Nevertheless, it is clear from all surveys (including the fertility-based DHS series) that use of condoms is still low throughout sub-Saharan Africa (Tables 4-6A and 4-6B).

In multivariate analysis of WHO/GPA data, age is negatively related to condom use, while use rises with both education and level of risk behavior. However, knowing that HIV is transmitted sexually and feeling personally vulnerable to infection[16] are not associated with condom use. Messersmith et al. (1994) confirm the negative correlation with age and the positive correlation with risk behavior (including contact with sex workers). They show a linear rise in condom use with the number of lifetime partners. They also show positive associations with knowledge of AIDS and a history of STDs. Using DHS data for Tanzania, Rutenberg et al. (1994) show that although condom use is scanty, it is concentrated among those with multiple partners.

Although around one-quarter of men reporting "commercial" sex in Burundi and Lusaka, Zambia, claim always to use a condom in such encounters, proportions recorded in the other WHO/GPA surveys are far lower. A consistently higher proportion of women than men reporting "commercial" sex said they never used a condom. These women are not likely to be full-time sex workers. A study of just such women in The Gambia (to whom condoms are freely distrib-

[16]This relationship might be expected to run either way: a person might feel at risk and so be more likely to use condoms, or be more likely to feel at risk as a consequence of not using condoms.

TABLE 4-6A Percentage of Sexually Active Men Who Have Ever Used Condoms

Age	Burundi	CAR	Côte d'Ivoire	Guinea-Bissau	Kenya	Lesotho	Tanzania	Togo	Lusaka, Zambia
15-19	18	34	42	46	10	23	14	9	55
20-24	29	34	45	50	28	17	11	18	59
25-39	21	16	33	47	18	19	17	17	38
40-49	9	11	13	20	17	19	12	12	15
50+	n.a.	12	3	7	2	9	10	12	3
All	18.5	21.0	30.3	33.0	16.4	16.1	14.0	14.8	36.3

n.a. = not available
CAR = Central African Republic

SOURCE: Cleland and Ferry (1995).

TABLE 4-6B Percentage of Sexually Active Women Who Have Ever Used Condoms

Age	Burundi	CAR	Côte d'Ivoire	Guinea-Bissau	Kenya	Lesotho	Tanzania	Togo	Lusaka, Zambia
15-19	11	10	16	21	11	9	5	8	31
20-24	10	8	15	11	12	7	10	9	29
25-39	8	5	7	14	9	10	10	6	20
40-49	4	3	1	4	6	5	8	2	14
50+	n.a.	n.a.	n.a.	n.a.	3	5	2	3	n.a.
All	7.3	6.8	9.3	12.3	8.7	8.0	8.5	5.9	24.2

n.a. = not available
CAR = Central African Republic

SOURCE: Cleland and Ferry (1995).

uted) gives limited grounds for hope (Pickering et al., 1992). Although in urban areas women reported using condoms with four clients out of five (a higher rate than that reported by the clients themselves), condom use fell as the number of clients per woman rose. At peak periods such as holidays, when women were recording over 11 clients a night, condom use fell below 50 percent (Pickering et al., 1992).

Condoms and STD and HIV Prevention

Notwithstanding Messersmith's finding that more people knew of condoms as a contraceptive, a substantial majority also knew of their properties in preventing STDs. The proportions of the latter were highest for single men and for single and separated women. Even in multivariate analysis, men with five or more partners were far more likely than those with fewer partners to know that condoms could prevent STD transmission. The number of partners was not an independent predictor of that knowledge in women (Messersmith et al., 1994).

For both sexes, there was a strong correlation between those who had heard of AIDS and those who knew that condoms could prevent the spread of STDs. This result is not, however, necessarily a cause for great optimism. A range of studies show that if a person knows of AIDS, knows that it is sexually transmitted, and knows that condoms can protect against STDs, it does not seem to follow that he or she will also believe that condoms protect against HIV. Indeed, the STD connection may be a dangerous one. Kisekka (no date) notes that commercial sex workers in Nigeria dismiss the need to adopt condoms because they already self-medicate to protect themselves from STDs. In fact, fewer than half of those who reported knowing of condoms in the WHO/GPA surveys in all the countries except Guinea-Bissau believed condoms were effective in preventing HIV transmission. In focus groups, people frequently scoffed at the idea that something as flimsy as a condom could protect against a disease as deadly as AIDS (Irwin et al., 1991; Konde-Lule, 1993; Kisekka, no date). Orubuloye et al. (1991) report that in Nigeria this view was common even among bar girls. It is worth considering whether this perception arises from overkill in AIDS awareness campaigns. Virologists have shown that HIV is not very infectious; while it is important to stress that, once contracted, AIDS is lethal, it would be wrong to suggest that it is all-powerful and cannot be kept at bay by fairly simple precautions.

Attitudes Toward Condoms

In strongly pronatalist societies, the fact that condoms prevent conception may weigh heavily against their use to prevent transmission of STDs and HIV/AIDS. Other barriers to condom use, expressed both in surveys and more clearly in qualitative studies, are rife. The single most common feeling expressed was that condoms reduce sexual pleasure. Both sexes surveyed in WHO/GPA study areas were more likely to say that condoms made sex less enjoyable if they had used them than if they had no experience of condom use. In all countries but one, over half of all men who had ever used a condom said doing so made sex less fun (Mehryar, 1995). The exception was Lesotho, the country with the highest prevalence of condom use among those who had ever heard of the device.[17] Annoyances such as the interruption of spontaneity, especially among those professing a habit of serial ejaculation, and the problem of disposal contributed to a distaste for condom use (Konde-Lule, 1993; Kisekka, no date; Preston-Whyte, 1994).

There is a general association of condoms with prostitutes and promiscuity (possibly engendered by AIDS awareness campaigns). Both men and women say that asking a partner to use a condom is tantamount to admitting one's own promiscuity or accusing one's partner of sleeping around (Irwin et al., 1991; Hogsborg and Aaby, 1992; Kisekka, no date; Preston-Whyte, 1994). Konde-Lule (1993) reports that some bar girls in Uganda said they were loath to suggest condom use for fear of getting a reputation as a prostitute. Although reports of condom use with "commercial" partners were infrequent in the WHO/GPA surveys, over three-quarters of men who reported ever using condoms said they thought them appropriate for casual partners (Figure 4-4A). Women with a history of condom use and male respondents who knew of condoms but had never tried them were only slightly less likely to agree. Not surprisingly, the percentage of people reporting that condoms were suitable for use within marriage or a regular partnership was correspondingly low, not rising much higher than one-third of male condom users; the exception was Lesotho, where over three-quarters of respondents were happy to use condoms with their wives (Figure 4-4A). Those who had never used condoms were consistently less likely to think use with a regular partner appropriate.

Women did not differ substantially from men in their views except in Togo and Burundi, where female users (Figure 4-4B) and nonusers were both substantially more willing than men to contemplate condom use with their spouses. However, women in Togo were also far more likely than men to think that their regular partners would be offended by condom use; in all other study areas, men were more likely than women to think condom use would offend their partners. The results suggest that there is substantial lack of communication between regular partners on the issue of condom use.

Some people also reported in group discussions that they believed condom use might encourage promiscuity, especially among the young (Irwin et al., 1991;

[17] It is tempting to infer that, whatever the direction of the relationship, the more men have experience of condom use, the less disdainful they are on the count of reduced pleasure. However, the country that follows Lesotho in prevalence of condom use among those who know of condoms, Guinea-Bissau, had the highest proportion complaining that condoms reduce pleasure.

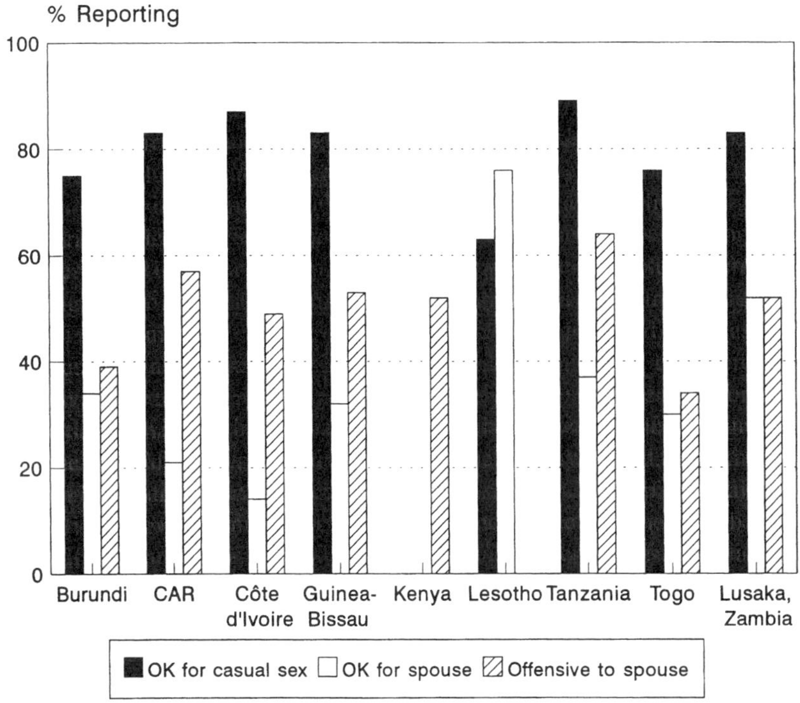

FIGURE 4-4A Attitudes Toward Condoms Among Men Who Have Used Them.
SOURCE: Cleland and Ferry (1995).

Preston-Whyte, 1994). It will be important to address these concerns when designing socially and politically acceptable programs targeted at adolescents.

Concerns over the safety of condoms, particularly for women, surfaced in study after study (Irwin et al., 1991; Lindan et al., 1991; Kisekka, no date; Hogsborg and Aaby, 1992; Konde-Lule, 1993). In focus groups, people frequently tell the story of a friend or local woman known to have died because of a wayward condom. The WHO/GPA surveys showed that a high proportion of people who had used condoms still believed they could "climb up into the womb or stomach." In Côte d'Ivoire, for instance, 61 percent of condom users believed this myth, while in Togo the figure was 46 percent (Mehryar, 1995). Orubuloye et al. (1991:71) report that in Ekiti district in Nigeria, "many believe they [condoms] are as dangerous as AIDS."

Erroneous health concerns aside, the social stress on fertility and the consequent quest for pregnancy can be important in determining women's propensity to disdain condoms. In areas where STDs are common, women may have to choose between not using condoms and exposing themselves to STDs (and

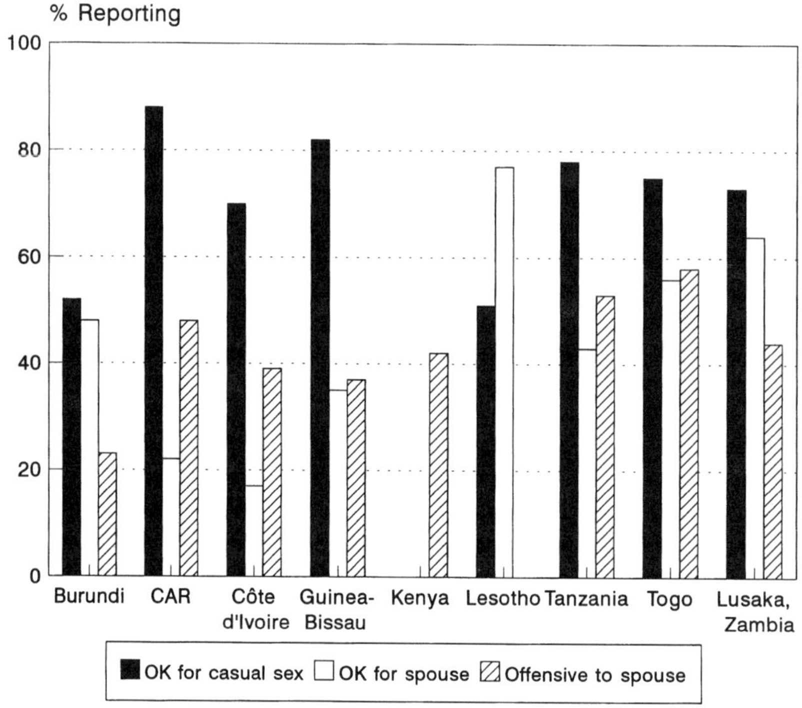

FIGURE 4-4B Attitudes Toward Condoms Among Women Who Have Used Them. SOURCE: Cleland and Ferry (1995).

thereby the possibility of sterility) or using condoms and foregoing the chance of pregnancy in the short term (O'Toole Erwin, 1993; Preston-Whyte, 1994).

Obviously, condoms are useful only if they are within people's means. In the WHO/GPA surveys, cost was considered a barrier to regular use by fewer than one-quarter of men who had ever used them, except in Côte d'Ivoire, where two-fifths thought them too expensive. In most study areas, female users were slightly more likely than men to consider regular use financially out of reach; this differential may be a reflection on women's relatively lower earning power in the areas in question. In Rakai district, Uganda, the availability and affordability of condoms have been shown in four annual surveys to have little effect on the decision to use them (Kivumbi, 1993).

BEHAVIOR CHANGE

As this chapter demonstrates, measuring sexual behavior is no straightforward matter and is a science in its infancy. Without a large body of evidence accumulated by measuring current behavior over several years, it is almost impossible to determine what changes have taken place.

The WHO/GPA surveys represent a step in establishing such a body of evidence. Although they do include questions on changes in behavior, single-round cross-sectional surveys are singularly inappropriate for establishing the causality of any changes that may have taken place in the past. Given that the section on behavior change in the WHO/GPA surveys comes after a long section focusing on the threats and dangers of AIDS, replies are quite likely to reflect what respondents perceive the interviewers want to hear. That said, the answers may give some indication of the types of behavioral change that people consider most plausible.

Over half of all men in every country surveyed by WHO/GPA (and up to 90 percent in the Central African Republic and 70 percent in Côte d'Ivoire) reported having changed their sexual behavior in response to the HIV/AIDS epidemic. Women reported lower levels of change in all populations but Lesotho. No clear link emerges between a sense of personal vulnerability and reported behavior change. Cleland (1995) maintains that risk reduction is usually incomplete, so some risk behavior will remain, and a positive correlation should be expected. It might equally be argued, however, that people would bother to reduce their risk behavior only if they thought doing so would be effective and would in consequence feel less vulnerable. The survey data show a positive correlation between risk behavior and reported risk reduction over the last 12 months. If this association were interpreted as a change from previous higher levels of sexual activity to a level still considered high risk in the survey classification, it would provide support for Cleland's hypothesis. An alternative explanation of the empirical evidence might be that behavior changed very recently and was thus not fully captured in the 12-month reference period.

Of behavior changes reported, few were related to casual transmission beliefs, with reduction of partners the most frequently reported measure. Nowhere except Guinea-Bissau was condom use reported as a specific change by more than 7 percent of those who reported any change.[18] However, some of these respondents had reported earlier in the survey that they had never used a condom. Certainly the level of potentially effective behavior change reported is not reflected in other markers of safer sexual activity, such as a decrease in the prevalence of STDs.

In-depth interviews conducted in Guinea-Bissau revealed that only two of seven men who had reported in surveys that they had started using condoms because of AIDS turned out to have done so (Hogsborg and Aaby, 1992). The

[18]In Guinea-Bissau, 25 percent of men and 23 percent of women reporting change said they had increased use of condoms. However, no details are given on the content of public health campaigns in the country in the period preceding the survey.

researchers further reported that men who said they would use condoms with casual partners did not in fact do so, explaining in each case that the circumstances were special because the woman was respectable. The researchers concluded that focusing campaigns on condom use with unknown partners who are assumed to be strangers is useless in a context in which people do not consider any partners to be unknown.

In focus group interviews conducted in Rakai district, Uganda, after several years of vigorous campaigns to promote AIDS awareness and behavior change, people in rural areas did believe that risky sexual activity was on the wane. Optimists might think this finding reflects a new, lower-level, post-AIDS norm. In urban areas, however, people thought their neighbors were just as active as ever but more discreet, a change that might also translate into an increasing tendency to underreport the numbers of partners in surveys (Konde-Lule, 1993). Adolescent groups were especially unlikely to think sexual activity had diminished. Working in the same area, Obbo (1993b) reports an interesting attempt to "map" sexual networks.[19] The work shows that even if people reduce their partner numbers to a small band of people they know well, such as old classmates, they are still at considerable risk of infection. Of 15 people in two interlinked urban networks in 1989, only 2 had survived by 1992.

The failure of awareness programs and interventions to effect more substantial change in condom use should be judged in context. Despite initial willingness among adolescents in Durban, South Africa, to try condoms with their partners, few had positive experiences, challenging widely held notions of male sexual prowess, love, and accepted patterns of interpersonal communication between the sexes (Preston-Whyte, 1994). In a culture where condoms are uncommon and have a rather sordid image, such an outcome is hardly surprising.

Focus groups illuminate the frightening possibility that behavior change may be in the wrong direction. An overwhelming majority of schoolchildren involved in an essay-writing exercise in Uganda thought it likely that those who found out they were seropositive would deliberately go out and spread the disease (Obbo, 1993a). Konde-Lule (1993) reports similar findings, and IRESCO (1995) describes the same dynamic in relation to STDs in Cameroon.

Authors frequently observe that knowing how to reduce risk effectively is not in itself enough to change behavior; people must have the power to make the required changes. Ulin (1992) suggests that the failure of AIDS campaigns to recognize this fact can be fatal to their impact. The WHO/GPA surveys attempted to determine how "empowered" people felt by asking whether they believed AIDS could be avoided by behavior change. Consistently high propor-

[19]The networks are discovered through what amounts to gossip (albeit from several sources), so it is difficult to judge how accurate the information is.

tions of those who had heard of AIDS said yes. However, since the question was asked impersonally, a positive response does not tell us whether people felt they were in a position to make those changes themselves, much less whether they felt able to urge changes on their partners.

In the HIV/AIDS literature, the discussion of power within a relationship usually turns on women's ability to refuse sex or enforce condom use. Women may have more chance of taking either action where a strong tradition of postpartum abstinence allows them to refuse sex at certain times, such as in West African societies, where a woman can rely on her natal kin for support if her insistence on behavior change results in the breakdown of the relationship (Awusabo-Asare et al., 1993; Orubuloye et al., 1993; O'Toole Erwin, 1993). Women are often in a fairly strong position to refuse sex with regular partners if they know their partner has contracted an STD, but attempts to "punish" men for infidelity are viewed with less sympathy. For instance, for women in Zambia, a husband's infidelity is not grounds for divorce, but women can and do seek divorce if they contract an STD from their husbands (Parapart, 1988, quoted in Standing and Kisekka, 1989). Women who rely on sex or sexual attachments for all or most of their income are among those who have least leverage over their partners. If they are commercial sex workers, they are also those most frequently exposed to the risk of infection.

CONCLUSIONS

What, then, have we learned from the WHO/GPA surveys and other work on sexual behavior in sub-Saharan Africa, and what are the implications? The following conclusions can be drawn:

- There is considerable diversity among African countries in reports of nonmarital sex.
- Multiple partnerships remain common, and marriages are in many places inherently unstable. A high proportion of regular partnerships are noncohabiting, even at older ages; noncohabitation is associated with casual sexual contacts.
- While there is generally more casual sex occurring in towns and cities than in villages, levels of sexual activity are remarkably similar across the urban/rural divide in a given country, and rural areas should not be neglected in planning campaigns to arrest the spread of HIV.
- AIDS is widely known and feared, and governments should not assume they will encounter opposition if they put the issue high on the national agenda.
- People know that HIV is sexually transmitted, but many still believe that mosquitoes and social contact can spread the disease as well. The concept of infection by an apparently healthy person is poorly understood and should be stressed in educational campaigns.
- From the point of view of program planners, health beliefs fall into three categories: those that are likely to prove supportive to interventions and behavior

change, those that are merely benign or neutral, and those that are dangerous. An example of this last category is the belief that links sex with a "cleansing" of sexual diseases. If such views are determined to be common, ways must be found of eroding them without spreading them further through suggestion.

- Levels of condom use are low and access is limited in many countries, although this picture is changing rapidly across the continent as governments and international organizations commit more resources to social marketing, family planning, and the control of STDs. Where condoms are known, their image is often still poor, sometimes for reasons that are inherent to the product and sometimes based on misconceptions. One of the most common of the latter, that condoms are dangerous to women, should be urgently redressed.
- AIDS awareness campaigns have focused on use of condoms with strangers and casual partners. This focus may jeopardize their use with regular partners, as well as with acquaintances who may belong to high-risk groups.
- There is no shortage of evidence that coercive sex, including rape, takes place and that schoolgirls are especially likely to be victims. As a human rights issue, this should stand alone; in areas where STDs and HIV/AIDS are prevalent, it is also a public health issue. Work should be initiated to determine the magnitude of the problem and address the forces that promote it, including silence.[20]
- Women consistently report fewer sexual partners than do men. Ways must be devised of discovering whether this discrepancy is the result of normative underreporting; if so, alternatives to survey methods of data collection for quantification of women's sexual activity must be developed.

RECOMMENDATIONS

The discussion in this chapter and the conclusions offered above lead to the following recommendations for future research related to sexual behavior and HIV/AIDS.

Recommendation 4-1. Research on sexual networks is critical.

Population-based research is needed to collect and analyze data on both the variables that describe individual sexual behavior and the possible socioeconomic determinants of the decision to have sex with a new partner or forgo protection. Since the details of interconnected sexual networks are difficult to

---

[20]In July 1991 at St. Kizito school in Kenya, 19 girls were killed and 71 reported raped by their fellow students. Following the incident, the deputy headmistress commented that "the boys did not mean the girls any harm. They only wanted to rape" (Okie, 1993:A15).

deduce from the answers to individual questionnaires, there is also an important role for social network research.

Recommendation 4-2. Researchers need to develop more reliable ways of collecting information on sexual behavior and to find ways of testing its validity.

There appears to be a much greater willingness to report sexual behavior than was believed until recently, but this field of research requires sensitivity. The challenge is to develop definitions and appropriate vocabulary, such as for categories of relationships, that are both specific enough to be clear to respondents and generalizable enough to be useful to analysts and program planners. The challenge is likely to grow as information about high-risk behavior spreads, increasing the likelihood that respondents will seek to give the "right" answers on questionnaires and in interviews. Hybrid research strategies involving both qualitative and quantitative approaches are essential. Where appropriate, and when both privacy and confidentiality can be ensured, biological markers of sexual activity (such as HIV or STD status) should periodically be incorporated into behavioral surveys to allow assessment of the validity of questionnaire responses and the extent to which the latter provide adequate information on risk.

Recommendation 4-3. Research is needed on patterns of sexual initiation and on the formation of sexual norms and attitudes.

The sexual habits of a lifetime may well be influenced by a socialization process that starts at or before puberty, often before sexual activity begins. A better understanding of the early influences on sexual norms and attitudes and of patterns of sexual initiation may prove essential to promoting safer behavior. For this recommended research to be successful, studies must include children and prepubescent youths, as well as sexually active adolescents and their partners. Recognition that sexuality is socially constructed and changing rapidly is essential to broadening the research agenda and improving interventions.

Recommendation 4-4. More work is needed to clarify the frequency of specific sexual practices.

Because the epidemic in sub-Saharan Africa is being sustained by heterosexual transmission, information on sexual behavior is needed to help develop more effective prevention strategies, as well as to provide baseline data to evaluate their effectiveness. Specific sexual practices—dry sex, oral sex, and anal sex being but a few examples—may impede the success of particular interventions, yet information about such practices is necessary for encouraging behavioral change.

Recommendation 4-5. Research on coercive sex, especially among adolescents, is critical.

The magnitude of the problem of coercive sex is all but unknown, as are the circumstances under which forced sex or rape takes place. How frequently does it happen and why? Do the aggressors or the victims share characteristics that might suggest a path for preventive or protective interventions? Research on community attitudes, mores, and gender expectations that may serve to encourage or inhibit coercive sex is urgently needed in order to determine how to enlist community support for the curtailment of such practices.

Recommendation 4-6. Research aimed at achieving a better understanding of perceptions about the dual roles of condoms is required.

Condoms help prevent the spread of HIV/AIDS; they also prevent pregnancy. How aware are people of these dual roles, and what weight do they give each when deciding whether to use condoms? How often are these roles in concord and how often in conflict? Do partners discuss this issue, and if so, what are the negotiating mechanisms used?

Recommendation 4-7. Research on attitudes and beliefs about and behavioral responses to sexually transmitted diseases is required.

To develop effective strategies for the treatment of STDs, understanding is needed about social and cultural responses to STDs, including stigmatization. Much more knowledge about the health-seeking behaviors of people infected with STDs, and whether their sexual habits are altered by knowledge of infection, is also needed.

Recommendation 4-8. Research on acceptance of and behavioral responses to HIV vaccination is urgently needed.

Because vaccine trials are likely to begin with vaccines of limited efficacy, there is an urgent need to learn whether individuals who are vaccinated increase their exposure to HIV through riskier behavior, and if so, to determine how to mitigate this response.

5

Primary HIV-Prevention Strategies

Over the past 10 years, African governments—through national AIDS control programs international development agencies, private voluntary organizations, and other nongovernmental groups across Africa have devoted resources, time, and energy to developing low-cost interventions to arrest the spread of HIV and AIDS. Many different programs have distributed AIDS leaflets, badges, stickers, and other paraphernalia. Messages informing people about the danger of AIDS are regularly broadcast on radio and television, published in newspapers, displayed on billboards, and performed by local entertainers. Hundreds of peer educators across the continent visit local bars, beer gardens, hotels, STD clinics, and work sites to provide AIDS- prevention education and distribute free condoms. Millions of other condoms are being made available at very low cost through social marketing programs.[1] At the start of the epidemic, when many of these interventions were first conceived, the hope was that they would induce a sufficiently large behavior response to contain the epidemic.

How successful have these efforts been at preventing new cases of HIV infection? Despite the many limitations inherent in attempting to evaluate the effectiveness of interventions aimed at HIV prevention, clear evidence is emerging that such efforts can be successful, particularly among higher-risk groups

[1] Social marketing is the application of commercial marketing techniques to achieve a social goal. Condom social marketing programs make condoms more accessible and affordable. At the same time, condom social marketing programs promote the use of condoms in an attempt to make them more acceptable to target populations.

(World Health Organization, 1992c; Coates, 1993; Lamptey et al., 1993; Choi and Coates, 1994; Stryker et al., 1995). At the same time, however, data from various surveillance systems indicate that current interventions are probably not yet having a significant impact on the epidemic at the continent or even the country level (Lamptey et al., 1993; see also Chapter 3). Despite the fact that levels of AIDS awareness are extremely high across the continent (see Chapter 4), getting people to change their behavior is difficult. Denial, fear, external pressures, other priorities, or simple economics can sometimes keep people from adopting healthier life-styles.

There are many reasons why prevention efforts in Africa have not had as large an impact on the spread of the epidemic as desired. AIDS has struck the continent at a time when it is undergoing its worst financial crisis since independence. In some countries, other catastrophes—such as wars, droughts, or famines—have been more immediate and taken precedence over AIDS-prevention efforts. Throughout the continent, the overall magnitude of the response has been inadequate, and expectations about what could be achieved quickly have been unrealistic. A lack of indigenous management capacity and chronic weaknesses in the public health system have hindered the development and implementation of AIDS control programs. Individuals and organizations working against the spread of AIDS have had to face discrimination, complacency, and even persistent denial in the community. Many AIDS workers have become exhausted after struggling for so long against impossible odds; many others have died (Mann et al., 1992). Myths surrounding modes of transmission hinder the dissemination of correct knowledge and sustained behavior change (see, for example, Krynen, 1994; Nature, 1993; Ndyetabura and Paalman, 1994; Ankomah, 1994).

But getting people to change their behavior is not impossible. Indeed, health educators in Africa have had a fair amount of success in the recent past. For example, broad-based education campaigns have persuaded large numbers of people to have their children immunized against various childhood diseases and educated mothers to give their children oral rehydration formula during episodes of diarrhea. Of course, attempting to modify more personal behavior, such as sexual practices, is more challenging. Yet, family planning programs have been successful even in some of the most disadvantaged countries of the world (see, for example, Cleland et al., 1994). Even the most cautious reviews of behavioral interventions aimed at slowing the spread of HIV conclude that although most have not been rigorously evaluated, some approaches do seem to work (e.g., Oakley et al., 1995). It is important to have realistic expectations about what can and cannot be achieved. Behavior change will never be 100 percent effective: some individuals will never choose to protect themselves, while others will relapse into old patterns of behavior after just a short period of time (Cates and Hinman, 1992; Lamptey et al., 1993).

To increase the likelihood of success, interventions need to be culturally appropriate and locally relevant, reflecting cognizance of the social context within which they are embedded (see Chapter 2). They should be designed with a clear idea of the target population and the types of behaviors to be changed. In turn, impediments in the social environment to behavior change probably need to be removed or weakened (Turner et al., 1989). Therefore, behavior-change interventions should include promotion of lower-risk behavior, assistance in risk-reduction skills development, and promotion of changes in societal norms (Lamptey, 1994). In Africa, as elsewhere, HIV-prevention messages have included promotion of partner reduction, postponing of sexual debut, alternatives to risky sex, mutually faithful monogamy, consistent and proper use of condoms, better recognition of STD symptoms, and more effective health-seeking behavior.

The purpose of the discussion in this chapter is to delineate opportunities for effecting beneficial behavior changes and to discuss how these opportunities might be realized. The discussion is based on an examination of interventions to achieve behavior change, an effort that has led to the development of a set of basic principles for successful strategies and programs. The remainder of this chapter is organized as follows. First we examine principles and issues in the design and evaluation of behavior-change intervention programs. We then examine the issues that challenge the design of effective interventions targeted to African men, women, and youth, respectively, and highlight strategies that have been implemented to address these issues. Each discussion is followed by an illustrative case study. Lessons learned from these programs are then highlighted. Next follows a discussion of strategies to prevent perinatal HIV transmission. The chapter ends with a set of recommendations for prevention research, which are made in light of the experiences of strategies and programs implemented in Africa to date.

BEHAVIOR-CHANGE INTERVENTION PROGRAM DESIGN AND EVALUATION

The rapid spread of HIV in sub-Saharan Africa since the early 1980s is a result of a multiplicity of factors, many of which have been discussed in previous chapters. Table 5-1 summarizes much of this information. As the table shows, it is analytically convenient to distinguish among four types of factors: (1) individual-level factors (i.e., ones the individual has some control over changing), (2) societal factors that may serve to encourage or discourage high-risk behavior, (3) health infrastructural factors that directly or indirectly facilitate the spread of HIV, and (4) structural factors related to development issues over which the individual has very little control. As the last column in Table 5-1 shows, each of these sets of factors requires a different length of time to bring about positive change.

A basic comprehensive HIV-prevention program should aim to address the

TABLE 5-1 Factors Contributing to Sexual Transmission of HIV in sub-Saharan Africa

Level	Definition	Examples	Changes Required	Comments
Individual	Factors that directly affect the individual and that the individual has some control in changing	*Biological:* • History and/or presence of STDs • Lack of male circumcision • Anal intercourse • Sex during menses • Traumatic sex • Cervical ectopy	• Prevention/treatment of STDs • Avoidance of sex during menses • Prevention of traumatic sex	Achievable in the short term
		Behavioral: • Frequent change of sex partners • Multiple sex partners • Unprotected sexual intercourse • Sex with a commercial sex worker • Sex with an infected partner • Lack of knowledge of STDs/HIV • Low risk perception	• Abstinence • Mutual fidelity • Consistent condom use • Knowledge and skills of STD/HIV prevention	Achievable in the short term

Societal	Factors related to societal norms that encourage high-risk sexual behavior	• High rates of prostitution • Multiple partners by men • Gender discrimination • Poor attitudes toward condom use • Social status of women • Extended postpartum abstinence	• Improvement in status of women • Job opportunities for women • Promotion of mutual fidelity • Changes in societal attitudes toward condom use	Achievable in the short to medium term
Infrastructural	Factors that directly or indirectly facilitate the spread of HIV, over which the individual has very little control	• Poor availability of condoms • Poor STD services • High prevalence of STDs • Poor communication services	• Changes in health infrastructure • Improvement in STD care, behavior-change communication, and condom provision	Achievable in the short to medium term
Structural	Factors related to developmental issues, over which both the individual and the health system have very little control	• Underdevelopment • Poverty • Rural/urban migration • Civil unrest • Low literacy rates for women • Laws/policies, including lack of human rights • Unemployment	• General economic development programs • Enactment of appropriate laws/policies • Income-generating opportunities • Improvement in education of women	Feasible in the long term

four types of factors cited above as contributing to the spread of HIV, particularly those related to health. Steps in a comprehensive strategy include epidemiological and behavioral formative research to help design programs; implementation of behavioral interventions to facilitate individual, group, and societal behavior change; condom provision; structural/environmental strategies that support individual, group, and societal change; and program evaluation to assess success in program implementation, intermediate outcomes, and ultimate impact. In addition, evidence that STDs may facilitate HIV transmission and the interconnectedness of STD and HIV transmission modalities and prevention (see Chapter 3) strongly suggest an important role for STD treatment, control, and prevention in AIDS prevention (Laga et al., 1991; Grosskurth et al., 1995).

Guiding Principles for Behavior-Change Interventions

Interventions designed to modify people's behavior need to be based on sound principles of behavior change. Many behavioral theories are described in the literature and have been applied to understanding HIV risk behavior.[2] However, no single theory sufficiently explains individual behavior changes or provides all the essential tools to change behavior (Coates, 1993). As a result, current thinking calls for a complementary combination of theoretical approaches that incorporates the key principles of behavior change into program design.

Seven guiding principles for effective behavior change interventions targeted at HIV/AIDS prevention have evolved. These principles, which are consistent with the behavior science literature and with experience in program development in Africa (Family Health International/AIDSCAP Project, 1995), are as follows:

- Targeting—Interventions should focus on well-characterized, specific target audiences.
- Skills development—Interventions should include components that encourage individual acquisition of skills and tools that will help to prevent the transmission of HIV.
- Support—A supportive social environment needs to be created to foster HIV-prevention interventions and reinforce individual behavior-change efforts.
- Maintenance—HIV-prevention interventions need to include strategies that will foster the maintenance of behavior change over time.
- Collaboration—Every effort should be made in the development and de-

[2]These include the Health Belief Model, Social Learning/Social Cognitive Theory (including the self-efficacy construct), the Stages of Change Model, the Theory of Reasoned Action (including the behavioral intention construct), Motivation/Protection Theory, Social Inoculation Theory, Cognitive Behavior Modification Theory, the Harm Reduction Model, and the AIDS Risk Reduction Model.

livery of prevention interventions to work collaboratively with other sectors, ministries, and communities so that the potential for synergistic program effects is enhanced.

- Monitoring and evaluation—Programs must be monitored and evaluated in order to determine intervention implementation integrity, effectiveness, and cost-effectiveness.
- Sustainability—Because resources are limited and donor support is intermittent, HIV-prevention programs should be designed for sustainability by building capacity to pursue alternative resources.

Evaluation is discussed in detail in the next section. Here we comment further only on the principles of sustainability and of targeting.

For HIV/AIDS-prevention programs to be effective and sustainable, it is critical to build local capacity in both the public and the private sectors. The chronic shortages of human and fiscal resources in most of sub-Saharan Africa often make program design, implementation, and management difficult. Major deficiencies include poor infrastructure and paucity of management and technical skills in both research and intervention programs (see also Chapter 7). Special efforts should be made to improve the technical, organizational, management, and financial skills of individuals, as well as to strengthen institutional infrastructure.

With regard to targeting and audience segmentation in HIV intervention programs, the primary objective is to obtain effective and rapid results by intervening with groups that are at the greatest risk of acquiring and spreading HIV infection (Lamptey and Potts, 1990). Although it would be highly desirable to design prevention programs that are based on a good understanding of the target population and the sociocultural, environmental, and structural context, few prevention programs are based on preliminary, or formative, research findings.

As noted earlier, the groups most commonly targeted are those traditionally seen as at particularly high risk, such as truckers, uniformed service workers, commercial sex workers, or STD patients. Targeting can also extend to other at-risk populations, including out-of-school youth, school children, university students, male and female factory workers, women in the general population, and men away from home. The target audience may be defined by (1) epidemiological risk factors (e.g., HIV prevalence among commercial sex workers); (2) behavioral risk factors (e.g., clients of commercial sex workers); (3) occupation (e.g., factory workers); (4) geographic location (e.g., urban adults); (5) access points (e.g., truck stops); (6) demographics (e.g., gender, age); or (7) relevant sociocultural factors (e.g., widows, street children). In later sections of this chapter, interventions targeted principally to men, to women, and to youth are discussed; although restricting our consideration to these particular groups, we recognize that all interventions should include some attention to the sexual partners of the target group.

INTERVENTION EVALUATION

Just as the stages of an intervention program can be described as design, implementation, and outcome, so can evaluation accompany or follow each of these stages to determine how successfully the program has met its stated objectives. The corresponding stages or types of evaluation are formative, process, and outcome (Coyle et al., 1991).

Formative evaluation of the design of an intervention addresses the question of whether the proposed intervention has the potential to achieve its goals. It considers structural factors that may affect the program. For example, are policies in place to facilitate implementation of the intervention strategies (e.g., a policy requiring sex education in the schools that includes HIV/AIDS prevention)? Formative evaluation also assesses the content, nature, and design of the proposed intervention strategies in terms of success potential. For example, are they skills-based? Are they derived from preliminary, formative research? Do they match the target audience's needs? Are they built on the characteristics of other successful programs?

Process evaluation techniques are used to monitor the program as it is being implemented. The goal is to determine how well short-term program objectives are being met. For example, are condoms being distributed? Are people tested for HIV returning to obtain their results? Is the number of patients attending STD clinics declining?

Outcome evaluation is the last and ultimately the most important stage. It addresses questions about the success of the intervention. For example, has the program succeeded in changing behavior? Has that behavior change been sustained? And finally, has that behavior change succeeded in reducing the incidence of HIV? This assessment of behavioral outcomes should be performed only when there is reason to expect that such outcomes could have occurred and can be measured (i.e., earlier formative evaluation has confirmed that the intervention was well designed, process evaluation has corroborated that the intervention is being carried out well, the observation period has been substantial, behaviors have been measured, and the sample size has been sufficiently large to detect behavioral differences). Good outcome evaluation is rarely feasible unless it is planned as an integral part of the intervention and usually is possible only in the context of studies with adequate research funding and undertaken by research institutions such as universities. Interventions evaluated in this way can serve as models for others that will not undergo as rigorous an outcome evaluation.

While the logical program evaluation sequence outlined above is time-consuming, expensive, and rigorous, following these steps can help avoid wasting scarce funds on evaluations that are limited in their ability to yield useful results and repeating or continuing intervention programs that are limited in their ability to achieve the desired goals (Oakley et al., 1995).

For Africa, as elsewhere, we have limited information on what works well because of the difficulties in carrying out rigorous evaluations, particularly outcome evaluations (Oakley et al., 1995). While the goal of rigorous evaluation must be maintained over the longer term, there is also demand for a faster, more pragmatic approach. Insistence on pure scientific rigor may be counterproductive for HIV/AIDS-prevention interventions, where innovative methods and program designs are urgently needed, and prevention efforts must rely almost exclusively on behavior change (Coyle et al., 1991).

Examples of programs that have been implemented in sub-Saharan Africa and reported in studies are described briefly in Annex 5-1 and referred to in subsequent sections of this chapter. This is not a comprehensive listing; rather it illustrates recent interventions that have used a variety of strategies and programs in trying to effect positive changes in the behavior of targeted audiences. Many have attempted to conduct modest evaluations with the limited funds available to them. Some of these evaluations suffer from methodological weaknesses so that the results must be interpreted with caution; yet all contribute to the growing effort to evaluate programs, with the twin goals of improving continuing intervention programs and designing new programs that are more effective in achieving results and at lower cost.

Even where the "gold standard" of an intervention that consists of a randomized trial with high-caliber formative, process, and outcome evaluation cannot be met, there are practical guidelines for program developers. First, at the formative stage, it should be recognized that programs are most likely to achieve desired outcomes when their design is based on the characteristics and principles of existing effective programs, past program experience, formative research, and sound theoretical underpinnings. Even when existing programs have not undergone a gold standard evaluation, if there is consistency and convergence in results from multiple programs in different places and/or over time and/or from multiple measures of results, synthesis and interpretation of findings can guide the design of new programs. Planners must be cautious in applying such findings, maintaining awareness of the potential for biases that can influence the results. Second, while rigorous outcome evaluations are desperately needed, not all programs should attempt to implement them. However, all programs should be required to conduct process evaluation to assess program integrity. Finally, evaluation results should be translated and synthesized into new programmatic guidelines and materials and new training activities so that programs can be improved.

A TYPOLOGY OF INTERVENTION PROGRAMS

HIV-prevention strategies can be classified according to the foundation on which they are based: (1) formal institution-based programs (e.g., at the workplace, school, or clinic); (2) community-based programs (e.g., among informal youth groups or informal women's groups); and (3) population-based programs (e.g., national media campaigns or policy development). These categories are not mutually exclusive. For example, the same individuals may be reached at work, in special community-based initiatives, or at home through the mass media.

The following sections describe each of these program types in greater detail and illustrate them with studies included in Annex 5-1. Although, as already mentioned, most of these studies lacked the resources to carry out definitive evaluations, we summarize the investigators' reports of quantifiable impacts.

Institution-based Programs

Both institution-based and community-based programs are designed to reach individuals and small groups, with the aim of teaching and reinforcing protective behaviors. They are intended to give individuals the opportunity to acquire information, assess their own risk of HIV, interact with a provider, and obtain relevant behavioral and communication skills that can help in reducing high-risk behavior; they also generate notions of peer norms that are conducive to risk reduction (Lamptey and Coates, 1994).

Institution-based programs include interventions in the workplace (factories, prisons, commercial farms, mining communities, military bases); in schools; and in health facilities, such as STD and family planning clinics, hospitals, and HIV counseling and testing clinics (see studies [4], [5], [7], [8], [10-12], [14-16], [18], and [20-24] in Annex 5-1). Targeted groups within these institutions may not be homogeneous in terms of individual behavior or social norms, and may or may not exhibit more high-risk sexual behavior than the general population. The relative ease of access to these institutional populations renders such programs attractive and potentially cost-effective.

Several institution-based programs in Africa have demonstrated changes in risk behavior (Ngugi et al., 1988 [4][3] ; Loodts and Van de Perre, 1989; Kamenga et al., 1991; Allen et al., 1992b [7]; Mwizarubi et al., 1992 [12]; Williams and Ray, 1993 [20-24]; Wynendaele et al., 1995). In Rwanda, for example, the initiation of an education, STD treatment, and condom distribution program for all military recruits led to a reduction in the incidence of urethritis (Loodts and Van de Perre, 1989; World Health Organization, 1992c [11]). In Rwanda, 1,458 women attending antenatal and pediatric clinics at the Centre Hospitalier de Kigali received pre- and post-test counseling, were shown an educational video, and were given free condoms. One year later, HIV seroconversion rates had decreased significantly (from 4.1 to 1.8 per 100 person-years among women whose partners were tested and counseled) (World Health Organization, 1992c [10]). Preliminary results from other ongoing programs in Tanzania and Zimbabwe also are encouraging (Mwizarubi et al., 1992 [12]; Williams and Ray, 1993 [20-24]; World Health Organization, 1992c [14]). In Tanzania, a workplace

[3]Numbers in brackets immediately following certain references are the numbers assigned to the studies in Annex 5-1.

intervention targets truck drivers, their assistants, and their sexual partners (Mwizarubi et al., 1992 [12]). In Zimbabwe, a workplace-based intervention program targets 4,500 factory employees and their families (Williams and Ray, 1993 [20-24]). This program provides STD treatment, behavior-change intervention, and condoms. The intervention employs a combination of drama, printed materials, group talks, and interpersonal counseling by 64 peer educators.

Although evidence about the impact of counseling and testing on risk behavior is mixed (Higgins et al., 1991), a few evaluations conducted to date in developing countries suggest that such efforts may be effective, at least in the short term, in changing sexual practices under certain circumstances or among certain groups (such as couples) (Higgins et al., 1991; Kamenga et al., 1991; Allen et al., 1992a [7], 1992b [8]; Wynendaele et al., 1995 [5]). In Rwanda, for example, results of an HIV counseling and testing program demonstrated an increase in condom use (Allen et al., 1992b [8]). HIV seroconversion rates were also reported to have decreased among seronegative women whose partners were tested, but not among women whose partners were not tested. In Uganda, an evaluation of a counseling and testing intervention found significant reported decreases in risk behaviors among both seronegative and seropositive individuals (Moore et al., 1993).[4]

Community-based Programs

Community-based programs use group interventions to reach communities. These interventions include the use of peer educators to reach sex workers or school-aged youth, use of traditional health providers to reach rural communities, or programs targeted to other community groups (see studies [1], [6], [9], [13], [25], and [26] in Annex 5-1).

Community participation can sometimes be a critical factor for program success and sustainability (Lamptey and Coates, 1994; Population Council, 1995). According to the guiding principles described earlier, HIV/AIDS-prevention programs should be designed at the outset with attention to their acceptability within the community and target groups, the external or institutional support required to develop and sustain the skills and talent needed to make them work, and the infrastructure support and the individual and collective commitments needed to maintain them over time (Lamptey and Coates, 1994). Community involvement is often only an empty slogan in programs without any real involvement of the community in decision making.

[4]In 1994, Family Health International/AIDSCAP and WHO/GPA initiated a multisite clinical trial in which those seeking HIV counseling and testing were randomly assigned to receive either counseling and testing or health information (De Zoysa et al., 1995). It is hoped that rigorous evaluation of this project will resolve outstanding questions about the impact of HIV counseling and testing on the frequency of risk behaviors,

Few intervention programs implemented to date in Africa have involved such community participation. Notable exceptions are in Uganda (Seeley et al., 1991; Katende and Bunnell, 1993), where, for example, participatory planning and evaluation workshops are being held at the district level so that district health officers, community members, and AIDS educators can participate in the joint planning and evaluation of programs (Barton, 1993).

Evidence of the success of community-based interventions, as reported by various authors, is summarized in column 5 of Annex 5-1. In Accra, Ghana, a pilot educational community-based intervention used local health workers to train and support selected prostitutes as health educators and condom distributors to their peers. Six months after the intervention had begun, reported condom use had increased dramatically (Asamoah-Adu et al., 1994). In Cross River State, Nigeria, a community-based prevention program among full-time prostitutes and their clients resulted in greater use of condoms (Williams et al., 1992 [6]). In a follow-up questionnaire administered 12 months after the baseline survey, 24 percent of prostitutes reported always using condoms with their clients/partners, as compared with 12 percent in the baseline survey. And in Zimbabwe, similar interventions resulted in a dramatic increase in the proportion of sex workers who reported consistent condom use with clients (World Health Organization, 1992c [26]).

Population-based Programs

Population-based programs, using mass media, aim to change societal norms, and provide information as well as individual behavior-change messages to large segments of the population. They may also encourage the enactment of policies to support HIV/AIDS-prevention efforts. Examples include media education programs, condom social marketing programs, and policy changes such as a regulation requiring condom use in brothels. Population-based programs may be targeted to such large segments of the population as adolescents, sexually active males, men and women with multiple partners, or all sexually active men and women (see studies [2], [3], [17], and [19] in Annex 5-1).

Undoubtedly the best known and most widely cited example of a population-based intervention is condom social marketing. For example, a program in Zaire subsidized the price of condoms, increased their distribution, and used innovative commercial marketing techniques to increase condom sales from around 10,000 in 1987 to around 18 million in 1991 (Population Services International, 1992 [17]). Not surprisingly, this model of social marketing has been quickly replicated through the continent.

INTERVENTIONS TARGETING SEXUALLY ACTIVE MEN

Sexually active men have played a critical role in the rapid spread of HIV in sub-Saharan Africa. Despite the fact that more women than men are now infected (World Health Organization, 1994a), the risk behavior of sexually active men remains the key vector driving the continuing spread of HIV in Africa. The epidemiological parameters of HIV and HIV-related risk behaviors among men are described in Chapters 3 and 4, respectively.

Issues

Perhaps the most significant issue in HIV-prevention in Africa relates to gender inequality. Because men play the dominant role culturally, socially, and economically, they also dominate sexual relationships. Sex is often initiated and controlled by men in both marital and nonmarital relationships. Women have less power in sexual relationships and are often unable to influence sexual relations.

A second and related issue is that in many African cultures, multiple partners and extramarital sexual relationships by men are either accepted or tolerated, and the data show high frequencies of multiple partners. There is higher risk in these situations. A person in a polygynous union in which all partners are supposed to have sexual relations only within that union is at somewhat higher risk of HIV infection than a person in a couple union, simply because there are more people who could potentially fail to stay faithful to that union. However, a person in such a polygynous union is at much lower risk than a person with multiple partners who themselves have multiple partners.

A third issue is that most family planning programs have traditionally targeted women who are married and ignored the role of men. Women have therefore been responsible for initiating behavioral changes related to reproductive health; as a result, female-controlled methods account for the vast majority of contraceptives used (Robey et al., 1992). In 1990, only 0.3 percent of married women of reproductive age were using condoms in sub-Saharan Africa, as compared with 4 percent in all developing countries (Liskin et al., 1990).

A final general issue that influences male sexual risk taking is that, up until recently, condoms had have a poor reputation in Africa. They have been widely regarded as making sex less enjoyable, as well as being a poor disease-prevention method and an ineffective and unreliable contraceptive (see Chapter 4). Condoms are frequently seen as linked to promiscuity and prostitutes and often connote a violation of trust (Ngugi et al., 1988 [4]; May et al., 1990; Allen et al., 1992a [7]). It is not surprising, therefore, that up until very recently condoms have been poorly promoted by family planning providers. Furthermore, access to condoms is a significant problem, especially in rural areas of Africa. Nevertheless, African men have in the past 10 years shown marked changes in attitudes toward condom use for disease prevention. In particular, demand for condoms has grown steeply since 1988, with more than 110 million condoms being distributed in 1994 through social marketing programs alone (Figure 5-1).

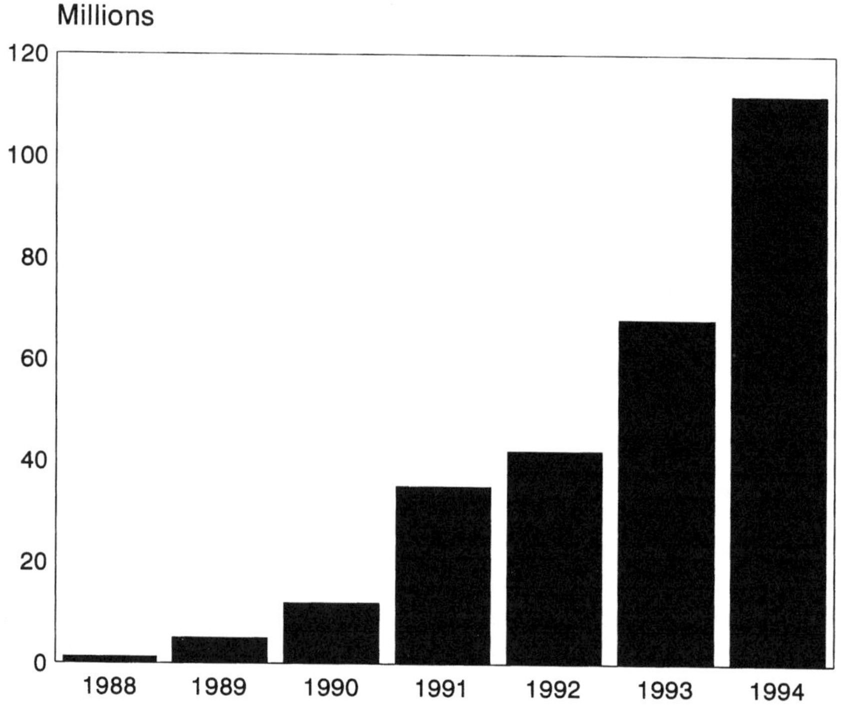

FIGURE 5-1 Population Services International (PSI) Condom Sales in Africa, 1988-1994. SOURCE: Adapted from PSI (1994c, 1995).

Target Population

Sexually active men who are not in mutually monogamous relationships or men in polygynous relationships where each member of the relationship has no outside partners are potentially at risk of HIV infection. This risk is especially acute in countries such as Tanzania, Uganda, and Zambia, where in certain areas well over one-half of urban commercial sex workers are HIV-positive (U.S. Bureau of the Census, 1994a, 1994b; see also Figures 3-3). HIV-prevention programs in such high-prevalence countries need to reach all sexually active men and women, but special attention still needs to be focused on particular groups of men who are high-risk transmitters. These population subsets include clients of sex workers, male STD patients, men in the uniformed services, truckers or other transport workers, men away from home, prisoners, and fishermen. In some parts of Zambia, for example, the prevalence of HIV among males attending STD clinics ranges from 33 to 60 percent (U.S. Bureau of the Census, 1994b).

TABLE 5-2 Objectives of HIV-Prevention Programs Targeted to Men

Individual Behavior Change:

- Reduce the number of sexual partners.
- Reduce the frequent change of sexual partners.
- Learn to recognize STD symptoms, and seek early appropriate treatment.
- Accept and use condoms properly and consistently.

Structural/Environmental Changes:

- Render condoms available, accessible, and affordable.
- Improve treatment of bacterial STDs.
- Change the social acceptability of multiple partners by men.
- Make STD treatment facilities accessible and affordable.
- Reduce the consumption of substances (alcohol) that enhance high-risk behavior.
- Promote public policies that enhance low-risk sexual behavior (e.g., condom-only brothels).

Types of Strategies and Programs

HIV-prevention strategies for men should aim to change individual sexual behavior, improve STD treatment services, provide condoms, change societal norms, and ease structural and environmental impediments to reducing risky behavior (Table 5-2). However, most programs targeted to African men to date have focused only on behavior-change interventions and the provision of condoms. The quality of the interventions varies widely. In some programs, only information services are offered; changes in behavior are not emphasized, and condom supply and availability are intermittent. In others, genuine attempts are made to change behavior; improve STD treatment; and make condoms readily available, accessible, and affordable by the target population (Mouli, 1992 [18]; Williams and Ray, 1993 [20-24]; Laga et al., 1994 [16]).

The following case study from Zaire illustrates a population-based intervention targeted to African men in which behavior change was promoted, and condoms were made available, easily accessible, and affordable.[5]

Case Study

The Zaire AIDS Media and Condom Social Marketing Project was initiated in 1988 (Population Services International, 1992 [17]). The program developed specific messages targeted to youth aged 12 to 19 and young adults aged 20 to 30.

[5]Throughout this chapter, we use case studies to illustrate representative intervention strategies, although few interventions have received rigorous evaluation.

However, the major beneficiaries were an estimated 13 million sexually active adult males in urban areas, as well as youth of both sexes in rural areas. The objectives of the program were to change attitudes about HIV, to promote behavior change (i.e., increased use of condoms), and to alter social norms regarding safer sexual practices. Innovative media materials were developed based on formative research. AIDS messages were presented in television and radio spot announcements, dramas, music videos, talk shows, interviews, and contests through the country's extensive media network. Condoms were advertised and sold at traditional outlets, such as markets, pharmacies, drug stores, and health clinics, as well as nontraditional outlets, such as hotels, bars, brothels, and village kiosks. In one year, the program produced 28 feature programs about AIDS that were broadcast by radio in 13 local languages, 22 TV spots with AIDS messages, 8 radio dramas that promoted AIDS awareness and safer sexual behavior, 2 songs about AIDS, and 5 AIDS knowledge radio contests. Knowledge, attitude, and practice (KAP) survey results from one target region (Sud-Kivu) were compared with KAP survey results from a nontargeted or "control" region (Equateur). Populations in the target region showed more correct knowledge about AIDS and significantly improved attitudes about risk-taking and risk-taking practices as compared with those in the nontarget or control region. For example, there was an 18 percent difference in the level of knowledge regarding AIDS transmission between those in the target group and control regions as compared with a 2 percent difference in level of knowledge between two groups in the targeted region. The study also demonstrated that only 16 percent in the control region were able to name methods of AIDS prevention, whereas 39 percent in the targeted region knew that postponing of sexual debut, mutual monogamy, and condom use are the most effective methods of AIDS prevention.

In 1991, 18.3 million condoms were distributed through the program, as compared with only 900,000 in 1988. Three-quarters of the condom buyers reported purchasing condoms for AIDS prevention as well as for family planning. Although their estimate can be debated, the project investigators concluded that the program's 1991 condom sales prevented about 7,200 primary cases of HIV/AIDS (Population Services International, 1992 [17]). This estimate does not include a much larger number of secondary infections (infections acquired from the primary cases) prevented.

Several strengths of the Zairian program contributed to its success. First, marketing principles of price, promotion, place, and product were successfully adapted to HIV-prevention strategies and sales of condoms. Second, Zaire's extensive satellite network of TV and radio contributed to impressive national coverage of both urban and rural areas; a major drawback to most HIV-prevention programs is their limited coverage—and subsequent limited impact—as a result of regional, not national, approaches. Third, marketing of condoms through numerous nontraditional outlets greatly expanded the reach of the program and enhanced condom accessibility. A fourth strength was the use of multiple innovative and culturally relevant marketing approaches to sell condoms and increase purchase behavior. Some of the most popular communication approaches were the use of renowned and persuasive local musicians to present key HIV-prevention messages; the use of theater through radio, television, and play presentations to confront attitudes about HIV; and the use of student notebooks to correct "AIDS myths" and present accurate HIV information to school children. Another strength of the program was partial program cost recovery due to condom sales. The income generated from condom sales was used to meet packaging and marketing costs. It also provided a profit motive for the sale of condoms through shops and bars, a key to establishing a comprehensive distribution network. Although not financially self-sustaining, the intervention was unique in that it generated resources.

Finally, this program is an example of the successful use of the private sector in AIDS prevention. African governments have been slow to admit that they alone do not have adequate human, fiscal, and institutional resources to arrest the epidemic without assistance. Participation by external donors, the commercial sector, private voluntary organizations, nongovernmental organizations, and other community-based organizations is vital to any country's AIDS control program.

Comparable levels of condom sales using mass media and social marketing have been achieved in several African countries, including Ethiopia, Cameroon, Côte d'Ivoire, Burkina Faso, and Zambia (Population Services International, 1994a). Cumulative sales of condoms—the main indicator of success in condom social marketing programs—are shown through 1994 for all of Africa in Figure 5-1 (Population Services International, 1994c, 1995).

Some weaknesses were inherent in the Zairian program. First, an STD treatment component was absent. As discussed in Chapters 2 and 3, STDs play an important role in the sexual spread of HIV in sub-Saharan Africa (Grosskurth et al., 1995). AIDS-prevention programs that exclude STD treatment will have limited impact on the epidemic. Mathematical modeling of the epidemic shows that the combination of partner reduction, STD treatment, and condom use has the greatest impact in slowing the spread of the epidemic (Sokal et al., 1991). A second weakness was inadequate evaluation of the program. Some process and outcome data, such as condom sales and pre- and post-KAP results, are available as indicators of the success of the program. However, a program of this magnitude should have included better behavioral outcome evaluation. Additional data—such as a profile of who was buying the condoms and for what reasons, the proportion of condoms actually used with the aim of preventing HIV infection, and the effect of the program on STD prevalence or incidence—would allow better measurement of the impact of the program. A third weakness of the program approach is the targeting of the general population as opposed to particular groups. Small-group interventions encourage the involvement of the community in program design and evaluation, and give individuals opportunities to interact more closely with the provider. Finally, the primary focus on safer sex through condom use is a realistic approach for most sexually active men, but other messages—such as postponing of sexual debut, mutual monogamy, and nonpenetrative sex—should be targeted to youth and young adults.

Despite the above weaknesses, condom social marketing interventions such as this program in Zaire are effective channels for condom distribution and behavior-change communication.

Lessons Learned

The strengths and weaknesses of the Zairian condom social marketing program point to several lessons that can be applied in developing future HIV intervention programs.

First, comprehensive and integrated interventions should be developed. Programs targeted to men typically include behavior-change interventions and condom provision. STD treatment, however, is often nonexistent, as in the case of the Zairian program. Given the role of STDs as a cofactor in facilitating HIV transmission, their continuing high prevalence in several African countries underscores the need for integrating STD treatment into future intervention programs.

Second, men are not as difficult to reach with intervention programs as is often assumed. Condom social marketing programs in Africa have been very successful in reaching men at home, at work, in bars and hotels, and at truck stops (Mwizarubi et al., 1992 [12]; Population Services International, 1994a). Other programs have reached men through the workplace, health clinics, prisons, brothels, HIV testing and counseling centers, and community-based initiatives (Mouli, 1992 [18]; Mwizarubi et al., 1992 [12]; World Health Organization, 1992c [10, 11, 14, 26]; Wilson et al., 1992 [25]; Williams and Ray, 1993 [20-24]; Population Services International, 1994a, 1994b, 1994d [19]).

Third, successful programs focus on changing not only individual behavior, but also social norms and other structural and environmental factors that enhance the spread of HIV (see Chapter 2). Interpersonal channels are more important in changing attitudes and social norms concerning the adoption of new behaviors among a large audience, while mass media channels are often more effective at creating awareness and enhancing knowledge of a new idea (Lamptey and Coates, 1994). Consequently, individual and small-group interventions should be combined with general population-based programs.

A fourth lesson to emerge from this case study is that multiple and repeated messages via various media are important in changing behavior. A combination of media programs—such as mass education programs, small media (brochures, posters), interpersonal approaches (STD/HIV counseling and testing, peer education) and educational entertainment (theater, music, and folklore)—has been effective in Zimbabwe, Tanzania, and Ghana (Mwizarubi et al., 1992 [12]; Wilson et al., 1992 [25]; Williams and Ray, 1993 [20-24]; Asamoah-Adu et al., 1994 [1]).

Finally, HIV-prevention programs in Africa desperately need good evaluation data for assessing program effectiveness and cost-effectiveness.[6] Studies showing the behavioral impact of various intervention programs are in particularly short supply.

INTERVENTIONS TARGETING SEXUALLY ACTIVE WOMEN

More than half of the estimated 11 million adults infected with HIV in sub-Saharan Africa are women (World Health Organization, 1994a, 1995). This section addresses HIV-prevention programs targeting sexually active adult women; the following section addresses programs targeting adolescents, including adolescent girls.

In a recent review article, Heise and Elias (1995) argue convincingly that current HIV/AIDS-prevention efforts are not well suited to meeting the needs of many of the world's women. Indeed, none of the three central elements of HIV/AIDS-prevention efforts in developing countries—encouraging people to reduce their number of sexual partners, promoting the widespread use of condoms, and treating concurrent STDs in populations at risk of HIV—are appropriate for women, whose vulnerability stems from their inability to protect themselves because of their lower cultural and socioeconomic status or their lack of influence in sexual relations (see also du Guerny and Sjöberg, 1993, and Ulin, 1992). For example, results from studies indicate that many infected African women have only one sexual partner (Heise and Elias, 1995). Hence, the greatest source of HIV risk for most sexually active women is their husbands or stable partners, who have multiple other sexual contacts. Heise and Elias (1995) conclude, "Women need both a new commitment to addressing the underlying inequities that heighten their risk, and new technologies that provide them with a means of HIV protection within their personal control" (Heise and Elias, 1995:931).

Early accounts of the epidemic suggested that the disease in Africa was an urban phenomenon, confined to commercial sex workers and their clients (Van de Perre et al., 1985; Kreiss et al., 1986; Ngugi et al., 1988 [4]). This finding led to the development of intervention programs that focused only on these two groups. Such programs continue to be appropriate because of the high-risk nature of commercial sex. But at the same time, these groups cannot be the sole focus of prevention programs because recent data from antenatal clinics indicate that the prevalence of HIV/AIDS among the general population is rising. Recent data from several countries in Central and Southern Africa reveal that there has been

---

[6]See Over and Piot (1993) for preliminary estimates of the cost-effectiveness of alternative interventions.

a dramatic rise in prevalence of HIV among both urban and rural women attending antenatal clinics (Stanecki and Way, 1994).

Research on HIV infection among women has been insufficient and poorly targeted (Faden et al., 1991; Herdt and Boxer, 1991; Hankins and Handley, 1992). When such research is undertaken, it often focuses on women's reproductive function and their role as mothers. Hankins and Handley (1992:967) emphasize the need for more epidemiological and clinical research in HIV progression among women:

> Concerted effort on the part of clinicians, researchers, funding agencies, and decisionmakers is required for redressing the inequities in both the gender-specific knowledge of the natural history, progression, and outcome of HIV disease and the adequacy of medical and psychosocial care for women with HIV infection. The unique features of HIV infection in women have been subject to both scientific neglect and policy void, situations that can and should be rectified with dispatch.

Some of the controversy regarding research on women stems from concerns about having women of childbearing age participate in drug trials or in intervention trials involving physical or biological agents, such as the female condom or vaginal viricides. There is no evidence that participation in such research harms women (Levine, 1991). Even if there were grounds for excluding women from research with biologically active agents, there is little justification for omitting women from social and behavioral research centered on questions that can help determine the level and nature of HIV risk and inform the development and evaluation of life-saving prevention strategies.

Among researchers, particularly in the developed world, there is growing consensus on the importance of research on disease prevention and progression among women. Reducing the spread of HIV among women is critical to slowing the epidemic. However, complex issues remain.

Issues

One issue is the way in which women have been narrowly categorized in studies. For example, although individual women typically have multiple social roles and functions, research has tended to classify them into discrete social categories, such as prostitute or mother (Caravano, 1991; Herdt and Boxer, 1991).

Rigid male-dominated sexual relations remove much of female sexual behavior, directly and indirectly, from women's own control, so that it is not subject to rational decision making. Holland et al. (1994:223) note the deleterious effects of dominant paradigms on research about women:

> The official conceptions of sexuality and models of behavior . . . were largely based on a view of behavior as a matter of choice by free individuals. . . . Women's ability to choose safer sexual practices or to refuse unsafe (or any

other) sexual activity was not a question of free choice among equals, but one of negotiation within structurally unequal social relationships.

The perception of unequal roles in sexual decision making has affected the design of behavioral interventions. Across Africa, one sees reliance on a male-focused HIV-prevention strategy that includes condom programs for prostitutes and men, partner-reduction programs for men, and STD treatment programs for men (Heise and Elias, 1995). Even programs targeted to women are limited in focus, addressing solely certain roles women assume, rather than the full range of women's issues and needs (Herdt and Boxer, 1991).

As discussed earlier, few programs have focused on sexually active women in the general population, but rather target high-risk women and men. There are several reasons why such programs have had very little effect on HIV risk for most sexually active women. First, in some circumstances, a woman's exposure to HIV and STDs depends less on her own risk behavior than on the behavior of her sexual partner, over whom she has little control. Second, most women do not possess the necessary negotiating skills and power to ensure condom use. Third, women's access to STD treatment services is very limited, syndromic diagnosis of STDs by women is difficult, and clinical testing of STDs is expensive and not widely accessible.

Gender-specific research that investigates women, their experiences, and their many roles has been deemed ill-defined and impractical by many health researchers. Many researchers and policy makers are skeptical of indirect effects, indirect interventions, and the social research methods required to measure these effects. Clearly, comprehensive research strategies that combine useful information from both qualitative and quantitative research are needed to identify what works in HIV prevention for women as well as men. However, many of the approaches to preventing HIV among the general population of women upset tradition. Public discussions of women's sexual behavior appear to be more sensitive and less open than acknowledgment of men's needs and desires. Women are seen as guardians of culture, as preservers of tradition, and as agents of socialization; in these capacities, they are regarded as the inviolable moral center of many cultures.

While acknowledging that fundamental social change takes time, Heise and Elias (1995:931) argue that the HIV/AIDS epidemic has created two imperatives:

> . . . to begin in earnest to work on changing the underlying causes of women's vulnerability *and* to pursue vigorously every means possible to strengthen women's immediate ability to protect themselves in the face of the economic and cultural forces currently allied against them. This, in turn, means placing greater emphasis within existing AIDS programs on empowering women and committing major resources to developing new prevention technologies—like vaginal suppositories or foams lethal to the virus—that women can use without their partner's knowledge or consent.

Target Population

Although not mutually exclusive, the following three groups should be considered when designing HIV-prevention strategies and messages targeted to women: (1) sexually active women with multiple partners, such as commercial sex workers; (2) single sexually active women; and (3) sexually active women in formal or informal unions. The vast majority of interventions targeted to women tend to focus on sex workers (who are at highest risk) while ignoring the rest of the population. Even these programs are neither as extensive nor as intensive as those in Thailand, for example, that target commercial sex workers (see, e.g., Hanenberg et al., 1994, and, Visrutaratna et al., 1995). The largest and most difficult group to work with are women in marital unions, whose desire for pregnancy and lack of control over their spouse's sexual behavior pose a challenge to the design of effective interventions.

As with men, HIV-prevention programs that target women should not be designed solely on the basis of risk behavior and epidemiological data. Programs need to address the multiple roles played by women and be cognizant of women's competing statuses and obligations. In thinking systematically about these roles, program managers as well as researchers need to consider individual, social, and environmental factors, such as location of residence, marital status, current and future desires for children, generational status, socioeconomic status, cultural expectations, and religious beliefs.

Types of Strategies and Programs

Programs targeted to women should include the basic program components provided to men—behavior-change interventions, STD treatment, and condom provision—as well as relevant structural changes. Table 5-3 shows the desired objectives of programs that target sexually active women. Some structural interventions that are unique to women include empowerment interventions, policy/legal interventions, and interventions that enhance access to nonhealth sectors.

Empowerment interventions are programs directed toward promoting women's increased skill in self-direction, often through self-organized, peer-led groups. It remains unclear whether these groups produce the anticipated benefit. We know little about how to create conditions that permit women to be empowered in Africa and what it means to be "empowered" in different settings.

Although policy changes and legislation are clearly needed to address status inequalities, women's rights may clash with clan, familial, or other roles. A fundamental issue is that even if laws and policies are changed, the impact of these changes at the local or personal level may be minimal.

Female access to education, other skills, and jobs is essential to redress status inequities. However, reduced expectations regarding schooling for females on the part of men, families, society, and women still persist. Some income-genera-

TABLE 5-3 Objectives of HIV-Prevention Programs Targeted to Women

Individual Behavior Change:

- Reduce the number of sexual partners.
- Reduce the frequent change of sexual partners.
- Learn to recognize STD symptoms, and seek early appropriate treatment.
- Improve sexual communication and negotiating skills for safer sex.
- Encourage partners to use condoms properly and consistently.

Structural/Environmental Changes:

- Render condoms available, accessible, and affordable.
- Improve diagnosis and treatment of bacterial STDs in women.
- Change the social acceptability of multiple partners by men.
- Make STD treatment facilities accessible and affordable.
- Reduce the consumption of substances (alcohol) that enhance high-risk behavior.
- Promote public policies that enhance low-risk sexual behavior (e.g., condom-only brothels).

Gender-related Objectives:

- Research the multiple roles of women as related to their risk of HIV infection.
- Improve the role and status of women to reduce their susceptibility to HIV.
- Change cultural practices detrimental to the health and status of women.
- Improve access to education.
- Improve skills and economic opportunities.
- Improve the involvement of women's groups in the design and implementation of interventions.

tion programs for women have been successfully attempted (Delehanty, 1993; Leonard, 1994).

Finally, because HIV transmission to women occurs in the context of a dyadic relationship between a man and a woman, strategies that influence this relationship are needed. Interventions targeting women have attempted to include men, but these attempts have been complicated and problematic. Further research will be needed to understand how to facilitate productive and effective intervention strategies that involve both men and women. This research will need to explore the role of the relationship between men and women and its impact on HIV-prevention strategies at the individual, group (e.g., family or kinship), and societal levels. Much of the prevention research issues for women remain largely unexamined. As mentioned earlier, current efforts to reduce HIV transmission among women in Africa have focused on interventions targeted to commercial sex workers. The first case study below describes such an intervention; it is followed by discussion of an innovative empowerment program targeting women in Botswana.

Case Study:
An Intervention Targeted to Commercial Sex Workers

In 1988, Projet SIDA[7] initiated a research study at the Matonge Women's Health Center in Kinshasa, Zaire (Laga et al., 1994 [16]). The objectives of the project, known as the Women's Health Project, were (1) to determine the prevalence and incidence of STDs, including HIV, among female sex workers in Kinshasa; (2) to study the interactions between STDs and HIV; and (3) to determine the impact of condom promotion and STD detection and treatment on the incidence of HIV and STDs.

A cohort of 531 initially HIV-negative female sex workers was followed for 3 years. The participants were surveyed to determine sexual behavior and practices, health-seeking and preventive-health behavior, and history of STDs over a 2-year period. Participants were screened every month for the presence of syphilis, gonorrhea, chlamydia infection, trichomoniasis, chancroid, and candidiasis and every 3 months for HIV-1; all STDs were treated free of charge. Individual and group counseling was provided to promote condom use, and free condoms were distributed during counseling sessions.

Reported regular condom use with clients increased from 11 to 52 percent and then 68 percent after 6 and 36 months of intervention, respectively. The decline in the monthly incidence of trichomoniasis and gonorrhoea is shown in Figure 5-2. The most significant finding, however, was a decline in the incidence of HIV-1 over time, from 11.7 per 100 woman-years during the first 6 months to 4.4 per 100 woman-years over the last 6 months, 3 years later (Figure 5-3). The risk factors for HIV-1 seroconversion included irregular condom use, gonorrhea, trichomoniasis, and genital ulcer disease. Among women who attended more than 90 percent of their clinic appointments, the HIV-1 incidence was 2.7 per 100 woman-years, compared with 7.1, 20.3, and 44.1 per 100 woman-years among women who attended 76 to 90 percent, 50 to 75 percent, and less than 50 percent of their monthly appointments, respectively. That this gradient remains after controlling for the effects of reported condom use and number of clients implies that STD treatment was a key factor in the decline in STD incidence.

This program demonstrates that a comprehensive prevention program of behavior-change intervention, STD treatment, and condom provision can lead to a reduction in the incidence of both STDs and HIV. Despite the impressive impact of the intervention, however, this type of project is not sustainable or replicable because of the high cost of the intensive research effort involved. A

[7]Projet SIDA is a collaborative effort of the Centers for Disease Control, Atlanta, Georgia, USA; the National Institute for Allergy and Infectious Diseases, Bethesda, Maryland, USA; the Armed Forces Institute of Pathology, Bethesda, Maryland, USA; the Institute of Tropical Medicine, Antwerp, Belgium; and the Zairian Ministry of Public Health.

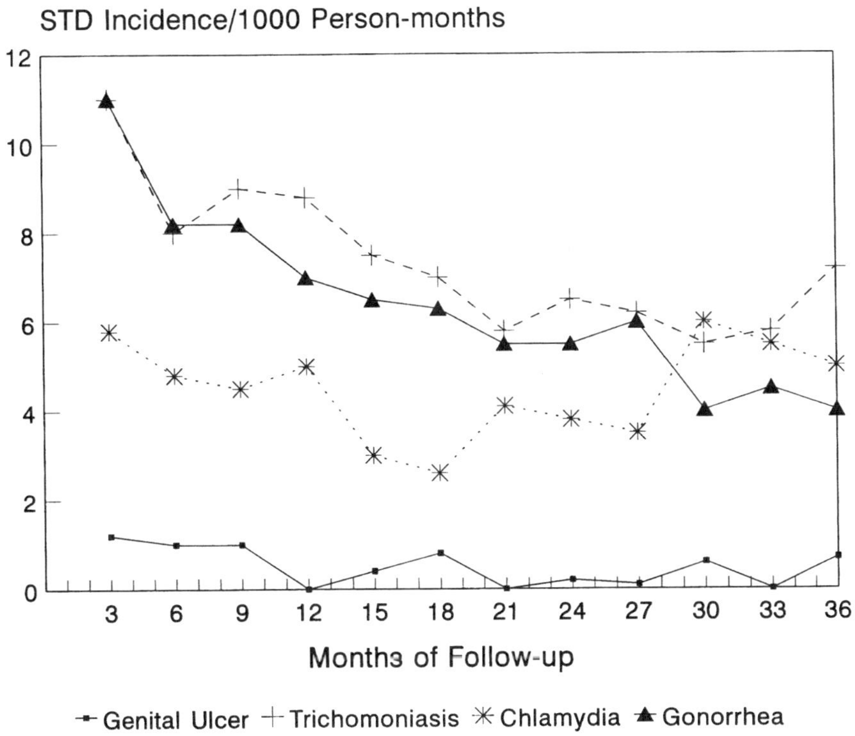

FIGURE 5-2 STD Incidence Among Prostitutes, Kinshasa, Zaire. SOURCE: Adapted from Laga et al. (1994).

further drawback of this intervention was its focus solely on women; male clients and steady partners were neither targeted nor involved. This omission may be one of the reasons why average condom use with clients did not exceed 60 percent.

Case Study: A Community-based Intervention

A two-stage study of the effectiveness of nurse-managed peer education and support groups for AIDS prevention among women was initiated in Botswana in 1990 (Norr et al., 1992; Tlou, 1995). The objective of the intervention was to heighten women's awareness and knowledge about AIDS and to enhance their communication skills and assertiveness in negotiating for safer sex with their partners.

In the first year of the program, in-depth interviews were conducted with 56 women to explore content and service delivery mechanisms for a peer education

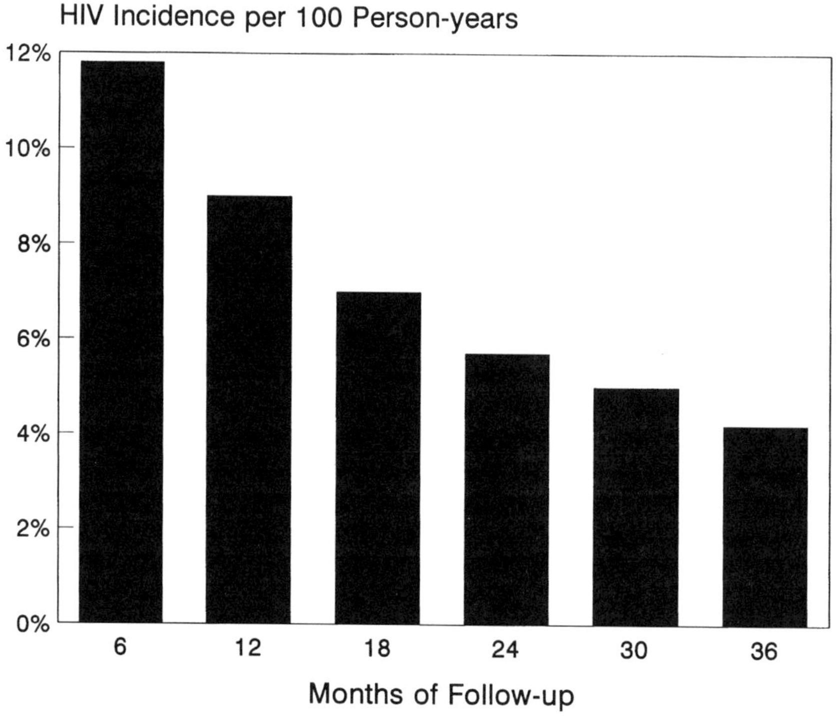

FIGURE 5-3 Trends in HIV Among Prostitutes, Kinshasa, Zaire. SOURCE: Adapted from Laga et al. (1994).

model appropriate to the culture, values, and resources of Botswana. Training sessions for women included condom skills sessions and practice in how to say "no" to unsafe sexual practices through role playing. In the second and third years, the intervention was extended to 600 women in 12 workplaces in Gabarone. The project is now expanding to 5 rural districts in the country using a training-of-trainers model and is being extended to include primary school teachers and university students.

Positive attitudes toward condoms and expressed confidence in correct condom use increased among the program participants from 35 to 76 percent. Those who reported always using condoms at each sexual encounter increased from 28 to 50 percent. Moreover, participants reported having increased their promotion of safer sex to others, including relatives, children, coworkers, and neighbors. Further evaluation of the program is under way.

There are several commendable elements of this intervention. First, it is a community-based intervention targeted to women in both urban and rural areas, rather than solely to groups traditionally seen as high risk (such as commercial sex workers). Second, it can be replicated at relatively little cost among other target populations, such as primary school teachers and university students. Third, it attempts to empower women with communication and negotiation skills for safer sex with their partners.

Nevertheless, two weaknesses of this program are evident. After participating in the program, married women still found it difficult to introduce condoms, probably because men were not targeted in the intervention. Moreover, available evaluation indicators were not adequately used to assess the effectiveness and cost-effectiveness of the program.

Lessons Learned

Among the lessons learned from the implementation and evaluation of prevention programs targeting African women to date, we can highlight the following:

- Programs need to reflect an understanding of, if not directly address, the multiple roles of women, which include wife, mother, housekeeper, and child rearer.
- Comprehensive models of programs for women are not available. A wider range of tested interventions is needed, including network, group, and community-based interventions; policy interventions; and interventions that focus on power and status. Women's STD programs must develop better ways of identifying symptoms and encourage care-seeking behavior, as well as enhance the provision of sensitive and appropriate medical care. Interventions also need to promote the use of condoms to protect against pregnancy. These interventions will be more effective if the status of women is enhanced through such means as legislation and social policies that protect and expand women's rights.
- Women are especially vulnerable to HIV. In many cultures, there is pressure to produce children to sustain a marital union. The fact that many men have partners outside of stable unions (see also Chapter 4) also makes women particularly vulnerable to HIV. Monogamous African women frequently report being exposed to HIV through their husbands' other sexual partnerships.
- Interventions based on individual decision-making models do not take into account women's low power. Low power and low self-esteem are not the same thing; low power in dyadic relationships with men is supported by tradition.
- Women are often entrusted with preserving traditions, a role that conflicts with social change and may restrict programmatic access to them. Successful design and implementation of interventions for women requires the tacit if not active support of political, religious, and community leaders. Women's roles cannot change in isolation. Male attitudes and behaviors, especially those of sexual partners, must also change.
- There is a need to develop new technologies and approaches to reach women since women's needs are not directly addressed by those that currently

exist. New barrier methods, especially nonspermicidal viricides, are needed. Moreover, new technologies need to be developed for STD diagnosis and new programs implemented to reach infected women.

- Women need to participate in the research and development of HIV intervention programs targeted to them. Their participation may lead to the identification of new prevention technologies that are responsive to women's needs.

INTERVENTIONS TARGETING YOUTH

Before discussing HIV/AIDS intervention programs that target youth, it is useful to define this group as it is referred to in this chapter. We adopt the WHO definition of adolescents, which includes persons from 10 to 24 years of age (World Health Organization, 1986) and use the terms "youth" and "adolescents" interchangeably.[8] People under 10 years old are referred to as children, and those aged 25 and older as adults. We adopt these definitions while acknowledging that in some African cultures, persons over 25, especially if not married, are still considered youth, and some younger than 25, especially if married, are considered adults.

It is imperative that HIV-prevention strategies reach youth before they become sexually active. Lives can be saved by educating youth before they acquire their attitudes about delaying sexual intercourse and about safe sexual practices such as condom use and nonpenetrative sex and by promoting a sociocultural environment that encourages these practices. These messages must be compatible with local mores and cultural beliefs. To the extent that prevention messages are realistic, clear, and expressed in language youth can readily understand, interventions are more likely to have a positive effect. Where social practices conflict with prevention needs, considerable dialogue among public health officials and parents, teachers, politicians, and religious and tribal leaders is needed. Multicomponent intervention strategies are important in targeting youth. Innovation, variety, and persuasive messages from respected sources such as peers and influential adults, as well as a supportive environment, play key roles in such programs.

Issues

Perhaps the most important task of adolescents is growing up. Integral to this process is the acquisition of adult skills and habits, including learning about

[8]Terms such as "children," "youth," "school-age youth," "young people," "adolescents," "teenagers," "young girls," "young boys," "young women," "young men," and "young adults" have been used to define target populations. Because they frequently are used as if referring to the same group but may be interpreted differently by different people, we have chosen to be quite precise in our definition.

adult sexual practices. To be accepted as an adult and a member of society in many African cultures, one must prove one's fertility—often in the context of marriage. Many cultures have strong expectations for early marriage and child-bearing soon after puberty, especially for girls. HIV-prevention messages must be developed with a recognition that postponement of sexual debut may be in potential conflict with local mores. Further, even where delay in sexual debut is considered possible or desirable, there is a paucity of information available to adolescents about responsible, safe expressions of sexuality once sexual relations have been initiated.

African adolescents, like adolescents elsewhere in the world, are often unable to discuss openly with their parents their questions, fears, and concerns about sex, marriage, and other adult topics. They also have poor negotiation skills when approached for sex by adults. With the exception of cultures that have adult female initiators,[9] youth have little opportunity for frank discussions with adults about sex. Youth therefore rely heavily on their peers for information. Unfortunately, peer information is often inaccurate. In addition, some youth may feel pressure from their peers to experiment with sex. Elders, who have traditionally been respected and whose guidance has been valued by youth, are now seeing their role and influence being eroded slowly by modern influences. The impact of these significant social changes remains unknown.

The escalating number of children and adolescents orphaned by parents who have died of AIDS is also a critical issue (see Chapter 6). The World Health Organization predicts that by the year 2000, more than 10 million HIV-negative children under age 10—90 percent of them in sub-Saharan Africa—will have lost their mothers to AIDS (World Health Organization, 1992b). Traditionally, orphaned children are absorbed by the extended family. But in many areas, such as the Rakai district in Uganda and the Kagera region of Tanzania, many heads of households have died of AIDS, leaving elderly grandparents to care for multiple sets of children. Inevitably, some children also slip through the cracks in the extended family network and find themselves living on the streets, where modifying high-risk behavior becomes secondary to satisfying basic needs, including food, shelter, and clothing.

Other issues relate to the subgroup of youth that attends school. On the one hand, schools are ideal vehicles for HIV education because they exist everywhere, even in rural areas, and provide easy access to youth. Moreover, schools can reach students daily, making critical reinforcement of prevention messages more practical. But schools as vehicles for HIV-prevention programs have their limitations. Many schools are overcrowded, and in some countries, such as Zambia, schools run double and sometimes even triple shifts per day. Conse-

[9]Initiators are female elders who teach pubescent young girls about sex, marriage, childbearing, child rearing, and other adult responsibilities.

quently, most youth do not spend more than a few hours a day at school, hours that are packed with learning the basics. Furthermore, schools as institutions are not homogeneous; there are public schools, private schools, and church schools, all of which have significantly different social climates, structures, and educational resources. In addition, student bodies in schools are heterogenous, ranging from the homeless to the elite. Thus, HIV education approaches need to be appropriate to the particular school environment. Finally, approximately half of all youth in many sub-Saharan African countries do not attend school (World Bank, 1993). These youth are not easily reached, organized, motivated, or tracked and are therefore difficult to target with intervention programs.

In some parts of sub-Saharan Africa, an increase in age at marriage has resulted in the creation of a new subset of youth: unmarried, postpubertal, adolescent girls or young women. This group may be especially vulnerable because the social norms relating to women their age in the past assumed they were married; there are few expectations to guide either the behavior of these girls or the behavior of others toward them. African adolescent girls often become targets of older men, but have few skills to control sexual relations. These girls may be at high risk of STDs, pregnancy, and abuse in addition to HIV infection. An added risk factor for HIV in this group may be biological, because of cervical ectopy (Bulterys et al., 1994). Worldwide, 70 percent of HIV infection among women is estimated to occur in girls between the ages of 15 and 25 (Ankrah, 1994). Adolescent girls in Zimbabwe are five times as likely to be infected with the HIV virus as adolescent boys (Ankrah, 1994).

Government ministries, nongovernmental organizations, and donors have called for long-term strategies to improve the subordinate status of and dearth of educational and employment opportunities for adolescent girls (Gupta and Weiss, 1993; Ankrah, 1994). Increased education, improved equity between girls and boys, and meaningful income-generating activities can help adolescent girls achieve economic security and higher social status, which may, in turn, enable them to avoid high-risk behavior. Intervention programs to date have focused almost exclusively on matters related directly to health (modification of sexual behavior, STD care, family planning-related activities, and condom use). A few notable exceptions have established links to organizations concerned with improving the social and economic situation of young women and shown promising results (Leonard, 1994; Delehanty, 1993).

Policy-based intervention strategies are also needed to influence social norms and change sexual practices that facilitate the spread of HIV in this group, such as the sugar daddy syndrome, child marriage, incest, and rape. Principally because of limited resources, however, virtually no prevention programs in Africa have linked advocacy for protective laws and policies for adolescent girls with program design and implementation.

Interventions to date (UNICEF, 1995; Annex 5-1 in this volume) point to several strategic approaches that should guide HIV-prevention programs targeted to adolescent girls. First, practical and culturally relevant information needs to be developed and disseminated through existing communication channels, including schools, radio, youth organizations, and traditional channels such as female initiators. Second, such communication should concurrently target adolescent boys and older men, a strategy that is seldom used. Finally, sustained efforts from multiple channels are critical to influencing social norms.

Target Population

Adolescents, like other age groups, are a heterogeneous group for which numerous multifaceted intervention strategies are required to achieve behavior change. Youth intervention strategies can target by access point (e.g., schools, clinics, media, street corners); by age of target audience (with different methods and messages for those aged 10-15, 16-20, and 21 and over); by marital status; and, as discussed earlier, by gender. Adolescents living in urban centers should be targeted differently from their counterparts in rural villages. Youth living in sparsely populated rural areas, such as the eastern province in Cameroon or the desert in Botswana, respond to different intervention approaches than youth living on the streets in large urban centers such as Lagos, Nigeria, or Dar es Salaam, Tanzania. Youth living on the streets have different needs and respond to different messages than youth living in families.

Types of Strategies and Programs

Prevention interventions targeted to youth should include not only individual behavioral but also structural/environmental components (Table 5-4). Yet most interventions targeted to African youth to date have typically focused on behavior-change intervention and the promotion and provision of condoms (UNICEF, 1995; Grunseit and Kippax, 1993). Strategies used have included setting up drop-in centers in the community that encourage youth to stop in on an ad hoc basis; sending outreach workers into markets, bus terminals, and truck stops; organizing community sports activities and clubs; initiating anti-AIDS clubs; and training adults—such as traditional initiators for coming-of-age ceremonies—who have regular access to youth.

HIV intervention programs need to expand beyond health-related components by linking with organizations that have the resources and expertise to incorporate economic, educational, and policy-based components into HIV-prevention programs. Examples are organizations that could improve access to education by providing school fee waivers or stipends or offer income-generating possibilities. Although such linked programs are admittedly difficult to implement, the few that exist have shown exciting results, albeit on a limited scale (Delehanty, 1993; Leonard, 1994).

AIDS care and management, especially coping with death and dying, should

TABLE 5-4 Objectives of HIV-Prevention Programs Targeted to Youth

Individual Behavior Change:

- Delay sexual debut.
- Decrease number of partners or frequency of sex.
- Increase consistent and correct condom use.
- Develop sexual communication and negotiation skills with regard to condom use.
- Develop risk-avoidance skills.
- Learn to recognize STD symptoms, and seek early appropriate treatment.
- Increase primary HIV-prevention knowledge (e.g., where to buy condoms).
- Increase risk perception.
- Increase risk-reduction motivation.

Structural/Environmental Changes:

- Render condoms available, accessible, and affordable.
- Improve diagnosis and treatment of bacterial STDs.
- Increase parent-child communication skills.
- Improve sexual communication, negotiation, and condom-use skills.
- Increase involvement of gatekeepers and youth in intervention program design.
- Advocate policies that support the advancement of youth.
- Increase access to education for out-of-school youth (e.g, waive school fees).
- Link income-generating components with HIV-prevention programs targeted to youth.

be an additional component of prevention programs targeted to youth, particularly in view of the large numbers of AIDS orphans projected in many African countries. Innovative responses to the burgeoning burden on families of AIDS patients and AIDS orphans are being developed (Delehanty, 1993). In Uganda, for example, orphaned children and adolescents are targeted in an intervention that links an economic development component to a basic comprehensive intervention package of behavior-change communications and STD counseling.

Comprehensive programs for youth should also include gatekeepers who shape and influence a group's culture. Such gatekeepers include community elders, parents, traditional healers, teachers, school administrators, the media, government officials, religious leaders, and adolescent heroes. The Family AIDS Education and Prevention Through Imams (FAEPTI) Project in Uganda, for example, successfully trained indigenous authoritative leaders in AIDS-prevention messages (Kagimu et al., 1995). The program's success was augmented by creating a community-chosen cadre of male and female family AIDS workers who supported and reinforced the imams' public messages on HIV/AIDS prevention.

Although the above examples highlight some of the more innovative approaches, strategies targeting youth to date have had several limitations. In general, comprehensive and integrated HIV-prevention models for African youth are virtually nonexistent. Instead, single-dimensional approaches have been advocated to address multidimensional problems (e.g., the disproportionate reliance on the "peer educator" approach for all adolescent HIV-prevention needs). In addition, little formative research has been done to tailor messages to specific youth subgroups. Moreover, inappropriate selection criteria have been used to qualify youth as peers, and peer programs have typically been neither well supervised nor well evaluated. Finally, youth have not been regular participants in the planning, design, and evaluation of programs.

The following case study highlights some of the issues and limitations discussed above and is representative of typical interventions targeted to African youth to date.

Case Study

In 1989, results from serosurveys in Addis Ababa, Ethiopia showed that 24 percent of female commercial sex workers between the ages of 12 and 16 were HIV-seropositive (Gebru et al., 1990). These results, while known to the Ministries of Health and Education, were not widely available to the public; a school-based HIV/AIDS education and prevention program was proposed. Before a new program of this type can begin, parents and other community members need to be educated about HIV prevention and the need for HIV education in junior and senior secondary schools. Focus group discussions with students and school teachers also help sensitize adolescents to the risk of HIV and build support and acceptance for the initiation of a strong school-based HIV/STD-prevention effort (Gebru et al., 1990).

A pilot HIV intervention project was implemented during 1990 and 1991, sponsored jointly by the Ministries of Health and Education. WHO/GPA assisted in the development and evaluation of educational materials and teaching methods that were incorporated into the curricular and extracurricular activities of Ethiopia's secondary schools.

The project had four specific objectives: (1) to teach students how to prevent HIV/STD transmission and enhance risk-reduction attitudes; (2) to reduce discriminatory attitudes toward HIV-positive fellow classmates and other community members; (3) to teach skills that would allow the students to disseminate HIV/STD-prevention messages to their families and the wider community; and (4) to train teachers to provide effective AIDS education and to stimulate student interest in becoming community health educators.

The project had multiple components. Innovative classroom curricula and teaching methods were developed that relied on role play, rehearsal of risk-avoidance skills, group discussions, drama, and peer educators. Sessions were held to train teachers and students to use these materials in class and in after-school clubs (such as drama, music, health education, and Red Cross clubs).

Students were also trained to become outreach educators for their family and local communities.

Five experimental schools were randomly selected from schools in Addis Ababa (two senior schools and one junior secondary school) and Debra Birhan (one senior and one junior secondary school). Two comparable junior and two comparable senior secondary schools were designated as controls. Most students in these schools conformed to the normal grade/age range, with 38 percent aged 12-14 and 33 percent aged 15-16, although reported ages ranged from 9 to 22. Examination of baseline data showed no significant differences between the experimental and control schools in terms of demographics, knowledge, and attitudinal variables. Other evaluation design features included a pre and post in-class questionnaire; in-depth student KAP interviews; and random surveys of parents and community members about their HIV/AIDS-related knowledge and opinions and their exposure to student educators and AIDS education materials. Monitoring of the project's implementation was performed by teachers and research assistants through checklists and observations. In addition to frequent supervisory visits by project staff, an evaluation workshop allowed teachers to provide feedback about the success or failure of the program.

Results from the project were positive. While rigorous statistical analysis was not performed, experimental students consistently showed the most knowledge gains. At the post-test, learning differentials between experimental and control groups ranged from 13 to 27 percent for items related to HIV-prevention facts (e.g., condoms reduce HIV risk) and correction of transmission myths (e.g., mosquitoes transmit HIV).

The experimental group also showed a greater change at post-test in their attitude toward classmates and others with HIV/AIDS. For example, at post-test, experimental students showed a 35 percent increase in willingness to care for someone with AIDS as compared with a 15 percent increase among the control students. Experimental students also showed a 26 percent increase in willingness to accept a teacher with AIDS, as compared with a 12 percent increase for control students. Statistical significance, however, was not reported. A "considerable effect" on attitudes toward risky sexual behavior was noted among the experimental students. At post-test, experimental students were more likely than control students to support abstinence (24 percent increase among the experimental groups as compared with a 10 percent decrease among the control groups), to report resisting pressure to have sex (20 percent increase among the experimental groups as compared with a 2 percent increase among the control groups), to think that sex with prostitutes increases the chances of getting AIDS (19 percent increase among the experimental groups as compared with 8 percent among the control groups), and to agree that proper use of a latex condom reduces the chances of getting AIDS (19 percent increase among the experimental groups as compared with an 8 percent increase among the control groups). Adolescent sexual behavior and condom use were not measured because of political and practical constraints.

The evaluation examined the effects of the peer outreach component in terms of the degree of student participation, coverage in the community, and the degree of change in knowledge and attitudes by those who were exposed to the student educators. Data were collected from 1,056 surveys conducted 3 months after the intervention took place in the community (357 experimental school parents, 349 control school parents, 350 members of the community). The results suggest that student educators were successful in the community. Evidence from the community surveys shows that a majority of the parents and community members surveyed had seen the AIDS textbook from the school and that a majority of the parents had discussed AIDS with their children.[10] Parent participation in school-based AIDS drama and music events and poster exhibitions also increased. In Addis Ababa, student presentations were videotaped by the Ministry of Information and then broadcast through its Youth Programme to the community.

This intervention is a good example of a multicomponent, skills-based, school-based HIV-education program that involves youth in the implementation of the program and targets youth early (at ages 11 or 12). The evaluation design lacked behavioral impact data, and the data analysis was simple, but trends in the results were consistent, suggesting that the program was able to achieve its objectives.

Lessons Learned

Several lessons can be learned from this case study and similar evaluations of school-based HIV-education programs in Tanzania (Klepp et al., 1994) and elsewhere in Africa (e.g., World Health Organization, 1994b). First, adolescents need to be reached before they become sexually active. Although some parents fear that an early discussion of sexual behavior may make adolescents prone to earlier sexual debut, a review of the HIV/AIDS-education literature shows that sex/AIDS-education programs do not increase sexual experimentation or promiscuity (Ford et al., 1992; Grunseit and Kippax, 1993; Kirby et al., 1994). In fact, some program planners in sub-Saharan Africa have been surprised to find that the majority of parents in their areas support AIDS education in schools (World Health Organization, 1994b). Furthermore, sex/AIDS-education programs, if well designed, can increase condom use among sexually active adolescents (Kirby et al., 1994). In particular, some African studies have shown that information about condoms can be delivered in schools with parental approval as long as

[10] It is not clear whether the "majority of parents" includes all parents or only those parents in the control group.

condoms are presented as the next best alternative to postponing sexual debut until marriage, followed by fidelity after marriage (World Health Organization, 1994b).

Needs assessments and KAP baseline surveys should be conducted with parents and educators, as well as students, before programs are initiated. Such instruments provide important information that helps enlist advocates for program implementation. In addition, they are necessary for designing programs to match local community values, an essential factor in garnering support for school-based HIV programs. In Uganda, for example, results from a KAP survey showed that parents supported AIDS education in the schools, but were not as comfortable with sex education (World Health Organization, 1994b). As a result, program planners presented AIDS education in the context of a comprehensive health-education program, a strategy that helped enlist support for and sustain the program.

Intensive training of educators in the design and delivery of feasible and effective curricula is essential. Training should include—but go beyond—biomedical factors and should address individual teachers' comfort levels in educating about HIV prevention in the classroom. For example, some African intervention programs have included speakers from local family planning organizations to help teachers explore their own values and comfort levels in teaching AIDS-prevention messages (World Health Organization, 1994b). Training should also focus on teaching skills in negotiation and condom use. In addition, interactive and participatory teaching methods should be used in tandem with didactic methods. Participatory methods might include drama, song competitions, poster drawings, games, group discussions, and role playing.

In conclusion, HIV-prevention interventions targeting youth should (1) be introduced throughout the school system and include explicit skills-based education; (2) reduce opposition to AIDS education by providing local information about the magnitude of HIV/STDs in the community to teachers, parents, religious leaders, and other community leaders; (3) include the family and enhance its role in AIDS education targeting youth; (4) provide education for both adolescent males and females regarding their responsibilities in human reproduction and HIV transmission; (5) include child-to-child (peer education) teaching methods, whereby older children share knowledge with younger children and those not attending school; (6) focus on preventing sexual transmission of HIV, with methods, information, and materials that are sensitive to the social context; (7) use interactive teaching methods; and (8) develop innovative strategies, such as teen drop-in centers, for reaching out-of-school youth.

PERINATAL TRANSMISSION

Perinatal transmission of HIV may occur during pregnancy via the placenta, during delivery, or after delivery through breastfeeding (see Chapter 3). Preventing infection in women has the addition benefit of preventing perinatal transmission. However, many women are already infected, and significant numbers will continue to be infected despite current intervention programs. For these women, other strategies are needed to reduce transmission of HIV to their newborns; several such strategies are described in the remainder of this section, although there are problems with each that limit their applicability in sub-Saharan Africa.

One approach may be the avoidance of breastfeeding by HIV-infected mothers. There are two problems with this strategy: large numbers of pregnant women would have to be tested and counseled for HIV infection and counseled as well in bottle feeding, and safe and affordable alternatives to breast milk would have to be easily available. This approach is not feasible in most countries in sub-Saharan Africa except for an elite urban minority, for economic and sociocultural reasons. The current recommendation by WHO/UNICEF is that all countries, irrespective of HIV infection rates, should continue to promote and support breastfeeding because of its impressive nutritional, immunological, and child-spacing benefits (World Health Organization, 1992a). In particular, WHO (1992a) recommends that in areas such as sub-Saharan Africa, where the primary causes of infant mortality are infectious disease and malnutrition, breastfeeding should be encouraged for all women, regardless of HIV status. The rationale for this recommendation is provided by studies showing that an infant's risk of becoming HIV infected through breast milk is lower than its risk of dying of other causes if deprived of breast milk.

Another approach to prevention of perinatal transmission is the provision of voluntary and confidential counseling and testing services to women who may then choose to avoid or terminate pregnancy. This alternative is unlikely to be feasible in African countries where access to HIV testing is poor, abortion is often illegal and frequently unsafe, and fertility is highly valued.

A third approach is the delivery by caesarean section of infants of HIV-infected mothers in order to minimize the risk of neonatal infection during vaginal delivery. While caesarean section delivery has proven effective in prevention of other viral infections (Minkoff and Duerr, 1994), no definite conclusions can be drawn on the basis of available data concerning its potential protective effect with regard to perinatal HIV transmission. Furthermore, even if the efficacy data were to point to caesarean section as an effective prevention strategy, the increased risk and high cost associated with the procedure render it an infeasible alternative in all but a handful of teaching hospitals in the region.

Another possible approach to reducing the risk of infection during vaginal delivery is vaginal lavage, or washing with a microbicidal agent during delivery. Vaginal lavage has been shown to lower rates of neonatal group B streptococcal infection in newborns and may prove to be helpful in the prevention of HIV transmission during delivery (Minkoff and Duerr, 1994). Potential problems, however, include fetal toxicity and genital mucosal irritation. More research is needed to quantify the risk of HIV transmission during vaginal delivery and to evaluate the efficacy of vaginal lavage in prevention of HIV transmission.

The most effective means of preventing perinatal transmission from HIV-infected mothers may be the administration of antiviral therapy such as Zidovudine (AZT) to the mother during pregnancy, labor, and delivery and then to the newborn during the first weeks of life. Data from a clinical trial involving 364 births to HIV-positive women showed a 67.5 percent reduction in the risk of HIV transmission attributable to AZT therapy (Centers for Disease Control, 1994). Efforts are now currently in progress to define the minimum dosage schedule for AZT in pregnancy. The trial results led the U.S. Public Health Service to issue new interim recommendations for care of pregnant women who meet the protocol eligibility criteria (Centers for Disease Control, 1994). However, there are several reasons why the therapeutic regimen in the trial (Protocol 076) will not be applicable to women in sub-Saharan countries. The main obstacle is the cost of the drug and sophisticated clinical equipment. Another obstacle is the requirement that babies be bottle fed with costly infant formula. Several studies are now under way to discover whether the trial results can be translated into a preventive strategy that can be used in developing countries, using either a shorter course of AZT treatment around the time of delivery or a lower dose of AZT (Cohen, 1995).

Vitamin A, dubbed "the anti-infective vitamin" as early as the 1920s, is currently under investigation as an alternative method to reduce vertical transmission. Several recent studies that have evaluated the impact of vitamin A on vertical transmission of HIV give reason for optimism that vitamin A can inexpensively and easily reduce the risk of vertical transmission. In a 2-year study of 338 HIV-positive mothers in Malawi, Semba et al. (1994) found that women with higher serum vitamin A transmitted HIV to their children significantly less often than their vitamin A-deficient counterparts. The results were dramatic: 32.4 percent of women in the most deficient group transmitted HIV, while only 7.2 percent of women in the group with the highest serum vitamin A did so. Unfortunately, the research was nonexperimental, and it is possible that other nutritional or behavioral factors associated with serum vitamin A (such as general nutrition) played a significant role.

Other studies have proposed that the usefulness of vitamin A is as a preventative measure for morbidity associated with HIV/AIDS in children, rather than an inhibitor of HIV transmission per se. This hypothesis posits that vitamin A serves to enhance the immune system, thus reducing the severity of opportunistic infections or the duration of specific illnesses, rather than the likelihood of infection per se. A randomized, placebo-controlled study of 118 children of HIV-infected women in Durban, Natal, found that all children showed improvements in morbidity (measured in child-months of ill health) with vitamin A supplementation and that children who were themselves HIV infected showed particular improvement for diarrhea-related illness (Coutsoudis et al., 1995). A recent review of the effectiveness of vitamin A supplementation in the control of morbidity and mortality among young children in developing countries concluded that "vitamin A supplementation can effectively reduce mortality rates in young children, and probably also reduce the risk of severe morbidity" (Beaton et al., 1993:66). Although the exact role of vitamin A remains unclear, further research into its effectiveness in inhibiting perinatal transmission and reducing the mortality and morbidity of HIV-infected children is clearly warranted.

RECOMMENDATIONS

Numerous interventions are being implemented throughout Africa, but most are still information-based health education campaigns. Many of the messages communicated are generic or vague and do not address specific risk behaviors. Innovative approaches are typically small scale and lack rigorous evaluation. Furthermore, it is not easy to demonstrate the success of a particular intervention because it is difficult to define and measure such outcome variables as "better health status" and to determine whether the intervention in question was the reason for a desired change. Consequently, the need for solid evaluation research is still urgent.

KEY RECOMMENDATION 2. An increase in research funding for the development of social and behavioral interventions aimed at protecting women and adolescents, especially girls, from infection deserves highest priority.

An important step in arresting the spread of AIDS in sub-Saharan Africa is to recognize that, although African women have relatively high autonomy by the standards of developing countries, their low and separate status remains a major obstacle to HIV prevention. In many societies, the presence of unmarried, postpubertal girls is a new phenomenon. Guidelines for their sexual behavior and that of others toward them are not well established; their low social status makes them particularly vulnerable. Moreover, in many areas of sub-Saharan Africa, high HIV incidence has been detected among adolescents and young adults, especially girls. Research on which to design culturally relevant programs targeted to adolescents and to adults who might be their sexual partners is an important priority.

KEY RECOMMENDATION 3. More evaluation research is needed to correlate process and outcome indicators—such as reported condom sales and behavior change—with reductions in HIV incidence or prevalence.

Rigorous designs, such as controlled intervention studies to assess the effectiveness of different prevention approaches, are needed. To date, few rigorous evaluations of intervention programs in sub-Saharan Africa have been conducted (see reviews in Choi and Coates, 1994, and Crump, 1995). Evaluations that have been reported often lack precision in their measurement of risk behaviors and are therefore not very informative. As a result, few strategies can demonstrate whether they are effective. Barriers to rigorous evaluation research include lack of human resources, expertise, financial resources, and equipment. Overcoming these barriers requires major changes in research infrastructure. Nevertheless, it is a priority to begin now a few large-scale behavioral interventions, including adequate baseline surveys, multiround surveys, and longitudinal studies with comparison cohorts, even if these interventions are relatively expensive. It is only with these types of studies that more definitive information on the effectiveness of various interventions, which is so desperately lacking for most studies in sub-Saharan Africa, can be obtained. The longer such studies are delayed, the longer will exist the uncertainty about which HIV-prevention strategies work best, for whom, and under what circumstances. In the interim, basic program evaluation and some formative and operational research can be completed, and such work should be required by donors as part of program implementation awards.

Recommendation 5-1. Interventions that promote gender equality deserve high priority as AIDS-prevention strategies in every country.

Women's primary source of risk is their society-wide subordination, not their lack of knowledge (Heise and Elias, 1995). Governments can effect change in many ways to empower women: reducing the financial necessity for multiple partnerships by changing laws to give women equal access to training and jobs, equal rights of inheritance and property ownership, equal access to education, and equal wage scales; enacting and enforcing laws against rape; building the capacity of women for collective action; and educating everyone about women's rights. Enhancing the status of women is a long-term strategy that would have many beneficial effects for development, in addition to the likely effect of reducing the transmission of HIV and other STDs.

Recommendation 5-2. In the short term, a female-controlled vaginal microbicide that would allow women to protect themselves without their partner's participation is an urgent research and development priority for international donors.

A microbicide is not a quick-fix substitute for the fundamental structural reforms necessary to achieve gender equality, but rather a temporary and partial response to this problem as it influences HIV transmission (Elias and Heise,

1994; Heise and Elias, 1995). Yet in the same way that the use of spermicides by women can reduce fertility, the use of a microbicide could, in and of itself, help arrest the spread of HIV.

Recommendation 5-3. Research is needed to address the HIV-prevention needs of several other populations with marked vulnerability, particularly the mobile and the disenfranchised.

There is a need to reach mobile individuals and groups with comprehensible and acceptable programs, particularly where linguistic and cultural barriers exist between migrants and the local population. Ways of effectively providing preventive services to the disenfranchised populations in the ever-growing urban slums and in refugee camps need to be developed; a major challenge to such programs is the lack of resources and social support for individuals in such settings.

Recommendation 5-4. Additional research should be conducted to determine the impact of specific STD interventions on the incidence of HIV infection within defined populations.

Research is needed to determine the extent to which STDs help cause HIV infection, to examine the importance of the behavioral synergy of STD and HIV transmission, and to design more effective intervention programs. There is a need for assessment of the relative efficacy and feasibility of various interventions for STD treatment and sexual behavior change in reducing HIV transmission. This research includes assessing the effects of programs that target individuals at high risk of acquiring and transmitting STDs, as well as the effects of community-based STD programs. The interventions themselves could comprise STD education, condom distribution, increased STD screening, and mass antibiotic therapy. Data on the effectiveness of these interventions, particularly those focused on decreasing STD prevalence, are essential for evaluating the impact of STD reduction on the spread of HIV. Behavioral research on ways of ensuring acceptance of various STD control strategies should be directly integrated into the epidemiological research.

Recommendation 5-5. Research is needed to assess the effectiveness and cost-effectiveness of the syndromic approach to STD diagnosis and treatment.

Clinical testing for STDs is expensive and not widely accessible. Therefore, research is needed on better ways to identify STDs more accurately through symptoms. In addition, new screening methods, including urine-based assays for chlamydia and gonorrhea and self-administered vaginal swabs for trichomonas culture and bacterial vaginosis gram stain, should be incorporated into research. Efforts are needed to make these techniques available and affordable in developing-country settings for surveillance, diagnosis, and validation.

Recommendation 5-6. For long-term program planning and resource allocation, cost-effectiveness studies should be incorporated in donor research work and the cost-effectiveness of HIV prevention compared with that of other health interventions.

Few intervention evaluations have adequately assessed effectiveness in terms of behavior change or seroincidence declines, much less cost-effectiveness. Results of evaluation studies currently in progress in several countries in sub-Saharan Africa (Family Health International/AIDSCAP, 1994) are expected to provide data on the cost-effectiveness of various HIV-prevention strategies. However, determining the effectiveness of HIV-prevention strategies is methodologically complex and will take several more years to complete. In the meantime, since resources are insufficient and may well decline further, efficient resource utilization is paramount. Thus, basic analysis of overall program costs and specific intervention costs is critical. Simple cost analyses and cost-effectiveness estimates could provide data that would be helpful for public health decision making and program design.

Recommendation 5-7. Operations research should be a high priority.

The growth of the HIV/AIDS pandemic in the past 20 years in sub-Saharan Africa has led to the development of institutional and community-based responses and a corresponding need for operations research to improve the effectiveness, cost-effectiveness, and quality of these responses. Primary research needs include scaling up successful experimental interventions, improving the effectiveness and reducing the cost of existing programs, examining the cost-effectiveness of linking HIV prevention with HIV/AIDS care, and improving the sensitivity and specificity of criteria for targeting interventions.

Recommendation 5-8. Research should be undertaken to measure the impact of female-controlled barrier contraceptive use on HIV transmission.

Studies should be undertaken to determine the effectiveness against STDs and HIV of female-controlled barrier contraceptives such as female condoms and spermicides. This research should encompass field-based studies of the acceptability of these methods. Moreover, greater efforts need to be made to integrate appropriate HIV/AIDS-prevention messages and programs for STD diagnosis, referral, and treatment into family planning programs.

Recommendation 5-9. Behavioral research is needed to develop effective pregnancy-related HIV counseling programs.

Given the rapid spread of HIV among women in sub-Saharan Africa, perinatal transmission continues to have a major impact on infant and child morbidity and mortality among populations with a high HIV seroprevalence. Studies using modified treatment regimens with Zidovudine (AZT), hyperimmune gamma globulin, vitamin A, vaginal washes, and other means of intervention should be undertaken to determine their overall effectiveness and cost-effectiveness in decreasing HIV perinatal transmission.

ANNEX 5-1 SELECTED AIDS INTERVENTION PROGRAMS IN AFRICA

Country (area)	Intervention Type	Target Population and Size	Program Components
1. Ghana	Community-based	Commercial sex workers	• Behavior-change interventions • Condom provision
2. Ghana	Population-based	Ghanaian youth	• Behavior-change interventions
3. Guinea	Population-based	500,000 couples in Guinea	• Behavior-change interventions • Condom provision • Family planning
4. Kenya	Institution-based	Female prostitutes and women attending clinics	• Behavior-change interventions • HIV testing and counseling • Free condom provision
5. Malawi	Institution-based (hospital)	General population (mostly married males)	• HIV/STD counseling
6. Nigeria	Community-based	Commercial sex workers	• Behavior-change interventions • Condom provision • STD services • Vocational and literacy programs
7. Rwanda (Kigali)	Institution-based (clinics)	53 HIV-discordant couples	• HIV testing and counseling • Free condom provision
8. Rwanda (Kigali)	Institution-based (clinics)	1,458 childbearing women in Kigali	• HIV testing and counseling • Free condom provision • Free spermicide provision • Behavior-change communications (videotape)
9. Rwanda	Community-based	5 rural communes, 100 km from Kigali	• Behavior-change interventions • Condom provision

Key Results	Reference
• Consistent condom use among sex workers rose from 6 to 71% in 6 months. • After the intervention, 64% of those followed up reported always using condoms with clients.	Asamoah-Adu et al., 1994
• The proportion of sexually active 15-year-olds fell from 44 to 27%. • Men reported an 18% decrease in sexual partners over 3 months.	Family Health International/ AIDSCAP, 1992
• In the first 6 months, 2.3 million condoms were distributed.	Hess, 1993
• The proportion of counseled women who use condoms increased from 10% at pre-test to 81% at post-test.	Ngugi et al., 1988
• STD treatment and control significantly improved (88% of those counseled were cured, 77% of those in the control still presented with STDs).	Wynendaele et al., 1995
• Post-counseling, the reported ever use of condoms increased from 41 to 71%.	
• Within the first year, the percentage of women never using condoms fell from 25 to 3%. • Post-test, >60% reported condom use in their most recent sexual intercourse act. • Post-test, "always" condom use doubled, from 12 to 24%.	Williams et al., 1992
• Condom use was associated with a lower rate of new HIV infections. • Discordant couples using condoms increased from 4 to 57% after one year.	Allen et al., 1992b
• Condom use increased from 7 to 22% of women. • HIV seroconversion rates decreased significantly among women whose partners were tested and counseled.	Allen et al., 1992a
• Condom use increased from 4 to 44%. • Reported ever use of condoms increased from 7 to 50%.	Mercer et al., 1993

ANNEX 5-1 Continued

Country (area)	Intervention Type	Target Population and Size	Program Components
10. Rwanda	Institution-based (clinics)	1,500 attending clinics in Kigali and their partners	• Behavior-change interventions • Condom provision • Free HIV testing and counseling
11. Rwanda	Institution-based (workplace)	Military recruits	• Behavior-change interventions • Condom provision
12. Tanzania	Institution-based (workplace)	Truck drivers and their partners	• Behavior-change interventions • Condom provision
13. Uganda (Rakai)	Community-based	Young adults aged 13-39 in rural communities	• Condom promotion and provision by trained peers and community health workers
14. Uganda	Institution-based (workplace)	The general population; 400,000 workers	• Behavior-change interventions • Condom provision
15. Zaire (Kinshasa)	Institution-based (textile factory and commercial bank)	149 HIV-discordant couples	• HIV testing and counseling • Free condom provision
16. Zaire	Institution-based (workplace)	Commercial sex workers in Kinshasa	• Behavior-change interventions • STD treatment • Condom provisions • Counseling and testing
17. Zaire	Population-based	13 million urban youth and their parents	• Behavior-change interventions • Condom provision
18. Zambia (Copperbelt)	Institution-based (workplace, school)	2 million people	• Behavior-change interventions • STD treatment • Policy component • Survival skills workshop
19. Zambia	Population-based	General population	• Behavior-change interventions • Condom provision

Key Results	Reference
• Consistent condom use rose from 7 to 22% in 1 year. • Prevalence of gonorrhea decreased from 13 to 6% among HIV-positive women. • HIV seroconversion rates decreased from 4.1 to 1.8 per 100 person-years among women whose partners were tested and counseled.	World Health Organization, 1992c
• Incidence of urethritis fell from 12 to 5% in 16 months.	World Health Organization, 1992c
• Condoms distributed increased from 60,000 to 700,000 in 6 months. • Condom use among women rose from 50 to 91%. • Condom use among men rose from 54 to 74%.	Mwizarubi et al., 1992
• Reported ever use of condoms increased from 7.6% in 1990 to 12.5% in 1992.	Konde-Lule et al., 1994
• Condom use rose from 3.5% in 1990 to 14.5% in 1991.	World Health Organization, 1992c; McCombie and Hornik, 1992
• Condom use increased from < 5 % to 71%, 60%, and 77% at 1, 6, and 18 months, respectively.	Kamenga et al., 1991
• Condom use among women rose from 8 to 60%. • Annual HIV incidence fell from 18 to 3% in 2 years.	Laga et al., 1994
• Condom sales rose from 100,000 in 1987 to 18 million in 4 years. • Fidelity rose from 29 to 46% in 6 months.	Population Services International, 1994d
• Three STDs treated at four clinics declined by 54, 53, and 42%, respectively.	Mouli, 1992
• In the first year of the program, 4.6 million condoms were sold. • Among condom users, 50% indicated they first used a condom within the months following PSI's condom launch.	Population Services International, 1994d

ANNEX 5-1 Continued

Country (area)	Intervention Type	Target Population and Size	Program Components
20. Zimbabwe	Institution-based (workplace)	4,500 factory, workers, families, and local community	• Behavior-change interventions • STD treatment • Condom provision
21. Zimbabwe (Marondera)	Institution-based (workplace)	Men, women, and youth	• Behavior-change interventions • Condom provision • Income generation for commercial sex workers
22. Zimbabwe (Eastern Highlands)	Institution-based (workplace)	15,000 male and female plantation workers and their dependents	• Behavior-change interventions • Condom provision • STD treatment • Home care & management
23. Zimbabwe (Rio Tinto)	Institution-based (workplace)	3,500 miners and their families	• Behavior-change interventions • Condom provision • STD treatment
24. Zimbabwe (Mutare)	Institution-based (workplace)	150,000 men, women and youth	• Behavior-change interventions • Condom provision
25. Zimbabwe (Bulawayo)	Community-based	General population and high-risk groups	• Behavior-change interventions • Condom provision • Income generation
26. Zimbabwe (Gabarone)	Community-based	Women in the community	• Behavior-change interventions • Communication and negotiation skills workshop

Key Results	Reference
• There was a decrease in the number of STD patients in 3 years. • There were 37,000 condoms a year distributed.	Williams and Ray, 1993
• Condoms distributed rose from 385,000 in 1991 to 962,400 in 1993. • There was an 80% decrease in STD treatment.	Williams and Ray, 1993
• There were 3,600 condoms/month distributed. • There was a 59% decline in the number of patients treated for STDs.	Williams and Ray, 1993
• Condoms distributed rose from 500/year to 56,000/year after 2 years. • STD patients at four clinics declined between 47 and 78%.	Williams and Ray, 1993
• The incidence of STDs decreased by 48% in 2 years. • There were 2.5 million condoms distributed in 1992. • The program was expanded to 10 additional workplaces.	Williams and Ray, 1993
• There were 2.5 million condoms distributed in 2 years • Consistent condom use in commercial sex workers rose from 5% in 1989 to nearly 50% in 1992.	Wilson et al., 1992
• Positive attitudes toward condoms and expressed confidence in correct condom use increased from 35 to 76%. • Those reporting "always" use of condoms increased from 28 to 50%.	World Health Organization, 1992c

6

Mitigating the Impact of the Epidemic

INTRODUCTION

As noted earlier, even if transmission of HIV were halted today, millions of Africans who are currently infected would still develop AIDS and die over the next 10 to 20 years. But transmission has not ceased. To the contrary, evidence from a variety of populations in Africa suggests that seroprevalence either is continuing to climb or has leveled off at discouragingly high levels (see Chapter 3). Approximately a dozen countries lying in a contiguous belt across central and eastern Africa account for more than 80 percent of all estimated HIV infections (see Chapter 1). For at least the next several decades, the HIV/AIDS epidemic will continue to ravage African prime-age adults and their children with death rates as much as 10 times higher than they would otherwise have been.

Although not immediately visible, the cumulative mortality effects of this "slow plague" will be substantial. Through the year 2000, the impact of AIDS will increasingly be felt on populations in the sub-Saharan Africa region, particularly those lying in the main AIDS belt. Increases in infant and child mortality will be accompanied by increases in adult mortality and reductions in life expectancy. Population growth will decline more rapidly than expected, and African populations in the year 2000 will be somewhat smaller than those projected in the absence of AIDS. In many of the worst-afflicted countries, deaths will more than double during the 1990s as compared with the number estimated without AIDS. These additional deaths will put increasing strains on already overburdened health-care systems and on individual households trying to manage with limited economic resources. Care and support for orphans will be a growing concern, and traditional inheritance and other legal rights will be challenged.

AIDS is one of many diseases with potentially great economic significance for developing countries. Diseases such as malaria and measles are far more prevalent in Africa, yet there are reasons to believe that the economic impact of AIDS will be greater. First, the fatality of AIDS and the duration of the illness increase its impact per case relative to other causes of morbidity. The long incubation period of HIV implies that the economic impact of existing levels of infection will be felt for 10 years or more, even if all infection were to cease today. The benefits of averting a case of HIV (19.5 discounted healthy life-years) are very high relative to other diseases (Over and Piot, 1993). By this measure, HIV ranks lower than neonatal tetanus, but higher than other widespread illnesses such as malaria, tuberculosis, and measles.

Second, HIV is likely to have a greater economic impact than other endemic diseases because it affects primarily adults in their economically most productive years (see also Chapter 3). In Africa, illness and death due to AIDS are concentrated among two age groups: newborn children, who acquire it perinatally, and adults between ages 15 and 50, who acquire it largely through sexual transmission. If one were to weight the years gained by averting a case of HIV by their productivity, HIV would rank highest among all diseases in terms of the value of preventing a case (Over and Piot, 1993). Adults aged 15 to 50 are usually the economic backbone of their families and their communities, on whom both young children and elderly parents rely for support. The illness and death of these economically active prime-age adults result not only in lower incomes for surviving family members, but also in all the other sequelae of poverty, including worsened health and reduced investment in the survivors' future productivity.

Third, unlike many other endemic diseases, AIDS does not spare the elite. Levels of HIV prevalence among high-income, urban, and relatively well-educated men and women are as high as those among low-income and rural groups, if not higher. Because wealthier, more-skilled, and better-educated subsets of the population have higher levels of consumption and investment, command higher wages, and are more likely to be employers, any disease affecting this group relatively more than other groups is likely to have a greater economic impact per case.

It is becoming increasingly evident that there is considerable divergence of opinion between industrialized and developing countries about the appropriate allocation of resources among various components of an African national AIDS control program. Industrial countries prefer to respond to the current and impending impact of the epidemic in Africa by donating their energy and resources to biomedical research and various prevention activities, while African governments feel an obligation to allocate resources not only to prevention, but also to mitigation of the direct impact on individuals and households already affected by the virus.

Whether directed at individuals with AIDS and their households or at other levels of social organization, mitigation interventions divert scarce resources from other uses, including efforts to prevent transmission. When individuals voluntarily devote their own time and resources to help persons with AIDS or their surviving family members, they demonstrate through their actions that they place a high value on these activities. However, if governments are to channel resources away from other useful objectives toward mitigating the impact of the epidemic, there must first be reason to believe that the value to society of the proposed government interventions is at least as great as the cost of the resources devoted to the effort.

Thus, research on this issue might improve the efficiency of current expenditures, as well as present a case for or against additional spending. Research questions arise about the degree to which resources should be diverted from efforts to prevent HIV infection or from other general development programs to finance mitigation interventions. On the one hand, these services provide access to basic human rights, such as an adequate standard of living, health care, and education. The obligation of governments and international organizations to support basic human rights need not be debated here. On the other hand, resources are limited.

There are two logical preconditions for adopting government interventions to mitigate the impact of the HIV/AIDS epidemic. First, certain social units or groups must have indeed been substantially harmed by the epidemic. Second, government programs designed to either limit the damage or target assistance to those who have been harmed must produce effects above and beyond any adjustments that would be made in the absence of any interventions. Assuming that such programs are feasible, policy makers need guidance in choosing which programs to implement and how much to spend on such programs in view of the many competing needs for government resources.

A great deal of attention has been devoted to attempting to limit the further spread of HIV; considerably less thought has focused on identifying solutions to the problem of coping with the millions of persons already infected with the virus. To date, the small amount of research effort devoted to the effects of AIDS on households and societies in Africa pales in comparison with the magnitude of the problem. There is an acute shortage of quality studies on the economic, demographic, and social impacts of the disease on families in Africa (Caldwell et al., 1993). Perhaps the most widely cited book on the impacts of AIDS in Africa is based on a sample of approximately 130 households in Rakai, Uganda, of which only 20 were affected either directly or indirectly by AIDS (Barnett and Blaikie, 1992). Several other studies have been based on findings from fewer than 50 households (see Caldwell et al., 1993, for a brief review). The Paris-based International Children's Center is analyzing the impact of AIDS on 200 households that are the homes of people with AIDS sampled at a few selected health facilities in Côte d'Ivoire, Haiti, and Burundi.

The largest study to date, and the only one based on a representative, population-based sample, is the World Bank/University of Dar es Salaam study of approximately 800 households in Kagera, Tanzania, which has not been completed as of this writing. This study promises to provide valuable information about the economic impact of fatal adult illness in Kagera and adjacent, culturally similar areas of Uganda, Rwanda, Burundi, and Zaire. The relevance of the study findings for Southern or West Africa, where modes of production, fertility and marriage patterns, female labor-force participation rates, and traditional gender roles are different, is unknown. Consequently, the field suffers from the continual recycling of a small number of research findings, liberally supplemented with enormous amounts of anecdotal evidence of varying quality (Caldwell et al., 1993).

In the rest of this chapter, we first consider the impact of HIV/AIDS in sub-Saharan Africa on people with AIDS, and then the impact on their extended family members and friends. We next consider the indirect effects of AIDS, both demographic and economic, on society at large. At each level of social organization, we review evidence regarding the magnitude of the epidemic's impact and explore the implications for the continent. We then examine the types of mitigation programs that are currently being implemented. Finally, we present recommendations on future research and data priorities. Annex 6-1 briefly surveys nongovernmental organizations currently implementing mitigation programs in sub-Saharan Africa.

IMPACT ON PERSONS WITH HIV

The ultimate fate of persons with HIV is well known. Virtually without exception, within 10 years of contracting the virus, individuals develop full-blown AIDS and die.[1] But before the symptoms of AIDS develop, people living with HIV infection face ostracism, poverty, physical pain, and fear of impending death. Many individuals refuse to believe that they could be infected, and many who suspect they may be seropositive refuse to be tested. Given the harsh reality of the disease, some researchers have identified a surprising "underreaction" to AIDS in Africa (Schoepf, 1988; Caldwell et al., 1994). There are numerous explanations for such an underreaction, including denial, shame, misunderstanding of the true risk of the disease, and a desire for silence because of the disease's association with illicit sexual behavior. These and other more obvious reasons for the silence about AIDS are discussed in detail in a seminal article by Caldwell and colleagues, who suggest that fatalism may also play a strong role:

---

[1]See below for a discussion on the length of the latency period from HIV infection to an AIDS-defining opportunistic infection in Africa. See Chapter 3 for a discussion of the differences in the voracity of HIV-1 and HIV-2.

> The most fundamental reason why the great majority of Africans are more sanguine than might have been predicted with regard to the AIDS epidemic is that they are not fully convinced that biomedical determinism is the only force operating in the world. . . . [The] African attitude toward illness and death rests on two partly related complexes of belief. The first is that there are different levels of causation. One is certainly the "natural" biomedical one, but this is triggered by other forces, chiding, punitive, or malevolent. The natural cause can be checked and reversed if the underlying force can be identified and appeased. The other is the belief in destiny, stronger in West Africa than in the East and South but probably not nonexistent in the latter areas. This, in its most extreme form, holds that the date of death is written and changes in lifestyle will not put off that event. The situation, even in most of West Africa, is usually more complex than this because of the concept of the employment of evil forces to cause premature death and the consequent need to identify this danger and take remedial action. AIDS can, and almost always does, result in premature death in that it occurs before old age, but such deaths predating the prescribed time are never solely biomedical. The HIV virus is merely the instrument (Caldwell et al., 1994:233-234).

Whatever the correct explanation, this underreaction has obvious implications for the speed with which African governments are forced to respond to the epidemic and for the probability of persuading Africans to change their behavior to contain the epidemic.

Stigmatization of the Seropositive

Despite the reports of an underreaction to the epidemic by some Africans, there is no doubt that many people with AIDS in the subcontinent have been subjected to trauma and isolation. In much of Africa, AIDS is still highly stigmatizing, in part because of beliefs concerning its association with illicit sex. In Ghana, for example, the disease has come to be widely viewed as a disease of women, and more specifically of female prostitutes (Porter, 1994). Even in countries hardest hit by the epidemic, such as Tanzania, AIDS is still very much perceived as a disease of sin in certain provinces (Kaijage, 1994b).

Discrimination against people with HIV/AIDS may be directed not only at those with the disease, but also at their families, friends, and caretakers and others with whom they have contact. In some cases, family members continue to be isolated, abused, or attacked after the death of the infected relation, partly because, as explained above, in many societies in sub-Saharan Africa the disease may be ascribed to supernatural causes, often associated with earlier misdeeds (Castle, 1994). Families who care for their chronically ill relatives may try not to let the nature of the ailment become known (Lwihula et al., 1993). A person with AIDS in Burundi explained:

> Now I am lonely, nobody comes to visit me except the doctor and the nurses. Yet, I have many relations here. I have many friends! But everybody has

abandoned me. I am disappointed! They certainly suspected that I had AIDS (Ministère de la Santé, 1992, cited in IRESCO, 1995:35).

Although the various dimensions and repercussions of stigmatization may be difficult to quantify, they are an extremely important aspect of the burden of AIDS in the region. Increasingly, counseling in preventing new infections and limiting the destructive forces of stigmatization and discrimination is being recognized as an essential part of caring for people with AIDS.[2]

Economic Hardship Due to HIV

Evidence about the magnitude of the economic impact of AIDS at the individual level is scarce and generally qualitative in nature (see below) (Ainsworth and Over, 1994a, 1994b). Certainly, people with AIDS face high medical bills and an uncertain economic future. As their health degenerates, illness results in the loss of income-earning potential, while at the same time many persons with AIDS spend their household savings in trying to treat various opportunistic infections or find a cure for AIDS itself.

Anecdotal reports of workplace discrimination have been documented in a number of African countries affected by the HIV/AIDS epidemic. For example, in some areas of sub-Saharan Africa, employers are reportedly subject to prison terms and fines if they hire HIV-infected people (Danziger, 1994). Government officials in another country have encouraged employers to test workers and dismiss those who are infected (Cohen and Wiseberg, 1990, cited in Danziger, 1994). The experience of AIDS-related discrimination can include social ostracism and exclusion from usual networks for accessing emergency resources. Ignorance of modes of transmission of the virus can result in abandonment of people with HIV/AIDS by their relatives and expulsion from the family safety net, leaving the infected completely destitute (Awusabo-Asare and Agyeman, 1993).

Care for People with AIDS

In those parts of Africa where the epidemic is already fairly advanced, AIDS has become a part of everyday life, and the need for care is most urgent. Extensive treatment protocols have been developed for people with AIDS in industrialized countries. However, these protocols are less relevant in Africa because of a shortage of manpower and resources for the treatment and care of people with AIDS and regional variations in the prevalence of certain opportunistic infections, such as tuberculosis and *Pneumocystis carinii* pneumonia (Schopper and

[2]See M'Pelé et al. (1994) for a recent review of the impact of counseling programs in Africa.

Walley, 1992). Diagnosing HIV-related diseases and providing care for people with AIDS in Africa is further complicated by the fact that HIV-related diseases often develop atypical clinical manifestations and may occur simultaneously, even in the same organs (Colebunders and Kapita, 1994). Furthermore, treatments are not available for some HIV-related diseases, and people with AIDS often experience serious side effects of drugs (Colebunders and Kapita, 1994).

A great deal of debate and controversy surround the level of appropriate care for people with AIDS (see, for example, Katabira and Wabitsch, 1991; De Cock et al., 1993; Biggar, 1993; Foster, 1994). For example, De Cock et al. (1993) set forth the treatment and care needs at different stages of the disease process: the seropositive person without symptoms of full-blown AIDS needs outpatient care and prophylaxes for opportunistic infections; the mildly to intermediately ill person needs to be actively treated for opportunistic infections as they arise; and those in the end stage of the disease need access to hospice care and continuing pain control. Unfortunately, providing extensive medical care to people at all stages of the disease would be prohibitively expensive in Africa (World Bank, 1992a; Biggar, 1993; Foster, 1994; Ainsworth and Over, 1994a). Given the magnitude of the problem and the corresponding amount of money that would need to be transferred into the health sector from elsewhere, the question of what constitutes adequate care for those with AIDS is, in all likelihood, more likely a political than a research question. The challenge for researchers and the medical community is to devise ways of treating people with AIDS at lower cost without seriously compromising the quality of their care.

Several African countries are already experimenting with various models of outpatient and home-based care as alternatives to hospitalization. Home-based care is also an effective way to involve families and communities in AIDS care and support (World Health Organization, 1991). Preliminary results from a study of the costs of home-based care in Zambia indicate that community-initiated care is considerably cheaper than hospital-initiated alternatives. Furthermore, the average duration of a visit by a health-care worker was typically longer with the community-initiated home care, indicating substantial variation in the types of service provided under alternative health-care models (Chela et al., 1994). A study of AIDS treatment costs in Tanzania found that a shift from inpatient to outpatient care can produce considerable cost savings to the health-care sector (World Bank, 1992a). In Rwanda, a training course designed to teach families how to care for people with AIDS at home appears to have enabled the families to do better with managing AIDS-related problems; moreover, the volunteer trainers seem to have provided family members with much-needed emotional support (Schietinger et al., 1993). A review of six home-based care programs in Uganda and Zambia seems to confirm the hypotheses that home-based care can improve the quality of life for people with AIDS and reduces pressure on hospital beds (World Health Organization, 1991).

At the same time, the results of a research project undertaken in South Africa indicate that a substantial proportion of the burden of caring for people with AIDS could be borne in primary health facilities (Metrikin et al., 1995).

The need for medical, economic, and emotional support implies that the best care might be provided by a "multidisciplinary team" (Brugha, 1994). Perhaps the best-known model of hospital-initiated outreach service is the Chikankata program in Zambia, initiated in 1987. (Chikankata Mission Hospital is a 240-bed general hospital run by the Salvation Army that serves a predominantly rural community of approximately 150,000 nearby residents.) The mobile home-care team consists of a clinical officer, a nurse, an assistant AIDS educator, and a driver who visits between five and eight people each day, three days a week (Chela and Siankanga, 1991).

Regardless of the level of outside medical attention that is available, however, much of the care received by people with AIDS is provided by household members. The largest portion of this burden is borne by women (Caldwell et al., 1993; Kaijage, 1994a, 1994b). Individuals, families, and communities need to be better educated about how best to provide safe and compassionate AIDS care at home. In this regard, WHO—in collaboration with The AIDS Support Organization (TASO), Uganda; the Nsambya Hospital, Order of St. Francis, Uganda; and the Salvation Army Chikankata Mission Hospital, Zambia—recently developed a handbook for AIDS home care for use in sub-Saharan Africa (World Health Organization, 1993).

IMPACT ON EXTENDED FAMILY MEMBERS AND FRIENDS

Early deaths due to AIDS are generating large numbers of people who are at increased risk of poverty. A death in the household or the family as a result of AIDS or any other illness can have profound implications for resource allocation, production, consumption, savings, investment, and the well being of survivors (Ainsworth and Over, 1994a).[3] As noted earlier, the age structure of the infected population is heavily weighted toward those in their most productive years (see Chapter 3), so that many of those who die are the sole breadwinners in the household. Therefore, AIDS has an unusually devastating effect on the entire household, both through loss of income and through dissolution of normal social relationships within the family. Adults aged 15 to 50 are usually the economic

[3]One of the most striking features of African social organization is that it downplays the role of the nuclear family and, in its place, stresses the importance of kinship and clan networks. Consequently, the interpretation of what defines a household or a family can vary considerably across societies. Obviously, one cannot do justice to the complete range of patterns of social organization in Africa here, but suffice it to say that the terms "household" and "family" in Africa often refer to quite different collections of individuals. This distinction is important to remember when comparing household- and family-level impacts across different societies.

backbone of their families and their communities, providers on whom both young children and elderly parents rely for support. Consequently, the illness and death of these economically active prime-age adults result not only in higher medical expenses and lower incomes for family members, but also in many other sequelae of poverty, including worsened health and reduced investment in the future productivity of their survivors. Because deterioration from AIDS is such a slow process, many families exhaust their entire savings before the person with AIDS dies. Furthermore, families lose income not only from the infected person, but also from other family members involved in his or her care. This loss is especially significant in families with more than one infected person. Finally, apart from losing a valuable contributor to household labor supply, survivors may also lose access to land, housing, or other assets.

Understanding and accurately predicting the long-term impact of HIV/AIDS on society depends critically on our understanding of how individual decision making is affected by the epidemic. For example, if individuals trust both in the future and in their fellow citizens, they are more likely to save a portion of their current income and invest those savings in risky, but potentially profitable, enterprises. Savings from current consumption can be invested (directly or through the intermediary of a savings bank or association) either in physical capital (e.g., a new irrigation pump) or human capital (e.g., a child's education or training). Thus, the HIV/AIDS epidemic makes immediately relevant the question of whether an individual's belief that he or she is or is likely to become infected causes that person to save or invest less.

Some economists have argued that one of the underlying causes of slow development in Africa has been the failure of states to develop dependable judicial and social mechanisms for enforcing contracts and thereby lowering the transaction costs for all concerned. Will people continue to choose to invest time, energy, and capital in social relations and the economy if they know that they, or others around them, are HIV-infected? Normal social relations, built on a degree of faith in the future and mutual trust, may be one of the most neglected casualties of HIV/AIDS in Africa. Relationships of trust that depend upon the participants' both knowing that they will be trading together for years to come may dissolve quickly if one or both of the participants become aware that either is infected with HIV. This observation raises the question of whether the epidemic, by reducing the willingness of individuals to trust one another, increases transaction costs and if so, whether government intervention could mitigate that increase.

Many AIDS researchers have indicated that people in Africa are unconcerned about HIV because of its long incubation period. Apparently, in the calculus of everyday life, the slow plague is a low priority for many (Caldwell et al., 1994). By the time one dies from AIDS, the logic goes, one could well have died from other things many times over (Schoepf, 1988). If a disinterest in long-term planning is independent of (or even partially causes) the sweeping prevalence of HIV, we would not anticipate transaction costs to increase perceptibly with the rising prevalence of AIDS. In this scenario, AIDS would not add significantly to all the other reasons for uncertainty or doubt already endemic to the continent.

Most of the evidence produced so far on the impact of the epidemic at the household level has been of extremely variable quality and often anecdotal in nature. In one of the few field studies of the economic effects of AIDS in Africa, Barnett and Blaikie (1992) describe the results of their fieldwork undertaken in 1989 on a sample of 129 households in the Rakai district of Uganda. The authors were able to provide many rich anecdotes of how the 20 households in their sample might have been affected either directly or indirectly by AIDS, including a reduction in the production of food crops, a gradual depletion of household assets, a withdrawal of children from school, and an increase in household malnutrition. However, they were unable to show that the epidemic had affected producer-consumer ratios in these households, or indeed that any of the supposed effects of AIDS were suffered more frequently or to a greater degree by the 20 AIDS-affected households than by other households. Furthermore, there was no discernible impact on total agricultural production in the Rakai district. The authors (Barnett and Blaikie, 1992:102) conclude that:

> . . . by 1989/90, AIDS had not yet drawn adaptive responses in production and consumption on a scale that dwarfed the many other adaptations households make all the time in response to other rapid processes of socioeconomic change. However, we believe that in certain localized areas AIDS is beginning to be the major determinant of socioeconomic change.

The ability of a household to cope with an AIDS illness and death is clearly a function of many factors, including the socioeconomic characteristics of the household, the economic role of the person with AIDS within the household (particularly how his/her illness affects household income), the household's access to alternative sources of income or support, the level of social and material support available to the household, and so forth. It is analytically convenient to divide the costs to the household of incurring a case of AIDS into three components: (1) direct costs associated with medical expenses; (2) indirect costs to the household directly afflicted with AIDS in terms of forgone earnings; and (3) indirect costs to other households, associated with contributing to funeral expenses or caring for orphaned children (Ainsworth and Rwegarulira, 1992).

Because AIDS manifests itself in a series of other diseases, the direct costs incurred by people with AIDS in seeking medical attention prior to their death can be considerable. The average cost of health care per HIV-seropositive patient admitted to Mama Yemo Hospital in Kinshasa, Zaire, was US $170, compared with US $110 per HIV-seronegative patient (Hassig et al., 1990). The direct costs of medical treatment of AIDS in Tanzania have been estimated at between US $104 and US $631 per person (Over et al., 1988). More recent estimates from

South Africa and Zimbabwe indicate that the direct costs of treatment can sometimes reach several thousand dollars per person (Ainsworth and Over, 1994b).

Besides the cost of medical care for the chronically ill, when the person with AIDS eventually dies, the household encounters further costs associated with the funeral and with lost production during a period of mourning. If the deceased lived away from the village, the family must usually pay for the body to be transported back to his or her home area, as well as for the transportation, food, and lodging of mourners. These costs can be considerable. For example, in Kinshasa, Zaire, families have been estimated to spend an average of US $320 for the funeral of a child who died of AIDS (Foster, 1993, cited in Ainsworth and Over, 1994a). In 1991, in the Kagera region of Tanzania, families were estimated to spend approximately US $60 for a single death, of which 60 percent was spent for the funeral (Over and Mujinja, 1993). Such expenditures are a substantial burden in a country where gross national product per capita was US $100 in 1991 (World Bank, 1993). Households in Kagera also contribute to expenses associated with the death of relatives who live outside the household. In 1991, this contribution was estimated to be approximately US $7 per death, of which 79 percent was for funeral expenses. At the same time, the period of mourning may have been reduced in Kagera from 7 to between zero and 3 days, a change implying that the annual cost of lost production has become quite high (Lwihula and Over, 1993).

Caring for Survivors: Children and the Elderly

Among the survivors severely affected by HIV/AIDS are dependents left without economic support. The increase in the number of orphans resulting from the HIV/AIDS epidemic may overwhelm traditional systems of adoption or institutional-care alternatives, so that the development of feasible and culturally acceptable models of child care for the minor children of people with AIDS will become a major challenge in upcoming years (Preble, 1990; Obbo, 1993). At the same time, elderly persons who have lost their adult children face potential economic hardship and the prospect of raising their grandchildren on their own.

Several studies have estimated the number of AIDS orphans that will result from the AIDS crisis. The reliability of these studies is uncertain, and the estimates they yield vary widely. Nevertheless, the bottom line is that no matter what the actual number, orphanhood as a result of AIDS will become an increasingly large problem (see Ainsworth and Over, 1994a, 1994b). In Africa, the extended family usually takes the place of the social welfare systems in industrialized countries. Furthermore, in some parts of the continent, but particularly in West Africa, there is a strong tradition of children being raised by people other than their biological parents (Page, 1989). These foster parents assume both the costs and the benefits associated with childrearing. In Sierra Leone, foster parents can be relatives, friends, neighbors, or patrons, and many may not even be related by blood or marriage to the children they rear (Bledsoe and Isiugo-Abanihe, 1989). It is unclear, however, whether extended families can cope with the large increase in orphans resulting from AIDS (Obbo, 1993). If they cannot, orphans will have little social and economic support. For example, in 1990, there were only 34 orphanages in the whole of Tanzania, sheltering a total of 1,083 children (Ainsworth and Rwegarulira, 1992). Compare this statistic with the fact that in 1988, in Kagera region alone, there were an estimated 47,000 children who had lost at least one parent and 8,000 who had lost both (Ainsworth and Rwegarulira, 1992).

One problem for researchers has been to distinguish between AIDS orphans and other orphans in societies where, for a number of reasons, orphanhood and fosterage are not uncommon. In Kenya, the number of AIDS orphans is estimated at about 250,000 in 1995 and is anticipated to rise to more than 1 million by 2005 (National AIDS Control Programme [Kenya], no date). In Uganda, estimates of the proportion of children orphaned range from 7 to 16 percent (Shuey, no date, cited in IRESCO, 1995). Some 40 percent of Zambian households are estimated to have at least one AIDS orphan in their care (Social Policy Research Group, 1993); those estimates are rising.

How will the loss of their parents early in life affect the lives of these unfortunate children? The short answer is that we do not know. Ryder et al. (1994) found no considerable health or socioeconomic effects of AIDS related orphanhood in a longitudinal study in Kinshasa, Zaire. The authors argue that the mitigation of additional hardship for orphans was due to the presence of concerned extended family members. However, as noted above, it remains to be seen whether this mechanism will continue to suffice as the numbers of AIDS orphans increase. Furthermore, societies may differ in the degree to which neighbors and relatives serve as an informal safety net to protect the survivors in an AIDS household. In Tanzania, a national assessment of families and children affected by AIDS found that some orphans received the same treatment at home as biological children, while others were distinctly disadvantaged (Tanzania AIDS Project, 1994). Some orphans face many social and economic problems, ranging from higher morbidity and mortality to a higher probability of dropping out of school (Tanzania AIDS Project, 1994). In Zambia, some orphans face food and clothing shortages, as well as a lack of access to education and health services (Social Policy Research Group, 1993). Furthermore, the frequently reported practice of property grabbing of the deceased's estate by the extended family results in the orphan's loss of property and household goods (Social Policy Research Group, 1993). While the available anecdotal evidence cites a range of serious problems that orphans may confront, there is a need for reliable estimates of the frequency—or rarity—with which orphans slip through informal safety nets to encounter these problems.

Orphanhood and the loss of traditional support mechanisms for the elderly as a result of AIDS will unquestionably become increasingly large problems. We need to know how many orphans and unsupported elderly there will be; what social mechanisms are being employed to care for them; what effects orphanhood has on children's own development and on the welfare of the nation; and what services could usefully be provided to these individuals, given resource constraints.

INDIRECT IMPACT OF AIDS ON THE REST OF SOCIETY

This section addresses the indirect impact of the HIV/AIDS epidemic on society at large, focusing in turn on demographic and economic impact.

Demographic Impact

AIDS has a number of demographic and related consequences. Among the more important are effects on future population growth, demand for health services, the size of the potential labor force, educational needs, and support for the elderly. Moreover, household composition and living arrangements are influenced by the AIDS pandemic through orphanhood and widowhood. To understand the consequences of AIDS, a wide range of data is needed. It is necessary to have baseline demographic information and to gather data on the progression of HIV, perinatal transmission, the process of incubation, and mortality risk.

Morbidity and Mortality

In several African countries in the main AIDS belt, AIDS has already become the major cause of adult mortality, doubling or tripling the adult mortality rates over levels that were already eight times higher than those in developed countries. AIDS is also a growing cause of infant and child mortality, threatening to reverse the reductions in infant and child mortality rates achieved to date. In countries such as Uganda, where an estimated 1.3 million persons out of a total population of 17 million are infected, AIDS looms as the predominant health problem for the entire population.

The excess female morbidity and mortality from HIV infection have important implications for the social and economic roles of women. The rising infection rates among women are accompanied by a corresponding rise in the number of children with perinatal HIV infection, estimated at around 1 million cumulative infections as of 1994 (World Health Organization, 1994) (see also Chapter 5). Transmission rates of HIV infection from an infected mother to her child in Africa are estimated to average about 30 percent, so the 70 percent of infants who remain uninfected are potential future orphans as the result of the premature death of one or both parents from AIDS (Chin, 1990).

AIDS has become the leading cause of hospital admissions in such cities as Abidjan, Côte d'Ivoire, and Kinshasa, Zaire. In Abidjan, where the first AIDS cases were recognized in 1985, AIDS has rapidly become the leading cause of death among men and the second leading cause of death, after complications related to pregnancy and abortion, among women (De Cock et al., 1990). In a 1990 study, 41 percent of male and 32 percent of female cadavers were found to be infected with HIV. AIDS kills people in their most productive years, and now ranks among the leading causes of potential healthy life-years lost in sub-Saharan Africa. In the Abidjan study, it was estimated that 15 percent of adult male deaths and 17 percent of male years of potential life lost resulted from AIDS, whereas among women, AIDS accounted for 13 percent of deaths and 12 percent of years of potential life lost. These figures probably underestimate the true mortality due to HIV infection. Factors leading to an underassessment of AIDS-related deaths include the exclusion of pediatric patients, the rigidity of the case definition used, a lack of clinical information concerning cause of death, and the desire of seriously ill persons who leave Abidjan to die in their home areas. Moreover, death due to pulmonary tuberculosis, the third-ranking cause of male adult death, was not specifically counted as caused by AIDS, although 50 percent of these cadavers were HIV-seropositive, and an important fraction of these deaths was probably attributable to HIV infection (De Cock et al., 1990).

In two community-based rural studies, in Masaka district and Rakai district, Uganda, mortality among HIV-infected adults, at over 100 per 1,000 person-years of observation, was found to be 10 times higher than that among adults not infected with HIV (Mulder et al., 1994b; Sewankambo et al., 1994). In both districts, which have an underlying adult HIV prevalence of 8 and 13 percent, respectively, HIV was found to be the leading cause of death among adults. For example, over 80 percent of deaths in the 20-29 age group occurred among those who were HIV-infected. In Rakai, HIV mortality was found to have resulted in substantial slowing in the rate of natural population increase, although the population continues to experience a positive growth rate, even in that stratum of villages where adult HIV prevalence exceeds 30 percent (Sewankambo et al., 1994).

Although data concerning mortality due to AIDS are scarce in other countries, it is likely that AIDS is the leading cause of adult death in several African cities and possibly some rural areas, especially those in the main HIV belt (Kitange et al., 1994; Nelson et al., 1991; Sewankambo et al., 1994; Mulder, 1994b; De Cock et al., 1990).

The demographic impact of AIDS will continue to expand in the remainder of this decade and into the next century as the epidemic continues to spread and mature. The deaths to date have occurred among those individuals infected relatively early in the epidemic, through the mid-1980s. In future years, those infected since the late 1980s will develop AIDS and die. In general, in the countries of sub-Saharan Africa, characterized by high population mobility and urbanization, high levels of STDs, and a doubling of infection rates in less than one year, there is a very limited time within which to curb the spread of HIV infection. AIDS has the potential to undo many of the current health, social, developmental, and political gains in Africa.

Anticipated Future Impact

Mathematical modeling can help us anticipate the demographic impact of the HIV/AIDS epidemic. The anticipated impact through the remainder of this decade would occur even if AIDS prevention and control programs were able to reduce the incidence of HIV infection drastically in the coming years. The vast majority of the excess deaths due to AIDS projected to occur in the 1990s will be among those who are now in the incubation stage of infection. Furthermore, WHO estimates that annual spending on AIDS control and prevention programs would have to increase by more than a factor of five to reduce by half the number of new HIV infections by the year 2000 (World Health Organization, 1993).

The results of several scenarios developed using the Interagency Working Group on AIDS (IWGAIDS) model (Stanley et al., 1989; Seitz, 1991) were applied to 13 sub-Saharan African countries in which low-risk urban seroprevalence was estimated to exceed 5 percent in the early 1990s (Way and Stanecki, 1994). For each country, the spread of HIV infection was projected based on recent trends, and the impact of each country's epidemic was estimated using the model (see Way and Stanecki, 1994, Appendix A, for a full description of the methodology). In the discussion that follows, the projected demographic impact for those 13 countries is presented for the year 2000.

In most African countries, the crude death rate is relatively low as the result of a young age structure and recent declines in mortality. By the year 2000, AIDS will double the number of deaths and the crude death rate in many of the countries most affected by the epidemic, as compared with the levels expected in the absence of AIDS (Figure 6-1). The magnitude of the impact varies because of both the severity of the projected epidemic and the underlying non-AIDS mortality levels.

As noted earlier, the HIV/AIDS epidemic in Africa is primarily heterosexual, with a consequently greater role for mother-to-child transmission. Although HIV transmission may occur in only one-quarter to one-half of births to HIV-infected women, the fact that most of the children thus infected die before age 5 implies a significant impact on the infant and child mortality rates. The impact is relatively larger on the child than on the infant mortality rate since many infected children survive beyond their first birthday, and since other causes of mortality under age 5 tend to be more severe under age 1 (Figure 6-2).

Life expectancy at birth, the single best summary measure of mortality, also shows a strong impact of the HIV/AIDS epidemic (Figure 6-3). Because AIDS deaths are concentrated among children and young adults, their effect is substantial, reducing life expectancy by over 20 years in several countries. The impact of AIDS on life expectancy at birth is not directly proportional to the severity of the

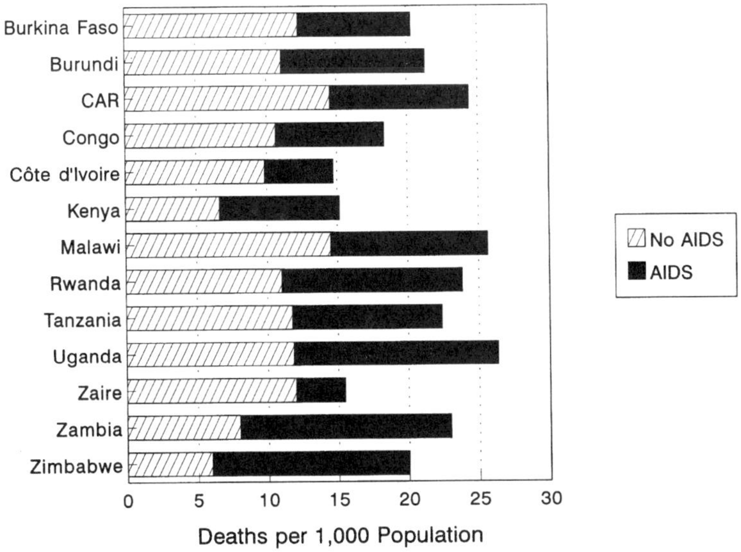

FIGURE 6-1 Crude Death Rate With and Without AIDS, for Selected Countries: 2000. SOURCE: U.S. Bureau of the Census, International Programs Center, personal communication, 1995.

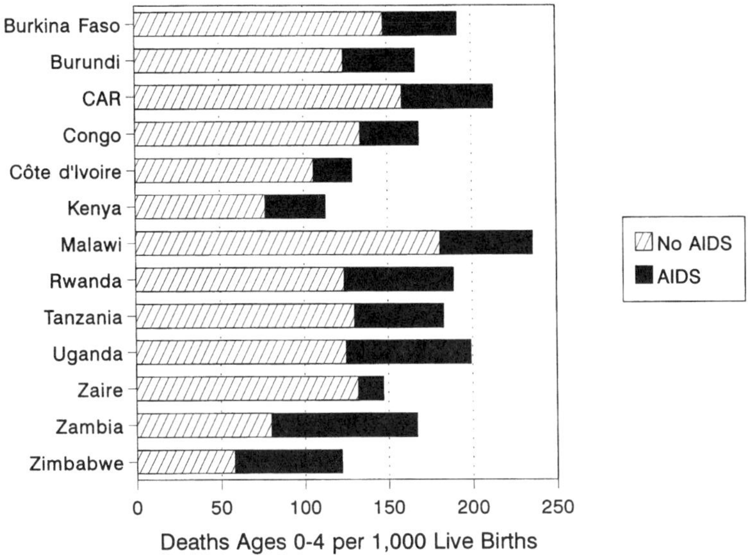

FIGURE 6-2 Child Mortality Rate With and Without AIDS, for Selected Countries: 2000. SOURCE: U.S. Bureau of the Census, International Programs Center, personal communication, 1995.

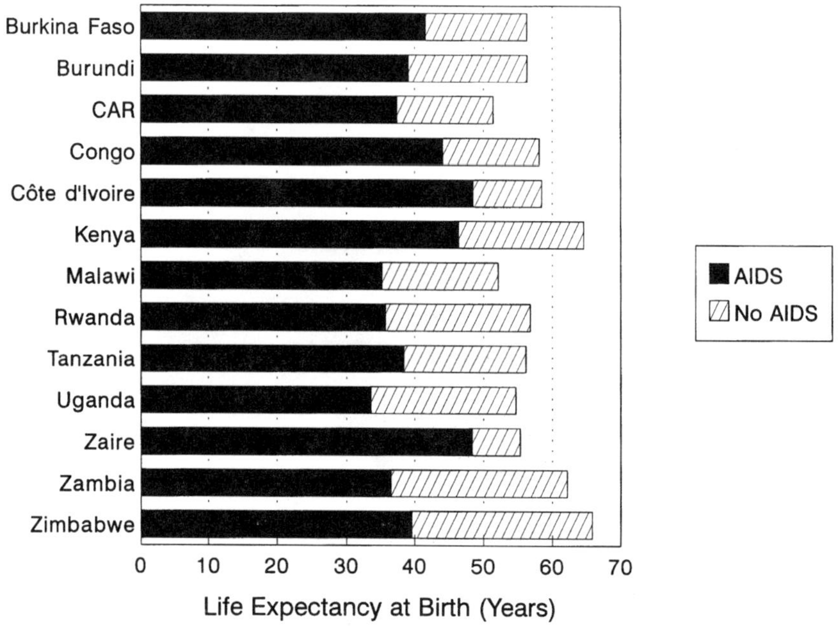

FIGURE 6-3 Life Expectancy at Birth With and Without AIDS, for Selected Countries: 2000. SOURCE: U.S. Bureau of the Census, International Programs Center, personal communication, 1995.

HIV/AIDS epidemic, however, since the number of years of potential life lost for a death at a given age varies. For example, the death of a woman at age 30 in Zimbabwe has a greater impact on life expectancy than the death of a woman of the same age in Malawi since Zimbabwean women have a higher life expectancy at that age, and hence more potential years of life are lost as the result of one death.

Clearly, then, the impact of AIDS on a number of mortality measures in affected countries will be great. Infant/child mortality and life expectancy, which had experienced a 30- to 40-year period of improvement in many of these countries, are already showing the impact of AIDS and will suffer further setbacks in coming years. Development programs and child survival projects, which have used such measures as indicators of program impact, will be forced to attempt to factor out the effect of AIDS or develop alternative indicators.

But will AIDS decimate the sub-Saharan region? Will family planning programs become redundant as the population of country after country begins to decline? All indications are that these extreme outcomes will not take place. Largely because of current high population growth rates resulting from high fertility levels, no country in sub-Saharan Africa is projected to experience a population decline (negative population growth) as a result of AIDS. Several factors will contribute to this result. Because of the long incubation period of HIV infection, relatively high HIV seroprevalence is required to overcome the 3 to 4 percent growth rate currently found in most African countries. For example, a national adult seroprevalence of 40 percent or higher would typically be required (Stover, 1994).[4]

As discussed earlier, HIV seroprevalence approaching this level is currently found in some urban areas. Thus far, however, no country has experienced, or is even projected based on our analysis to come close to, such levels of infection at a national level. Available data suggest that there are differences in sexual behavior between urban and rural populations and that even within urban areas, large proportions of the population do not engage in behaviors that put them at risk of infection. These factors will tend, especially in the long run, to limit the spread of the HIV/AIDS epidemic. In addition, AIDS intervention programs are under way in most countries of the region. Although these programs are limited in scope and resources, some evidence of behavior change is becoming available. It is likely that additional change will result as the mortality effect of AIDS is felt by increasing numbers of households in a country.

Projections indicate that population growth rates will be sharply reduced by the impact of the HIV/AIDS epidemic, as one would surmise based on the above data on crude death rates. In many countries, population growth rates in the year 2000 will decline by more than one percentage point as compared with those expected in the absence of AIDS. Nonetheless, growth rates in the affected countries will typically be around 2 percent, as compared with non-AIDS projected growth rates of about 3 percent (Figure 6-4). The lowest projected growth rate among these AIDS-affected countries is in Zimbabwe (about 1.2 percent).

How much effect will AIDS have on the future size of populations? As shown in Figure 6-5, population size is clearly affected by AIDS, but the resulting deficit in population is not too great. In the aggregate, the projected total populations of the 13 countries in the year 2000 will be about 16.7 million lower as a result of AIDS as compared with the non-AIDS scenario (224.8 versus 241.4 million). This difference, however, is not due entirely to AIDS deaths. Some of the difference is due to the deficit in births to women who would have given birth had they not died from AIDS (either as infants/children or as adults). In longer-term projections, there is also a cumulative effect of the deficit due to the lack of births to those potential offspring.

An additional, potentially important impact of the HIV/AIDS epidemic may also be noted: its possible impact on family planning programs. Populations

---

[4]In rural Rakai district, Uganda, trading centers with an HIV prevalence of 35 percent among adults had an annual rate of natural increase of 1.1 percent (Sewankambo et al., 1994).

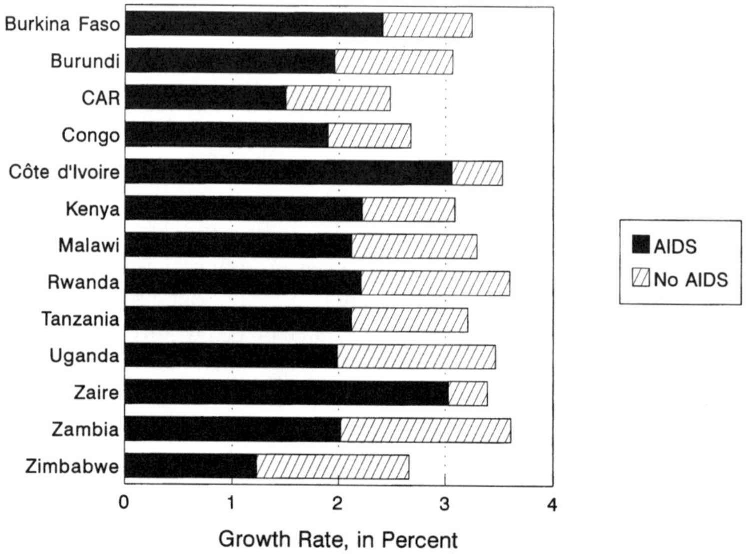

FIGURE 6-4 Population Growth Rates With and Without AIDS, for Selected Countries: 2000. SOURCE: U.S. Bureau of the Census, International Programs Center, personal communication, 1995.

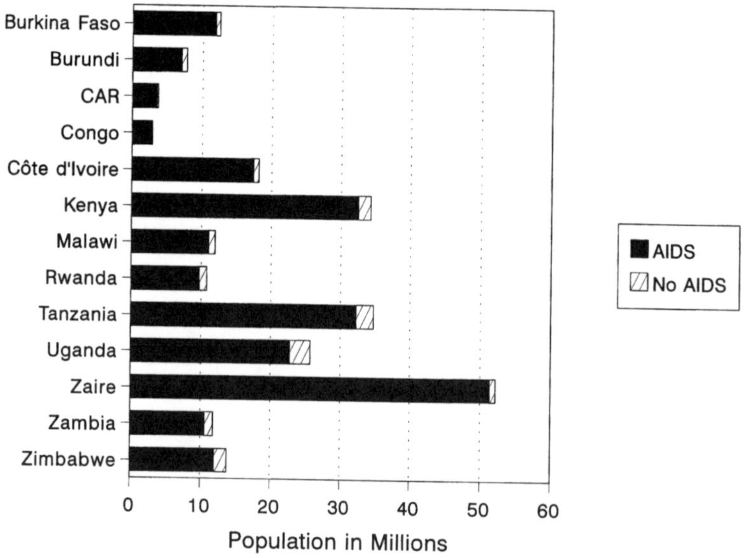

FIGURE 6-5 Total Population Size With and Without AIDS, for Selected Countries: 2000. SOURCE: U.S. Bureau of the Census, International Programs Center, personal communication, 1995.

experiencing elevated mortality as a result of AIDS may be reluctant to accept any services that may further reduce their completed family size (Wasserheit, 1989). There are as yet few formal data regarding this issue. However, in rural Uganda, community health workers have expressed some reluctance to distribute condoms, which were seen as further reducing birth rates in the face of population loss due to HIV (Joseph Konde-Lule, personal communication, 1995). In the same setting, an STD control project encountered concerns regarding STD medication because segments of the population were suspicious that the antibiotics were actually oral contraceptives being administered as part of an overall plan to reduce the local population through AIDS and family planning. These problems were successfully resolved through community education (Nelson K. Sewankambo, personal communication, 1994).

AIDS is not the only major health problem in sub-Saharan Africa, but in many countries throughout the region the impact of AIDS—at least until the year 2000 and perhaps well beyond—will increasingly be felt. Increases in infant and child mortality will be accompanied by increases in adult mortality, reducing life expectancy. Population growth will decline more rapidly than expected, and African populations will be somewhat smaller in the year 2000 than they would have been without AIDS. In many African countries affected by AIDS, deaths will more than double during the decade of the 1990s as compared with the number expected without AIDS. These additional deaths will put increasing strains on already overburdened health-care systems and on individual households trying to manage with limited economic resources. Care and support for orphans will be a growing concern, and traditional inheritance and other legal rights will be challenged. Although no country will experience an overall decline in population, the impact of AIDS—not only demographic, but also social and economic—will be enormous throughout the region.

Relationship Between Seroprevalence and Mortality Rates

In examining the impact of AIDS on society, it is useful to review the arithmetic consequences for adult mortality of what is known or believed about the epidemiology of HIV in sub-Saharan Africa. As discussed in Chapter 3, rates of prevalence of HIV infection among low-risk adults in sub-Saharan Africa range from zero among large portions of the rural populations of many countries to as high as 30 to 40 percent among the urban populations of Zambia and Rwanda. However, without careful attention to the arithmetic of this slow plague, it is easy to overestimate the effect of even these very high infection rates on adult mortality.

Table 6-1 presents the calculations required to approximate the mortality impact of various levels of seroprevalence on a cohort of 1,000 African adults aged 15 to 50. Column 2 of the table gives the number of adults in the cohort who would be infected at each rate of infection in column 1. Columns 3 and 4 present

TABLE 6-1 Impact of Seroprevalence of HIV on the Annual Mortality Experience of 1,000 African Adults, Aged 15 to 50

Seroprevalence (%)	Number of HIV+	Annual Deaths from HIV with Median Incubation Period		Deaths Without HIV	Total Deaths per Year with Median Incubation Period	
		10	5		10	5
0	0	0	0	5	5	5
5	50	2.5	5	5	7.5	10
10	100	5	10	5	10	15
15	150	7.5	15	5	12.5	20
20	200	10	20	5	15	25
30	300	15	30	5	20	35
45	450	22.5	45	5	27.5	50
90	900	45	90	5	50	95

NOTE: Annual deaths are estimated by assuming that (1) all infected individuals die of HIV within 2 × M years after their infection and (2) deaths are distributed uniformly from the first year of infection to 2 × Mth year, where M is the assumed median incubation period. Thus, if M were 10, 5% of the infected would die each year, and if M were 5, 10% of the infected would die each year. Adding the baseline deaths to the HIV deaths assumes that those who die of HIV are different individuals from those who would have died in the baseline scenario. This assumption that the risk of HIV does not "compete" with the baseline risks is approximately valid unless seroprevalence rates become extremely high.

the number of deaths from HIV infection that would occur under two different extreme assumptions regarding the median incubation period of the epidemic in Africa. Thus, with an HIV prevalence of 20 percent, HIV would cause the death of between 10 and 20 adults per year in this cohort. Column 5 presents the baseline mortality for African adults in the absence of HIV infection, which is assumed to be 5 per 1,000 in this age group. Columns 6 and 7 give the total deaths in the cohort obtained by adding the baseline deaths to the deaths caused by HIV under each of the two assumptions regarding the incubation period.

There is a good deal of uncertainty surrounding the length of time from HIV infection to AIDS-related symptomatic disease and from symptomatic disease to death for AIDS cases in sub-Saharan Africa. Some investigators have speculated that the latency period from HIV infection to an AIDS-defining opportunistic infection may be shorter in sub-Saharan Africa than it is in North America or Europe because of high levels of other infections that may occur concurrently, such as malaria, trypanosomiasis, and filariasis, and are also known to have a major effect on the immune system (Quinn et al., 1987). Furthermore, the time between an AIDS-defining illness and death is substantially shorter in sub-Saharan Africa than in North America or Europe because most Africans do not have access to or cannot afford drugs that prevent or treat AIDS-related opportunistic infections or slow replication of the virus (Ryder and Mugerwa, 1994). Consequently, the length of time from HIV infection to death in sub-Saharan Africa is shorter than it is in North America or Europe, and death rates are higher at every level of prevalence (see Table 6-1). Recent results from a prospective cohort study in rural Uganda suggest that progression from HIV infection to death in sub-Saharan Africa is extremely rapid (Mulder et al., 1994a).

Columns 6 and 7 of Table 6-1 demonstrate that a 20 percent seroprevalence is likely to cause a 3- to 5-fold increase in prime-age adult mortality, from 5 to 15-25 per 1,000. Among groups where the seroprevalence rises to between 45 and 90 percent, mortality might rise by a factor of 10. However, it is important to realize that, even with a 5-year incubation period, a 90 percent seroprevalence would result in no more than 95 deaths per 1,000 per year. Note in particular that a seroprevalence of 90 percent does not produce a mortality rate of 90 percent (or 900 per 1,000) in that year.

Economic Impact

HIV/AIDS and Per Capita Income Growth

The arithmetic of Table 6-1 has implications for the magnitude of the impact of the epidemic on various aggregates of the population. Using a range of sophisticated demographic models, demographers predict that the disease will slow the rate of growth of the population in sub-Saharan Africa by approximately one percentage point (Bongaarts and Way, 1989; Bos and Bulatao, 1992; Stover, 1993; Way and Stanecki, 1993; Bongaarts, 1994). While a reduction of one percentage point in the rate of growth of an African population will not halt population growth in countries that are currently growing at 3 percent per year, a one-third decrease in the population growth rate is sizeable. If a family planning program were to reduce the population growth rate of an African country by this much, it would be declared a resounding success and would be presumed to yield many benefits for the country.

It is obvious that a higher mortality rate is a terrible way to achieve a lower rate of population growth and that a decrease in population growth caused by the HIV/AIDS epidemic will generate immense human suffering that would not exist if the same decrease were caused by a voluntary family planning program. However, setting aside this difference, is it possible that the reduction in population

TABLE 6-2 Contrast Between the Impacts on National Economic Growth of Comparable Reductions in Population Growth Caused by a Family Planning Program and an HIV/AIDS Epidemic

Nature of Impact on Income Growth	Source of Reduction in Population Growth	
	Family Planning Program	HIV/AIDS Epidemic
Impact on growth of capital	A1. Fewer children will reduce schooling expenses. A portion of this reduction may be saved, financing physical investment, and a portion may be spent on lengthening the schooling of each child. Both of these results would increase the earnings of the next generation of workers.	B1. Increased expenditures on medical care may come partly from savings, slowing the accumulation of physical capital. B2. The presence of an epidemic may induce households to increase their precautionary saving in anticipation of future health problems. This effect offsets, to an unknown degree, the additional costs incurred at the time of AIDS sickness and death.[a]
Impact on growth of labor	C1. The growth of the labor force slows.	D1. The growth of the labor force slows.
Impact on productivity of workers	E1. Reduced child care per adult worker may reduce absenteeism and increase productivity. E2. Increased schooling per child may increase later productivity.	F1. When an HIV-infected worker converts to AIDS, productivity is reduced by sickness and absenteeism. F2. Increased health-care expenses per worker increase employer costs without improving workers' net remuneration. F3. The time of healthy workers is diverted to care for the sick family members. F4. Increased worker attrition due to AIDS sickness and death increases employer costs per worker. F5. To the extent that AIDS increases the morbidity and attrition of top-level managers and professionals, employers' costs rise more for the same number of deaths. F6. Children may be withdrawn from school to help at home, decreasing their future productivity.

TABLE 6-2 Continued

Nature of Impact on Income Growth	Source of Reduction in Population Growth	
	Family Planning Program	HIV/AIDS Epidemic
Impact on the mix of workers	G1. More-educated parents are usually more likely to adopt family planning. Thus, unless a national program reaches out to the poor with particular vigor, it may reduce the growth rate of educated workers more than that of uneducated workers	H1. The impact on the mix of workers depends on the epidemiology of the epidemic. In many sub-Saharan African countries, education is a risk factor for men and for their wives, while poverty is a risk factor for single urban women.
Impact on the efficiency of the production process	I1. None.	J1. Loss of a top manager may induce chaos in the organization and destroy it. J2. Lower life expectancy among the population may increase the rate at which even businessmen discount the future and therefore may reduce the enforceability of contracts and increase crime.

[a]Only if households fully anticipated future health costs from AIDS sickness and discounted those future costs at a relatively low discount rate would the precautionary saving of item B2 in this row offset the increased medical costs of item B1. This level of precautionary saving seems quite unlikely in poor sub-Saharan African societies.

growth caused by the epidemic could benefit the survivors? The differing consequences of the two processes in slowing population growth are worth comparing to see why the HIV/AIDS epidemic might slow per capita income growth, while the family planning program might speed it up.

Table 6-2 shows several differences between the impact on national income growth of comparable reductions in population growth caused by a family planning program and an HIV/AIDS epidemic. This table is based on a simple model of economic growth, which assumes that the growth rate of national income depends on the growth of the factors of production of national output—capital and labor—and on changes in the efficiency with which these factors are used and combined.

Both family planning and an HIV/AIDS epidemic are likely to slow the growth of total national output simply because they both slow population growth. However, Table 6-2 makes clear that the HIV/AIDS epidemic is likely to slow output growth more than a similar decrease in population growth caused by family planning. The first row of the table contrasts the positive likely impact of family planning and the negative likely impact of the HIV/AIDS epidemic on national savings rates. Although labor-force growth would be slowed in both scenarios, the third row of the table shows that the family planning slowdown would enhance labor productivity, while the HIV/AIDS epidemic will have six distinct negative effects on labor productivity, both now and in the future. By increasing employers' costs of labor relative to capital, the epidemic will bias employers toward labor-saving and away from labor-using technologies.

The fourth row of the table points out that family planning and HIV infection could both change the mix of workers in the same direction—toward a less-skilled work force. In the case of the family planning program, unless a national policy of targeting the program to the poorest households is extraordinarily effective, higher-income households will demand more family planning services and make more use of the program than will the poor. By slowing the growth of the educated labor force more than that of the uneducated, the program will have the unintended consequence of decreasing the proportion of the work force with more education.[5]

For HIV, the argument rests first on the ubiquitous observation that infection rates are higher in urban areas, where average levels of education are the highest, and second on the hypothetical link between male socioeconomic status and casual sexual activity. Evidence from recent surveys of sexual behavior supports the hypothesis that men of higher status (specifically, men with higher educational attainment) have more casual sex partners per year (Caraël et al., 1994). The finding holds for men throughout the world, and for eight of the nine surveyed African countries (Caraël et al., 1994). Thus it is not surprising that where data on male HIV prevalence by socioeconomic status exist, they often show higher prevalence at higher income or education levels (see Ainsworth and Over, 1994b, for a recent review of the evidence on the current rate of HIV infection in sub-Saharan Africa by economic group). Since African populations are known to have improved greatly their understanding of the causes of AIDS since the risk behavior that resulted in the higher infection rates at higher social levels occurred, it is possible that this relationship has since been reversed. However, no data have yet been collected to demonstrate that more highly educated African men have responded to their improved knowledge of the causes of AIDS by (1) having fewer casual sex partners than less-educated men, (2) having safer sex more often than less-educated men, or (3) becoming infected at a lower rate than less-educated men. Moreover, even if such changes have occurred, the pattern of the epidemic for the next decade or two has been set by past risk behaviors and prevalence patterns. Those patterns make it likely that HIV will kill relatively

[5]Of course, if the higher-income families reduce their children by a larger percentage than the poor, they will also save more educational expenses and will therefore have more resources available to be rechanneled into the education of the children they do have. This effect may partly offset the change in mix described in the text.

more of the more highly educated workers, thus changing the mix of the work force toward the less educated. Note that higher *prevalence and incidence* of HIV infection among the more educated are entirely consistent with higher *numbers* of HIV-infected being uneducated. For predicting the impact of the epidemic on economic growth, the rates are more important than the absolute numbers.

Finally, the fifth row of Table 6-2 points to two more speculative impacts of the epidemic. First, the loss of a top manager could cause his or her firm to collapse. This outcome would occur in any situation where the skills embodied in the departing manager were so rare in the country that they could not be replaced in time to save the firm. Second, high levels of seroprevalence may engender a reduced concern for the future, with potentially deleterious effects on all formal or informal, explicit or implicit contractual relationships in the economy.

Table 6-2 should make clear that similar declines in the rate of population growth caused by family planning and by the HIV/AIDS epidemic could be expected to have quite different impacts on economic growth. A few authors have attempted to quantify the effects of HIV on macroeconomic growth in sub-Saharan Africa by constructing simulation models of African economies and shocking them with HIV/AIDS epidemics that would reduce population and labor-force growth from about 3 to about 2 percent per year. Cuddington and Hancock (1994) and Cuddington (1993) have focused on the impacts of the epidemic on savings and on the reduced productivity of workers on the job. Over (1992) has modeled impacts on savings and the socioeconomic gradient of the infection, as the latter affects the mix of workers across and within the rural and urban sectors of the economy.

Cuddington and Hancock (1994) simulate the effect of AIDS in Malawi, assuming that population growth slows by 1.2 percentage points, treatment costs are financed entirely from savings, and workers with AIDS are half as productive as their healthy counterparts. The authors predict that gross domestic product growth rates would be between 0.2 and 0.3 percentage points lower in a medium scenario and between 1.2 and 1.5 percentage points lower in an extreme scenario. Under similar assumptions about treatment costs and productivity, but assuming a slightly smaller slowdown in population growth, Cuddington (1993) predicts that the epidemic would have a slightly smaller effect in Tanzania.

Over (1992) finds that the *distribution* of a one percentage point reduction in labor-force growth rate within a population will determine whether the epidemic reduces or increases the rate of growth of per capita income. Figure 6-6 presents the simulated impact of a one percentage point decrease in the growth rate of the population on the growth rate of per capita gross domestic product in 10 African countries (Over, 1992). Note that not only the magnitude but also the direction of the impact depend critically on which elements of the population are hardest hit. If the infection rate of the more highly educated is twice or four times as high as

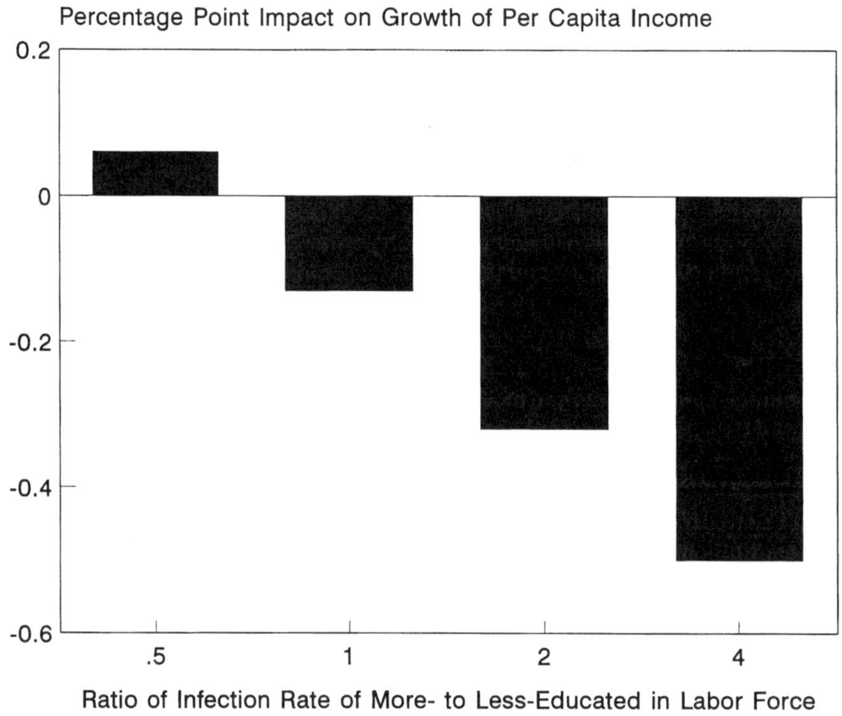

FIGURE 6-6 Sensitivity of the Estimated Impact of an HIV Epidemic with Respect to the Socioeconomic Gradient of Infection. NOTE: Assumes that half of AIDS treatment costs are financed from savings. SOURCE: Over (1992).

that of the less educated, as is likely to be the case while HIV/AIDS remains a predominantly urban epidemic, the disease may slow growth in gross domestic product by more than it slows population growth, thereby slowing the growth of per capita gross domestic product by as much as half a percentage point. In economies that are struggling to return to positive per capita growth rates after years of stagnation, this consequence represents a substantial additional handicap. On the other hand, if HIV infection follows the pattern of other endemic diseases in developing countries by infecting a higher proportion of the poor than of the nonpoor, the loss of these less productive workers will reduce growth in gross domestic product less than proportionately, leading to a net increase in the growth rate of per capita gross domestic product. This result, which is illustrated by the left-most bar in Figure 6-6, parallels exactly the effects of the twelfth-century European black plague: the death of approximately one-third of the population in approximately 3 years led to an increase in the ratio of land to labor, and thus increased the average productivity and wages of the remaining workers.

Both of the models described above show that the impact of AIDS will depend importantly on the nature and degree of reduction in savings caused by the epidemic. Estimates of the impact of HIV infection on individual savings behavior will inform future macroeconomic models of the impact of the epidemic. However, greatly improved understanding of the microeconomic dynamic coping behavior of households will be required before such macroeconomic models can fully capture the complexities of the effects the epidemic will have on the economy.

Effect of the Epidemic on Sectors of Economic Activity

Illness and death from AIDS will affect productivity, turnover, training costs, and resource allocation. Productivity is liable to suffer from absenteeism of both sick and healthy workers. Sick workers will miss work because of illness; healthy workers are liable to miss work as they care for the dying or attend funerals, the latter being a custom which in Africa often involves extensive travel and can take many days.

Policy makers sometimes inquire whether a few sectors of the economy are likely to be particularly vulnerable to the HIV/AIDS epidemic and therefore might benefit from sector-specific mitigation policies. In this regard, it is necessary to distinguish between the health sector and all other sectors of the economy.

The Health Sector There is little disagreement that the health sector faces a potential crisis. In the presence of a major HIV/AIDS epidemic, the health sector will experience a large rise in demand, which will continue to increase in the coming years, as well as decreased supply through increased worker absenteeism and attrition.

AIDS will certainly result in a rise in the demand for health care, although the magnitude of this increase is impossible to predict. Cost assessments of the impact of the disease on the demand for health care are complicated. First, AIDS increases the prevalence of opportunistic infections that are already widespread in the region, such as tuberculosis, pneumonia, and malaria, and it is difficult to recognize whether these diseases are symptoms of AIDS (Ainsworth and Over, 1994a). Second, there is a huge difference between the type of care that would be provided ideally and the type of care that is realistic in sub-Saharan Africa, where drugs for controlling opportunistic infections and skilled nursing staff are in such short supply. While we can be certain that Africans will seek some medical care for opportunistic infections and illnesses, research has yet to ascertain the percentage of Africans with AIDS who seek professional medical care, the type and amount of care they seek, or how much they pay for it. Nevertheless, the effects of an increase in the demand for medical care in sub-Saharan African countries, where this kind of service is already in short supply, cannot be welcome. In addition to increasing health-care costs on both a personal and a national level, services provided to persons with AIDS will further limit the availability of professional-service time, hospital space, and medications for other patients, some of whom will have curable maladies. In general, however, despite the obvious seriousness of the epidemic for the health sector in Africa, just how the epidemic will ultimately affect the supply, demand, and quality of health care on the continent is still unknown.

The public sector provides a substantial portion of all health care in Africa, and public health-care facilities can neither fairly raise prices in the short run nor realistically increase capacity in the longer run. The public health system may instead be forced to resort to rationing its hospital beds and to placing increasingly stringent service requirements on its publicly employed physicians in order to keep them from leaving to work in private clinics. Neither of these solutions is desirable. Whether the epidemic results in higher prices, as in a private system, or rationed beds, as in most public ones, the result will be to crowd out some patients suffering from curable ailments who have neither the money to pay for private care nor the connections to obtain care in the rationed public system.

The health-care sector will also be confronted with the increased mortality of health-care professionals due to HIV/AIDS. A recent study conducted in Zambia indicated that female nurses at two hospitals have experienced a 13-fold increase in mortality since 1980 (Buvé et al., 1994). Mann et al. (1986) found a seroprevalence of 6.4 percent among 2,384 hospital workers in Mama Yemo Hospital in Kinshasa, Zaire, although they found no difference in seroprevalence between nurses providing care to people with AIDS and other nurses. To the degree that health workers themselves succumb to AIDS, their greater scarcity will further increase the price of, or reduce access to, care for the poor.

The medical costs of treating a person with AIDS are considerable. Excluding associated costs such as transportation, medical care can cost hundreds or even thousands of dollars per case (Ainsworth and Over, 1994b; Shepard, 1991; World Bank, 1992a). Efforts at extrapolation are in their infancy and continue to rely on guesswork for major variables. The more affected nations—Zimbabwe, Kenya, Malawi, Tanzania, and Rwanda—may have spent between 23 and 66 percent of their 1990 public-health-care budgets on AIDS-related treatment alone (Ainsworth and Over, 1994b). The factors identified as determining the level of spending include the severity of the epidemic, the strength of the economy, and the availability of medical care. AIDS commandeered far less of the total health spending of these nations in 1990: between 3 and 30 percent (Ainsworth and Over, 1994b). In Zambia, average costs of visits for people with AIDS in 1993 ranged from US $17 for care in a rural health clinic to US $66 for care at a district hospital (Foster, 1993). Given that the demand for resources associated with caring for HIV-infected individuals competes with other similarly urgent health concerns, it is essential that we ascertain the most cost-effective approach to treating people with AIDS.

How the health sector will and should adjust to the increasing demand and decreasing supply resulting from the HIV/AIDS epidemic must be studied as the disease progresses.

Other Sectors For most other economic sectors, both demand and supply are expected to decrease as a result of the epidemic; furthermore, the slow nature of the epidemic will allow time for those sectors to adjust. The direct impacts of HIV/AIDS in most economic sectors may therefore be difficult to detect.

The Agricultural Sector Agriculture constitutes the primary economic sector of most of the African countries severely affected by the epidemic, employing a large percentage of the labor force and accounting for a major portion of gross domestic product and export earnings. For example, three of the sub-Saharan African countries hardest hit by the epidemic—Kenya, Tanzania, and Côte d'Ivoire—depend on agricultural products for over 70 percent of their exports; in four of the other most severely affected countries—Burundi, Malawi, Rwanda, and Uganda—that figure is over 90 percent (World Bank, 1992b). The effects of HIV/AIDS on the agricultural sector are therefore likely to reverberate throughout the national economy of these countries. As the epidemic progresses, agriculture, like most economic sectors in Africa, will be forced to adjust in some way to both the decrease in adult labor and the decrease in national demand.

Although there has been a great deal of conjecture about the impact of AIDS on the agricultural sector, the analyses to date have generally focused on the impact of an adult death on a given agricultural household; they ignore the possibility that a neighboring household that has not suffered an adult death can use the land that the affected household may not be able to use. In rural areas, where the vast majority of the labor force is engaged in subsistence farming and where migration to the city has already reduced the number of people of prime working age, the additional burden of AIDS-related morbidity and mortality may be significant. To the extent that agricultural labor is already fully employed, AIDS can be expected to result in declining agricultural production relative to predictions without AIDS. Yet analyses of the epidemic's impact on agriculture have also paid scant attention to the reduction in demand for food crops, especially from the urban sector. Insofar as AIDS-related deaths decrease national demand for agricultural products relative to a no-AIDS scenario—as indeed they must—the effects of a decrease in production may be mitigated. Data are not yet available to clarify the net result, although the loss of the main food-producing age group suggests that there will be a food deficit in the affected areas.

The ultimate impact of AIDS on production and exports will depend most heavily on how households respond to the crisis. Households continue to constitute the major agricultural production units in sub-Saharan Africa; their decision making about crop selection and labor inputs will shape the availability and prices of both domestic foodstuffs and exports. Some subsistence crops, such as maize, sweet potatoes, and cassava, are substantially less labor-intensive than export crops such as cotton or tobacco (Norse, 1991; Gillespie, 1989). Consequently, the epidemic may result in an increase in the production of subsistence crops relative to export crops as the agricultural labor crisis deepens. Research on the economic impact of AIDS in the agricultural sector is still too preliminary to indicate whether this substitution will occur and what further impact it will have.

It may also be noted that AIDS is just one of the many stresses on the rural labor force. Africans suffer from many tropical and infectious diseases, and identifying the distinct impact of any one presents enormous difficulties in research design.

Attempts to measure the effects of AIDS on agricultural production have found little conclusive evidence thus far. Barnett and Blaikie (1992) observe that the abundant rainfall and types of crops grown in the Rakai and Masaka districts of Uganda allowed even these heavily affected areas to adjust to the loss of adult labor to AIDS. Gillespie (1989) estimates the impact of AIDS on each of the five agricultural areas of Rwanda. He proposes that the impact of the epidemic on agriculture will depend on how labor is employed: the seasonality of labor demands, the degree of age and sex specialization, the independence of labor inputs, the economies of scale in labor, and the feasibility of employing labor-saving technology. More empirical research is needed to test his hypothesis.

A rapid assessment of the effects of HIV/AIDS on farming systems and rural livelihoods in Uganda, Tanzania, and Zambia was recently prepared by the Food and Agriculture Organization (FAO) (Barnett, 1994). Despite the high national seroprevalence and cumulative number of AIDS cases in all three countries, the research team had difficulty documenting the impact of the epidemic. In Zambia, they collected some evidence that the epidemic is affecting individual households in certain areas. It is also having an impact on the supply of skilled and educated workers in the estate sector, but this labor shortage does not have serious financial implications. Only in one part of Uganda—Gwanda—was the research team able to find significant impacts. Based on a study of only 14 households, of which 12 were either affected or afflicted by AIDS, the team hypothesized that in AIDS-affected agricultural areas, farmers will shift to more basic and less varied food and other crop production. It is unclear, however, how the larger economy is coping. Indeed, the study reports that in Kasensero, located a few kilometers from Gwanda, it is very difficult to acquire employment because there is a surplus of labor. Despite numerous deaths from AIDS in this fishing village, there is no shortage of fishermen; any fishermen who die are replaced quickly by new ones.

The Education Sector The education sector is likely to be affected by HIV/AIDS. Both the numbers of children enrolled in school and the numbers of teachers available to teach them are likely to decline as the epidemic proceeds. The paucity of careful studies of the education sector makes it difficult to assess the degree to which these declines will compensate and what other effects they will have on social organization.

On the demand side, the epidemic will reduce the number of children enrolled in school. As children become ill, cohort size can be expected to drop; as children are needed to care for ill family members, they may be withdrawn; as resource-strapped families can no longer pay school fees or buy uniforms, children can be anticipated to stay home. Similarly, households headed by the more educated, who have higher HIV infection rates, may view education as a risky investment and thus choose to keep their children home (Ainsworth and Over, 1994a). As school cohorts decline in size, total costs associated with education may also decline, although costs per student may reasonably be assumed to increase.

At the same time, the supply of teachers may decline. Insofar as teachers are infected and develop AIDS, there will be a reduction in supply; replacing them will be both difficult and costly. For example, the World Bank estimates that by 2020, Tanzania will have lost some 27,000 teachers to the disease, and training of their replacements will cost US $37.8 million (World Bank, 1992a). At the same time, the total population paying for education will increase more slowly than in a no-AIDS scenario.

Whether supply side and demand side factors will balance to maintain somewhat steady expenditures per capita for education is unclear. One recent study in Tanzania indicates that the net impact of AIDS on schooling expenditures per capita may be slight (World Bank, 1992a), but this study has yet to be replicated widely throughout the region.

Impact of the Epidemic on Firms

There are multiple anecdotal accounts of the impact of the epidemic on the labor costs of individual firms, but there has been no systematic study of the impact of AIDS on a random sample of firms in a severely affected African economy. Of course, it must be emphasized that the ultimate measure of the impact of the epidemic is not the effect on firms. If firms go out of business, but their employees are able to find alternative employment, and their owners are able to sell the firm's assets and reinvest those assets equally profitably elsewhere, then the impact of the firm closures will be very small. Conversely, if firms are able to adjust with impunity, but their adjustment is at the expense of individual workers and members of their households, then the damage caused by the epidemic may be great. For these reasons, the definitive measure of the impact of the epidemic is its effect on the well-being of households and individuals.

Nevertheless, firms are important because they provide employment and facilitate the production and distribution of goods and services. Thus their well-being does, in fact, have an impact on the well-being of individuals. Skeptics point to two reasons for doubting that AIDS is, or will soon be, a serious impediment to private-sector growth in Africa. First, even in the most severely affected economies, attrition resulting from illness and death due to AIDS may not be a large proportion of the total attrition in firms. Consequently, the additional cost of recruiting replacements for sick or dead workers will be small in the context of the recruitment that is necessary anyway. Second, even if attrition from AIDS is large relative to that from other causes, the total impact on the firm will depend on how difficult it is to replace the lost workers. Given the fact that most African economies are operating with labor surpluses, skeptics suggest that hiring a replacement worker with similar or superior productivity may be as easy as stepping to the front gate of the firm and taking the first person in line. To make a convincing case for a large impact of AIDS on individual firms, one would have to refute both of these hypotheses.

Here again, few published studies are available to address these questions. A study of the Zambian Sugar Company explicitly sought impacts of the virus on the company and found none (Ministry of Health [Zambia], 1994). A study of 21 companies in Lusaka, Zambia, found that mortality of workers increased significantly between 1987 and 1991, but the percentage of deaths or of total worker turnover attributable to AIDS was unspecified (Baggaley et al., 1994).

To examine the reality of worker attrition in sub-Saharan Africa, we exploit a new and unique survey of firms in Zimbabwe, Kenya, and Ghana. Coordinated by the Africa Region Private Enterprise Development (RPED) project of the World Bank, a team of economists selected a random sample of approximately 200 registered manufacturing firms in each of seven countries to learn how firms respond to changing market conditions, especially with respect to the outward- or inward-oriented policies of their respective governments. In the most recent round of the survey, the investigators added one page of questions designed explicitly to learn more about the two questions posed above. Results from only three of the seven countries were available at the time this report was prepared (World Bank Regional Program on Enterprise Development, personal communication, 1995).

Table 6-3 presents basic information regarding firm size and attrition in the three countries for which the relevant labor-force data are currently available from the RPED database. The countries differ dramatically in average size of firms, ranging from 300 workers in Zimbabwe to 50 in Ghana. Total attrition as a percentage of total workers also varies across the countries, with attrition as a percentage of total workers per annum estimated at 9.1 and 11.6 percent for Zimbabwean and Ghanaian firms, respectively. The higher attrition in the Ghanaian firms is clearly not related to the severity of the epidemic, since the latest data suggest a much less severe epidemic in Ghana than in the other two countries.

The explanation for this seeming paradox is that attrition obeys roughly the same statistical law in all three countries: small firms have high and unpredictable attrition rates. Regardless of the country, the larger the firm, the more

TABLE 6-3 Data on Worker Attrition in Zimbabwe, Kenya, and Ghana, 1994: Total and by Sickness or Death

Country	Percent Urban HIV+ (Low-Risk)	Total in Sample: Firms	Total in Sample: Workers	Attrition Due to All Causes: Number	Attrition Due to All Causes: Percentage of All Workers	Attrition Due to Sickness or Death: Total	Attrition Due to Sickness or Death: Percentage of All Workers
Zimbabwe	18.0	199	59,210	5,366	9.1	695	1.2
Kenya	15.0	214	17,126	1,325	7.7	151	0.9
Ghana	2.2	188	9,607	1,110	11.6	30	0.3
Total		601	85,943	7,801	9.1	876	1.0

SOURCES: Seroprevalence data from U.S. Bureau of the Census (1994). Other data from the Africa Region Private Enterprise Development Project (World Bank Regional Program on Enterprise Development, personal communication, 1995).

closely its annual attrition rate approximates 6 percent of its work force. Hence the explanation for the higher attrition rate in Ghana despite that country's lower HIV prevalence rate is simply that the average size of its firms is much smaller than in Zimbabwe and somewhat smaller than in Kenya.

Assuming that the HIV infection rates given in the first column of Table 6-3 apply to the work forces of the firms in those countries, we can apply Table 6-1 to estimate the attrition that would be expected as a result of HIV in each country. In Kenya and Zimbabwe, respectively, seroprevalence of 15 and 18 percent means that 1.2 and 2.3 percent of workers should be forced to leave the work force each year because of AIDS. On the other hand, Ghana's 2.2 percent seroprevalence suggests that fewer than 0.6 percent of workers should be forced to leave because of AIDS. The last column of Table 6-3 demonstrates that the ranking of attrition rates from sickness and death across the three countries does match their ranking by seroprevalence. However, the attrition rates due to sickness and death are systematically lower than would be expected based on the arithmetic in Table 6-1.

Thus, limited data suggest that there is a statistically measurable increment to the worker attrition rate associated with HIV infection. Furthermore, the differences among the three countries are statistically significant at the 99.9 percent confidence level. However, the magnitude of the effect is extremely small, perhaps only half of what one would expect based on national seroprevalence. Of course, the main effects may be yet to emerge as more HIV-positive people develop full-blown AIDS. Another possible explanation is that premature departures from a firm are hidden under another category, such as "fired" or "quit," when in fact the departure was due to AIDS. If people systematically return to their families in rural areas to receive care, this scenario is quite likely. In the countries in this sample, attrition due to illness and death ranged from 3 percent of all attrition in Ghana to 13 percent of all attrition in Zimbabwe. Any attrition is costly to a firm, but it seems unlikely that an increment of even 15 percentage points in the attrition rate would be enough to impede seriously a firm's growth. Further examination of this question would require combining the RPED data on worker attrition with data on firm profitability in order to study the impact of the former on the latter.

Unfortunately, the RPED data do not categorize all hires and departures by grade level. However, on the questionnaires for Zimbabwe, Kenya, and Ghana, an additional page of questions was added to gather more complete data on the first nine deaths in each firm. While compliance was not always perfect, of the 592 workers who had left because of death, some detailed information is available on 258 (44 percent).[6]

Table 6-4 presents information on the difficulty of replacing workers by four skill categories. Among the 229 workers for whom data on skill category and the result of the replacement process were available, only 8 were professionals, while the other 221 were grouped into the descending categories of "skilled," "operator," and "unskilled." Focusing on these last three groups, we note that the proportion of deceased workers for whom a replacement had been found as of the time of the interview decreased with increasing skill level, from only 59 percent for skilled workers and 56 percent for operators to 72 percent for unskilled. Conversely, the proportion of openings that the employer was still trying to fill declined from 12.1 percent for skilled workers to 2.4 percent for the unskilled. We must also note that the response "do not plan to replace" was more frequent than the response "still looking" for every skill category, sometimes by an order of magnitude. Whether these responses represent downsizing, a change of job description, an extended and expensive search, or a misunderstanding of the questionnaire is impossible to interpret. Yet the data tend to indicate support for the hypothesis that the labor market is tighter at the top of the skill spectrum than at the bottom.

The last column of Table 6-4 gives, for those positions for which a replacement was found, the number of weeks the employer reported searching until finding the replacement. Here again, though the sample size is small, there is evidence that more search was required at higher than at lower skill levels. There are a number of reasons to expect firms to spend longer searching for higher-

[6]Ghana provided information on 95 percent of its deaths, Kenya on 86 percent, and Zimbabwe on 35 percent. Zimbabwe's lower completion rate was due partly to the fact that some large firms had experienced more than nine deaths. Since the questionnaire had space for only nine questions, the form was not physically able to handle the other deaths.

TABLE 6-4 Relationship of Skill Level to the Ease and Speed of Replacement of a Deceased Worker

Skill Category	Number of Observations	Found a Replacement	Still Looking	Decided Not to Replace Employee	Average Weeks to Find a Replacement for Those Found
Professional	8	1 (12.5%)	1 (12.5%)	6 (75%)	n.a.
Skilled	58	34 (58.6%)	7 (12.1%)	17 (29.3%)	3.1
Operator	78	44 (56.4%)	4 (5.1%)	30 (38.5%)	3.0
Unskilled	85	61 (71.8%)	2 (2.4%)	22 (26%)	1.7
Total	229	140 (61%)	14 (6.1%)	75 (33%)	

n.a. = not available

SOURCE: Africa Region Private Enterprise Development Project (World Bank Regional Program on Enterprise Development, personal communication, 1995).

skilled than for lower-skilled workers, such as the desire for better matching of skills with job requirements among more important workers. Yet, firms in the sample are apparently not typically required to engage in an extended search for even a skilled worker. Of the 34 positions vacated by the deaths of skilled workers and later filled, 8 were filled within one week, and another 15 required only a second week of search. Based on these data, it is difficult to argue that the deaths of skilled workers will greatly impede the operations of sub-Saharan African firms.

It has often been conjectured that the loss of a small number of elite individuals in the economy can disproportionately disrupt economic and social activity. If the maturing cadre of younger leaders is too small or too inexperienced to fill adequately the roles of its deceased seniors, economic growth suffers. Table 6-3 presents data on worker attrition, but unfortunately these data do not permit a breakdown of attrition rates by skill category of worker. If, in the absence of AIDS, attrition among professionals and managers is much lower than the 6 to 12 percent attrition rates among the general work force, then a seroprevalence among managers of 45 percent would, according to Table 6-1, increase the mortality rate among this group by a factor of 10 (from 5 to 50 per 1,000). However, the results of the RPED survey reported in Table 6-4 demonstrate the difficulty of measuring the mortality rate among professionals through sample survey techniques: even in a survey of 600 firms, the total number of top-level professionals is so small that very few deaths are reported.[7]

Summary

The impact of HIV/AIDS on life in sub-Saharan Africa is fragmented. For individual people living with infection and all the social ramifications it brings, the disease is devastating. On the other hand, the epidemic may not have the drastic effect on economies that was first imagined. Unifying these disparate interpretations of the impact of AIDS is difficult. Clearly, preventing and assuaging human suffering is important. Yet not all people with AIDS are poor, and not all of the poor have AIDS, so there are numerous other ways to allocate scarce resources. With resources so precious, other poverty-alleviation intervention efforts compete with AIDS mitigation for attention. How can mitigation of HIV/AIDS be responsibly integrated into the general health-improvement/poverty-reduction package? We now turn to a discussion of mitigation programs, both actual and potential.

ATTEMPTS TO MITIGATE THE IMPACT OF HIV/AIDS

Many donors believe that government or donor intervention is unlikely to have much effect on the severity of the epidemic's impact, and that resources would be better spent on interventions designed to prevent the spread of HIV. These beliefs are unchallenged by any broad-based, representative, empirical information about what kinds of programs are currently under way to mitigate the impact of the epidemic on the survivors and how successful they have been to date. Current interventions to mitigate the deleterious effects of HIV/AIDS in sub-Saharan Africa are implemented by a variety of organizations, governments, local and national nongovernmental organizations, international aid organizations, and grassroots groups, and are targeted to a variety of recipients. Many of these groups are performing important and worthwhile work. Yet the question raised earlier of best use of resources returns: How can the negative impact of AIDS on sub-Saharan Africa best be assuaged?

---

[7]Suppose that each of the 601 firms in the sample had only one professional- or managerial-level employee, who was the head of the firm. Then the 8 deaths reported in Table 5-4 would constitute an adult mortality rate of 13 per 1,000, which would be consistent with a seroprevalence of between 5 and 10 percent. If the average were two professionals/managers per firm, the mortality rate would be only 7 per 1,000, a rate insufficiently high to show the effect of an HIV/AIDS epidemic. Of course, firms whose head had died in the last year would be under-represented in the sample if such firms were more likely than others to disintegrate.

Mitigation interventions can be classified along three dimensions: by the level of social organization of the intended beneficiary, by the type of social or governmental organization rendering support, and by the type of support rendered. This section examines the distinctions that can be drawn along each of these dimensions in turn and identifies associated issues.

Intended Beneficiary

Assistance can be provided directly to a person with HIV or AIDS, to the individual's entire household, to a village or community affected by AIDS, to a geographic region containing many villages, to a firm (whether it be in the formal or informal sector), to a government entity (such as a university or ministry), to a specific economic sector or industry (such as the trucking industry), or perhaps to an entire national economy.

Since the provision of any kind of assistance to everyone affected in a country would be prohibitively expensive, a key issue is how the recipients of assistance are selected. The assisting entity might choose beneficiaries informally and subjectively, or it might use a formal set of targeting criteria to determine eligibility. An alternative would be to provide a form of assistance that would have little or no value to people outside the class of desired beneficiaries. An example of such a "self-targeting" assistance program would be home care for people with AIDS, which would be neither needed nor desired by a household without a person having the disease.

The application of formal criteria for eligibility consumes resources that could otherwise finance more of whatever type of assistance is being rendered. Therefore, assistance agencies face the problem of designing criteria that will discriminate successfully between intended recipients and others on a relatively easy and inexpensive basis. Furthermore, all such targeting criteria, once known to the public, are vulnerable in varying degrees to opportunistic behavior intended to divert assistance to recipients who would otherwise not qualify.

Providers of Mitigation Assistance

Providers of assistance can be family members, neighbors, local communities, formal or informal financial institutions, local or international nongovernmental organizations, or government agencies. Any of these providers can operate with or without the support of bilateral or multilateral donors.

In view of the potential for opportunism discussed above, a critical issue in the implementation of targeted assistance programs is the ease with which providers of assistance can gather information on the characteristics of potential recipients. Generally speaking, providers of assistance that are located close to the potential recipients will have access to better information about recipients than will a more distant provider. For example, family members and neighbors are in a better position to judge the need of an individual or household for assistance than is a local nongovernmental organization, which in turn would have an advantage in this regard over a national government agency or a bilateral donor.

Types of Mitigation Help Being Provided

In evaluating the costs and effects of proposed programs, total program costs must be categorized as fixed or variable. Then, for each type of program, it is necessary to propose an indicator or output measure that can serve as the denominator in computing both types of costs. The institutional framework or context and its effect on costs, particularly on fixed costs, must be carefully specified as well.

The fundamental evaluation issue is how to compare the outputs of the different interventions. This comparison is relatively easy in the area of prevention because one can compare, at least theoretically, all the different possible interventions with respect to the number of (primary and secondary) cases of HIV each prevents per dollar. Not only is it difficult to compare the benefit of assisting an orphan to attend school with the benefit of averting a case of HIV infection, but it is even difficult to compare the benefits of two mitigation interventions. For example, how does one compare a program that assists a dying person with AIDS and another that helps the surviving household members? A related issue is how to weigh assistance to improve a household's well-being immediately after an AIDS death (for example, by providing food) against assistance that improves the future well-being of the surviving children (for example, by helping them to stay in school). One impact of the epidemic is an increase in the cost of insurance, both formal and informal. Thus, a potential type of assistance would be to subsidize insurance premiums. In the formal sector, this subsidy would help people prepare for the possibility that a family member would get sick, while also increasing the national saving rate. The comparable intervention in rural areas without formal insurance might be to subsidize rural credit programs that would help people self-insure ex ante through precautionary savings or cope ex post with the shock of a death in the household.

While informal information about AIDS support projects is widespread, databanks of "who does what" are rare and incomplete. Relatively little information is available about mitigation efforts, and certainly nothing is available about their effectiveness.

There is an urgent need for hard data on the cost-effectiveness of alternative mechanisms for assisting severely affected households. On the cost side, little is known regarding the unit cost of delivering a package of welfare services of known quality. A rather superficial investigation of nongovernmental organization social and economic support activity reported in the annex to this chapter indicates that large numbers of organizations are engaged in these activities and that many of the best-developed of these organizations do not exist primarily to respond to the epidemic. This suggestive information calls for a deeper investigation of the characteristics of the broad range of for-profit and nonprofit nongovernmental institutions involved, regardless of their previous connection to the epidemic, and of the links between these characteristics and the institution's capacity to implement various kinds of prevention and mitigation programs. Such research would inform, for example, the development of criteria to be used in judging the relative competence of alternative nongovernmental organizations bidding for a given contract.

RECOMMENDATIONS

The following are recommendations for future research in the area of mitigating the impact of the HIV/AIDS epidemic.

KEY RECOMMENDATION 4. Research on mitigating the impact of the disease should focus on the needs of people with HIV/AIDS.

A great deal more is known about designing and implementing HIV-prevention programs than is known about providing care to the millions of people in sub-Saharan Africa already infected with the virus. Simple, cost-effective solutions to daily living problems faced by persons with AIDS, such as palliative care, part-time home care, and group counseling, may make larger, more expensive interventions unwarranted.

Recommendation 6-1. Research efforts to evaluate the impact of HIV/AIDS on individuals, households, firms, economic sectors, and nations are badly needed.

Research on impact should incorporate both qualitative and quantitative approaches to data collection and should evaluate both short- and long-term effects. Of particular interest is research that would permit an understanding of the impact of HIV/AIDS on poverty and on individual decision making. Research is needed to ascertain whether decreased life expectancy reduces willingness to save or invest in financial and real assets, in human capital, and in the relationships necessary to maintain social interactions. In the long term, the impact of HIV/AIDS on sub-Saharan Africa will depend on the strength and malleability of social and economic networks in accommodating the changes that are occurring.

Recommendation 6-2. Since the attempt to assist directly every affected household would be financially nonsustainable, research is needed on

criteria for determining which households and communities should be targeted for assistance and which institutions should deliver that assistance.

The epidemic has already affected millions of households in sub-Saharan Africa and will continue to do so for at least the next 20 years. Efforts to mitigate the effects of the disease have been uncoordinated and poorly targeted, and their ability to provide solutions for those infected and their families remains to be proven.

Recommendation 6-3. Discovering the optimal roles of government, nongovernmental organizations, and donors in HIV/AIDS prevention and mitigation is critical and requires further study.

Governments are now moving to decentralize and privatize AIDS programs by contracting, licensing, or franchising activities to various types of nongovernmental institutions. Research is needed on the determinants of the effectiveness of nongovernmental organizations, including those not devoted primarily to AIDS prevention and mitigation, in a variety of AIDS prevention and mitigation activities. Care is needed in defining the technical assistance needs and the absorptive capacities of nongovernmental organizations, to enhance their roles in research and prevention and to avoid overload and inefficient use of scarce resources.

ANNEX 6-1: A BRIEF SURVEY OF NONGOVERNMENTAL ORGANIZATIONS IMPLEMENTING MITIGATION PROGRAMS IN SUB-SAHARAN AFRICA

In an attempt to alleviate partially the dearth of information on mitigation activities, the panel recruited consultants in each of six sub-Saharan countries to administer a standard questionnaire to a selected sample of nongovernmental organizations (NGOs) in each country. The first and second columns of Table 6A-1 list the countries that participated in the survey and the number of questionnaires received from each.

There was no attempt to define a formal sampling frame for each country, but the consultants were asked to sample a broad range of NGOs, not restricting themselves to those that were established explicitly in response to the HIV/AIDS epidemic. Because the consultants were themselves associated with the struggle against the epidemic in several countries, this strategy was successful only in Tanzania and Zambia, where few of the NGOs sampled are explicitly related to the epidemic (see column 3 of Table 6A-1). Ironically, in Cameroon, where the epidemic and the struggle against it are less advanced, all the examples in our sample of NGOs mention AIDS prevention among their objectives or goals. Column 4 of Table 6A-1 shows that among the NGOs that mention AIDS in describing themselves, approximately half also mentioned mitigation of the epidemic's impact.

TABLE 6A-1 Sample of Nongovernmental Organizations by Country, and Whether Prevention or Mitigation of the Impact of AIDS is Among Their Objectives or Goals

Country	Number of Questionnaires Received	Percent Naming as Goal or Objective	
		Prevention	Mitigation
Cameroon	25	100	32
Côte d'Ivoire	5	80	60
Kenya	5	80	40
Tanzania	22	45	27
Zambia	13	8	8
Zimbabwe	5	100	80
Total	75	65	32

TABLE 6A-2 Comparison of AIDS and Other Nongovernmental Organizations (NGO): Scale of Operations

Characteristic of NGO	General NGO	AIDS NGO	Total
Average year of origination	1973 (26)	1986 (49)	1982 (75)
Total workers (volunteer & salaried)	97 (26)	68 (49)	78 (75)
Percentage of workers who are volunteers	32 (26)	76 (49)	61 (75)
Monthly expenditure (in 1995 US dollars)	12,749 (14)	1,097 (28)	4,981 (42)
Total number of individual beneficiaries in last 3 months	3,661 (23)	37,094 (45)	25,786 (68)
Total number of household beneficiaries in last 3 months	55,057 (23)	28 (45)	18,640 (68)
Total number of community beneficiaries in last 3 months	26,538 (23)	2,739 (45)	10,788 (68)

NOTE: The number of responses to each question is given in parentheses.

Table 6A-2 presents the responses to several of the questions in the survey, classified by whether or not the NGO mentioned AIDS among its goals or objectives. Since most of the NGOs outside Tanzania and Zambia are connected to AIDS, the differences between the two groups might also be due to differences between NGOs operating in Tanzania and Zambia and those in other countries.

As might be expected, the NGOs established for purposes other than AIDS are on average about 13 years older than those whose objectives or goals mention the epidemic. Perhaps because these general-purpose NGOs are older, they seem to be better established by any of the other measures in Table 6A-2. That is, they have 43 percent more workers and four times as many salaried workers. The average dollar budget of the 14 non-AIDS NGOs answering the questionnaire is almost 12 times as large as the average budget of the 28 AIDS NGOs interviewed. The non-AIDS NGOs count more households, communities, and firms as beneficiaries. The AIDS NGOs exceed the other NGOs on only one dimension—the average number of individual beneficiaries—and this difference disappears if we drop one outlier that claims to serve 1.5 million individual beneficiaries throughout Cameroon.

Similarly, we can separately examine the 48 AIDS-related NGOs to discover that those which mention mitigation of the impact of the epidemic are about the

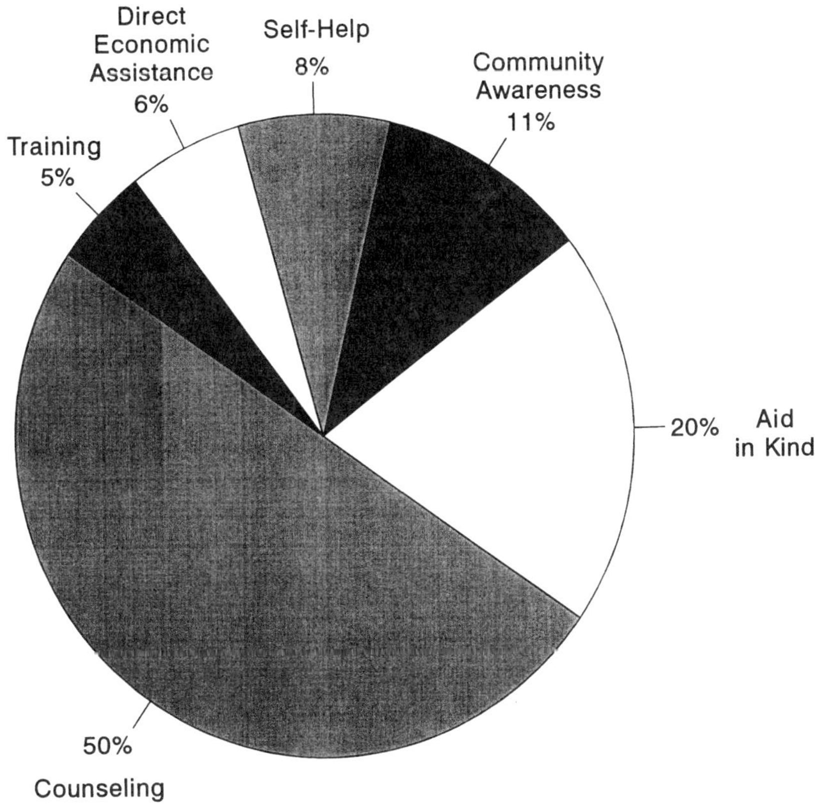

FIGURE 6A-1 Types of Mitigation Interventions Provided (total of all countries).

same age as those which do not. However, they have smaller budgets and fewer workers, use a smaller percentage of volunteers, and serve fewer individuals and firms, although they serve more communities and are more urban, than those which do not mention mitigation.

Figure 6A-1 presents the types of mitigation interventions offered by the NGOs in the sample. The question of intervention type is pertinent to the question of effectiveness, as discussed earlier in this chapter. Although the sample is small and not random, this graph demonstrates the diversity of projects loosely termed "mitigation." Surprisingly, economic assistance, whether in cash or in kind, constitutes only 26 percent of the mitigation effort. If self-help projects are added, the cumulative total is still only 34 percent. Counseling, which has both a supportive and preventative role, is the primary service provided by NGOs for people with HIV/AIDS in Africa; 50 percent of the program components described by the NGOs fit into this category.

Figure 6A-2 shows how many program components per NGO are dedicated

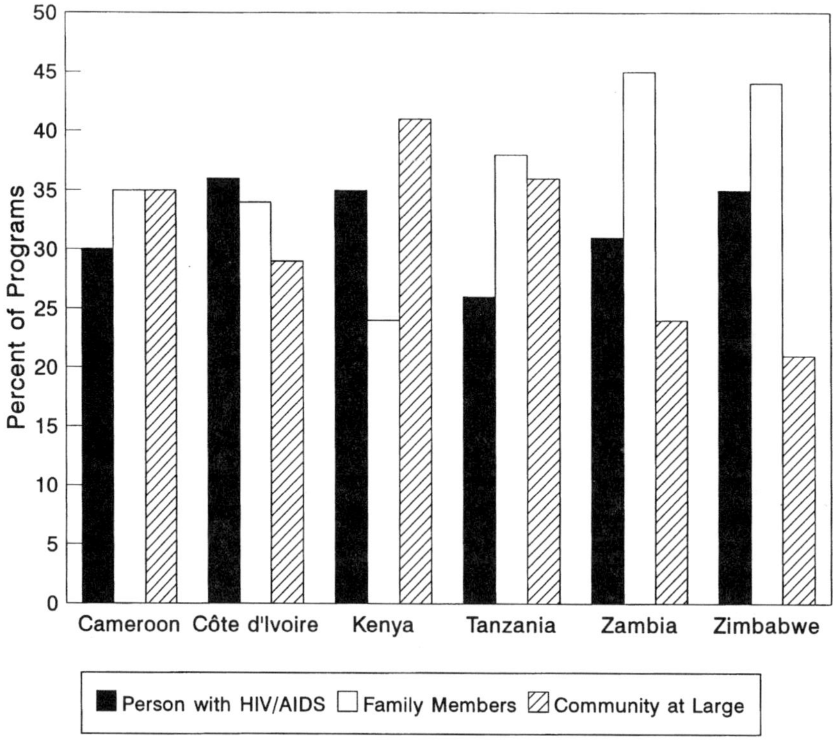

FIGURE 6A-2 Primary Beneficiary of Mitigation Efforts.

to providing services to each of three beneficiary groups: individuals with AIDS, their families, and the community as a whole. Each of the three groups is beneficiary of about one-third of the program components, but the families of people with AIDS are the intended beneficiaries of slightly more components than either the people with AIDS themselves or the community at large.

Table 6A-3 compares the sources of funding for AIDS and non-AIDS NGOs. Although AIDS NGOs are smaller and have smaller budgets than other NGOs, Table 6A-3 reveals that they take less advantage of every source of financing than do the other NGOs. With due regard to the small sample, which renders the differences statistically insignificant, and the fact that almost all the non-AIDS NGOs are in two countries, Table 6A-3 communicates the strong suggestion that AIDS-related NGOs are doing less than they could to raise funds. Similar analysis of only the AIDS NGOs shows that those which profess mitigation as one of their objectives are slightly more likely than those which do not to gain funds from both religious and nonreligious sources, while having equal access to bilateral donors and beneficiary fees. The mitigation NGOs are also slightly less

TABLE 6A-3 Comparison of AIDS and Other Nongovernmental Organizations (NGO): Funding Sources

Sources of Funding	Percent Receiving Funds by Type of NGO: General NGO	AIDS NGO	Multiplier[a] (t-statistic)
Fees charged beneficiaries	23	13	2.43 (1.6)
Member dues	77	71	0.19 (–2.5)
Government grants	42	2	3.25 (2.2)
Local groups	54	29	8.85 (3.9)
International religious organizations	27	20	1.15 (.27)
International nonreligious NGOs	81	33	2.64 (1.5)
International bilateral donors	54	31	3.71 (2.5)
Other	58	57	1.26 (.59)
N	26	49	

[a]Multipliers are the antilogs of the coefficients on the dummy variables for the indicated funding source in a regression explaining the logarithm of the monthly dollar budget. The R-squared is .83 on 41 observations, and the antilog of the estimated constant term is US $191, with a t-statistic of 8.3.

likely to fix membership dues, perhaps because many of the individuals they serve are destitute as a result of the epidemic.

The last column of Table 6A-3 explores the question of whether some of the funding sources are statistically more associated than others with (the logarithm of) the monthly dollar budget of the type of organization. The regression fits extremely well, with coefficients that are highly statistically significant on several funding categories. The figures listed in column 3 of Table 6A-3 are estimates of the multiple by which an organization could increase its monthly budget if it took advantage of one of these funding sources, having not previously done so. Note that organizations that are successful at tapping the resources of local community groups achieve monthly expenditures 885 percent larger than those which do not. The source of funds with the second-largest estimated impact on monthly expenditures is the bilateral agency representing a developed country, which is estimated to increase monthly expenditures by 271 percent. Local

TABLE 6A-4 Operation of Social and Economic Programs by Nongovernmental Organization Goals

	Type of Program		
Goal of NGO	Mitigation	Other	Total
Prevention	99 (58%)	72 (42%)	171 (100%)
Other	57 (50%)	57 (50%)	114 (100%)
Total	156 (55%)	129 (45%)	285 (100%)

government resources come next, with an estimated increase of 225 percent, while reliance on membership dues is apparently associated with a net decrease in total expenditures of 81 percent. A possible interpretation of this last finding is that members are quite parsimonious with organization resources when those resources come from their own pockets, but less so when the resources are raised outside.

The 75 individual NGOs in the sample operate a total of 288 separate programs or program components. Using the organization's description of the activities associated with each program, it is possible to score each component with a zero or a 1 on mitigation, depending on whether it includes any social or economic support activities. Such programs can provide substantial assistance to AIDS-affected households, regardless of whether the program was originally intended to address the impact of AIDS.

Table 6A-4 shows the percentage of programs capable of helping households and other social units cope with the impact of AIDS by type of NGO. Of the 171 programs operated by AIDS-related NGOs, 58 percent have a social or economic objective and thus can help individuals, households, or other social units cope with the impact. However, the proportion of the 114 components operated by other NGOs that includes social or economic activities is 50 percent, almost as large. The lesson here is that governments should not look only to AIDS-related NGOs as potential operators of mitigation programs. In fact, if the greater experience and resources of the non-AIDS NGOs in this sample can be generalized to other settings, a mitigation program may have more chance of success if it is implemented by a non-AIDS NGO.

7

Building Capacity for AIDS-Related Research

INTRODUCTION

In this report, the panel identifies research and data priorities intended to improve our understanding of the social and behavioral factors influencing the spread of HIV/AIDS in sub-Saharan Africa. In turn, this understanding can be used to inform the development of prevention and mitigation strategies designed to arrest the spread of HIV/AIDS. The panel realizes, however, that if effective research is to be undertaken and research results are to be applied appropriately and effectively, the necessary infrastructure must be in place, a prerequisite that is often lacking in sub-Saharan Africa. As a result, virtually all research undertaken on AIDS in sub-Saharan Africa to date has been made possible only with technical cooperation and foreign assistance from the international community.

Thus, beyond the immediate challenge of the panel's mandate—identifying the critical research questions—there remain enormous practical challenges of actually obtaining the answers: Who is going to do the research, where, and with what resources? The objective of this chapter is to identify the constraints on conducting research in sub-Saharan Africa and to offer a series of recommendations for addressing these constraints in the short term. It is worth noting that although the focus of this chapter is on capacity building for HIV/AIDS-related research, many of the obstacles identified here are also hindrances to optimal management and implementation of AIDS prevention and mitigation efforts.[1]

[1]For further discussion of the obstacles to implementing successful AIDS-prevention programs, see N'Galy et al. (1990).

Problem Statement

As noted above, undertaking effective research requires that a basic infrastructure be in place. Key aspects of this infrastructure include access to adequate funding, skilled labor, and appropriate technology, as well as sufficient managerial and administrative capacity to plan, execute, monitor, and evaluate a study. Even in developed countries, amassing the resources required to undertake complex research endeavors is difficult, but these difficulties are multiplied many-fold in sub-Saharan Africa. Many sub-Saharan African universities have been badly neglected in recent years. The poor preparedness of matriculating students, entirely inadequate salaries for all levels of professional and support staff, neglect of buildings and libraries, and a lack of core funds necessary to move institutions into the technological age have contributed to the universities' slow demise and the widespread flight of their faculties into the private sector.

When research has been conducted in sub-Saharan Africa, it has usually lacked a coordinated plan. Furthermore, many of the findings that have emerged from the research have not been adequately disseminated, so that results are not widely known across the continent. As a consequence, the contributions of social and behavioral scientists have not been fully utilized.

As noted above, the objective of this chapter is to consider constraints on designing, implementing, and disseminating AIDS-related research in sub-Saharan Africa. The basic constraints to be addressed are as follows:

- Insufficient/poorly allocated funds,
- Inadequate manpower,
- Unintended negative consequences of donor policies,
- Inadequate coordination of research efforts, and
- A harsh environment for conducting research.

There are no easy solutions to these problems, but after discussing each in turn, we make several recommendations that may marginally improve the situation in the short run and should be considered in developing any long-term strategies for conducting and applying research in sub-Saharan Africa.

Data Sources

This chapter draws on two types of information: (1) existing documents, including evaluations of national AIDS control programs conducted in the late 1980s and early 1990s; and (2) interviews conducted by members of the panel during site visits to Zambia, Tanzania, and Cameroon during January and February 1995 (see Appendix A for detail on these visits). These countries differ greatly with regard to HIV/AIDS infection rates, the extent and nature of their response to the epidemic, and the importance of social and behavioral research in prevention and mitigation strategies. In Zambia, where HIV/AIDS is widespread, the Ministry of Health has developed a strong and coordinated response to the epidemic. This coordination contrasts sharply with the situation in Tanzania, where the response is fragmented and implemented largely through the uncoordinated activities of nongovernmental organizations. In Cameroon, the epidemic is less advanced and has generated a lower level of government and nongovernmental organization response. Within each country, the panel interviewed individual researchers and representatives of various research units, nongovernmental organizations, donor agencies, and government offices. The panel acknowledges that this fieldwork does not provide an exhaustive assessment of the state of AIDS research and prevention and control programs throughout sub-Saharan Africa, but it does provide some indications of the pertinent problems.

CONSTRAINTS ON RESEARCH IN SUB-SAHARAN AFRICA

This section reviews each of the five constraints listed above.

Insufficient/Poorly Allocated Funds

The single largest barrier to conducting research in sub-Saharan Africa is grossly inadequate funding. As with most activities in developing countries, resources for research are in short supply; this is especially true for AIDS-related social and behavioral research in sub-Saharan Africa. Funding for salaries, facilities, equipment, and even basic office supplies is inadequate. In African universities, the limited budgets available are spent on wages, leaving very few resources for maintaining buildings or equipment, purchasing general office supplies, providing staff training and development, and initiating and sustaining a research program. At the same time, a lack of managerial and administrative capacity leads to inefficiencies in the way money is allocated and spent and results in a less-than-optimal utilization of existing resources.

Data on the total amount of money spent in sub-Saharan Africa each year on AIDS-related research from all sources are not readily available. However, a large share of behavioral and social science research in sub-Saharan Africa is being funded by international donors,[2] and some information is available about expenditures on AIDS research by the 10 major industrialized countries and the European Community. In 1991, these countries spent US $1.55 billion on HIV/AIDS-related research, more than in any year previously, although the pace of growth slowed after 1989, and spending has begun to show signs of reaching a

[2]A review of 559 AIDS-related research projects identified in Africa in 1989 found that 47 percent were funded from national resources alone, while 53 percent were collaborative projects with various external donors (Heymann et al., 1990).

plateau (Mann et al., 1992). Yet there is little correspondence between the severity of the epidemic and the allocation of research funding. For example, recent WHO estimates conclude that of the 18 million adult HIV infections that occurred from the start of the epidemic until the end of 1994, 11 million were in sub-Saharan Africa. Yet of the US $1.55 billion spent on HIV/AIDS-related research by developed countries in 1991, for example, only US $179 million (3 percent) was allocated to research on developing countries (Mann et al., 1992). An analysis of 10 years' worth of AIDS-related studies cataloged in MEDLINE, an electronic database of primarily medical journals, found that only 3 percent addressed AIDS in Africa (Elford et al., 1991).

Furthermore, social and behavioral research has received a relatively small share of the available resources, despite the fact that experts both within and outside the behavioral sciences agree that traditional health education messages are insufficient to induce widespread behavior changes (Mann et al., 1992). A recent review of all HIV/AIDS-related research cataloged on MEDLINE over the period 1983-1989 identified more than 20,000 papers on HIV/AIDS-related research, of which only 2,299 (11 percent) pertained to the social and behavioral sciences. Of these, 1,262 (55 percent) addressed studies of homosexuality and AIDS or substance abuse and AIDS, both of which have limited relevance as modes of transmission in Africa (Mann et al., 1992).

Researchers throughout sub-Saharan Africa often face a lack of basic resources. For example, Uganda is one of the countries in the epicenter of the AIDS epidemic. It was among the first countries in sub-Saharan Africa to report the presence of HIV and as of July 1993 had the second-highest cumulative total number of AIDS cases anywhere in Africa (World Health Organization, 1994). In a recent report, the National AIDS Commission in Uganda identified many research-related items for which funding is either unavailable or inadequate, including the following:

- Salary support,
- Rehabilitation of research infrastructure (e.g., laboratories, computer rooms, protected storage for data and various specimens),
- Capacity for data storage and retrieval,
- Maintenance capacity for new specialized equipment imported for AIDS-related research, including tools, spare parts, and skills (both in operation and in maintenance), and
- Low-cost HIV testing kits.

In all likelihood, the experience of Uganda is not unique.

The dominance of international donors in AIDS research in Africa is the consequence of a lack of domestic funding for such research in the region. Tragically, AIDS has hit sub-Saharan Africa at a time of severe economic crisis. Yet African governments appear complacent about the current and expected magnitude of the epidemic and to date have contributed little to HIV/AIDS research. In 1991, a WHO/GPA study that examined the mix of external support and domestic contributions to national AIDS programs in developing countries concluded that their "governments were not at all or very insignificantly sharing the resource burden for AIDS control" (World Health Organization, 1991:531, cited in Mann et al., 1992). Not surprisingly, therefore, a recent expenditure survey of national AIDS control programs in 24 sub-Saharan African countries reported that in 9 countries, no funding is allocated for research; in 6 countries, less than 3 percent of the national AIDS control program budget is allocated to research; and in 8 other countries, between 3 and 5 percent of the budget is allocated to research. Cameroon has designated 10 percent of its national AIDS control program budget for research, more than twice the amount spent by the next-highest country (Mann and Tarantola, forthcoming). Current spending levels on research within national AIDS control program budgets, both in absolute and in relative terms, appear not to be a function of the severity of the epidemic, the country's total national AIDS control program expenditure, or the overall size of the economy.

In reality, of course, sufficient funds will never be available to answer all the questions and address all the issues identified in this report, so they must be prioritized in some way. Moreover, even if sufficient funding were available, it would be impossible to implement all the research recommendations made in this report without technical assistance from outside Africa because of a shortage of well-trained African social and behavioral scientists (as discussed in the next section). Yet the dependence on international donors for AIDS research in sub-Saharan Africa raises a number of issues. Support from international donors for AIDS-related research in sub-Saharan Africa has not been able to meet demand, for a variety of reasons. First, the global political climate is characterized by a growing complacency; this in turn has resulted in shrinking donor budgets, particularly at WHO/GPA, which historically has been a significant funder of AIDS-related research (see also Chapter 1). Second, AIDS research priorities in sub-Saharan Africa must now compete with similar demands for funding created by emerging AIDS epidemics in other parts of the world, particularly Latin America and Asia. Third, the priorities of foreign donors may be inconsistent with those of a country's national AIDS control program, so that research priorities established in a country are either underfunded or not funded at all.

This last issue—the misalignment of donor funds and benefactor needs—is illustrated by information compiled on competing research priorities of three parties active in AIDS prevention in Tanzania (Susan Hunter, personal communication, 1995). The second column of Table 7-1 shows the research priorities of the Tanzanian national AIDS control program (which presumably reflect Tanzanians' perceptions of their own needs) alongside the research priorities identified by two sets of outside experts from agencies based in Washington (third column) and Tanzania (fourth column). All three groups of experts rated 12 potential areas for future AIDS-related research as being a high priority, a low priority, or

TABLE 7-1 Research and Data Collection Priorities in Tanzania

Area	Level of Priority		
	National AIDS Control Program	Washington (AIDSCAP)	Tanzania AIDS Project
Research			
Innovative behavior change and communication interventions	N	H	H
Links between prevention and care	N	H	H
Workplace structure and interventions	N	H	H
Women in stable relationships: approaches to sexual safety	N	H	L
Male responsibility in sexuality and family	N	N	H
Social and economic factors in HIV risk	H	H	L
Behavioral consequences of policy (e.g., medical barriers to STD care)	N	H	H
Female condom	N	H	L
Counseling and testing	H	H	L
STD screening in family planning clinics	H	N	H
STD interventions for high-risk groups	H	N	H
Family structure and adaptation to HIV/AIDS	H	N	H
Data Collection			
AIDS knowledge, attitudes, beliefs, and practices	H	H	H
Condom use availability	H	H	H
STD incidence	H	H	H
STD points of first encounter	H	H	H
Orphan and family composition data	H	N	H
National nongovernmental organization inventory and database	H	N	H

NOTES: H = high priority; L = low priority; N = not a priority.

SOURCE: Susan Hunter (personal communication, 1995).

not a priority for funding. No single area received a high rating from all three groups, although there was more consensus on priorities for data collection activities. In July 1991, the Tanzanians held a 4-day workshop to prioritize research areas in the country "so as to optimize research efforts in support of the objectives of the second Medium Term Plan . . . [by identifying research that] most closely relate[s] to the problems of, and may help answer questions relevant to, the National AIDS Prevention and Control Programme" (United Republic of Tanzania, 1991:1). However, research projects that had been funded were established outside Tanzania rather than in collaboration with Tanzanians, and their objectives were not always consistent with the priorities established by the national AIDS control program in 1991.

In Uganda, the Uganda AIDS Commission recently complained that funding of donor-driven priorities has led to an overemphasis on large-scale studies and an excessive concentration of resources in a small area of the country, leaving many other districts, cultures, and target groups understudied (Uganda AIDS Commission, 1992). Furthermore, some Ugandan researchers have complained that "several western-financed studies have not included a service commitment to the local population, and there is a tendency [for western researchers] to address problems more relevant to western populations rather than those felt most appropriate by local workers" (Serwadda and Katongole-Mbidde, 1990:843). In Cameroon, because several major donors each focus their efforts in one particular province, considerable research is done in some geographical areas, while in others there is none. In Zambia, the Director of the National AIDS/STD/TB & Leprosy Programme concluded that donors' assistance during the period 1986-1990, including funding for research, had not been as effective as expected because "most of the major donors, in particular the bilateral donors, insisted that the Government of Zambia follow the package of interventions that they [the donors] have defined" (Msiska, 1994:16).

Inadequate Manpower

A second fundamental constraint on implementing AIDS-related research in sub-Saharan Africa is the shortage of competent indigenous researchers. The few highly trained or exceptional African social or behavioral researchers currently working in the AIDS arena are in constant demand and are already involved in multiple projects. At the same time, AIDS itself has probably disproportionately affected the more-educated population (see Chapter 6), which may have affected the pool of professionals and researchers in African cities even further. Research capacity within Africa cannot be improved without an increase in the number of well-trained African researchers. Many sub-Saharan African institutions suffer from having few competent professionals, and those institutions that are well staffed have enormous difficulty retaining their best staff. Many of the best

African scholars are attracted abroad by higher salaries, greater job satisfaction, and better opportunities for their children and families.

A recent research needs assessment conducted by the Uganda AIDS Commission identifies behavioral researchers and interdisciplinary specialists as categories of professionals that are in short supply, particularly ethnomedical researchers, social scientists with qualitative research skills (e.g., anthropologists), and meta-analysts (Uganda AIDS Commission, 1992). The report also identifies the need for more basic research scientists and clinical and laboratory researchers. The lack of manpower results, in part, from the lack of emphasis placed on training AIDS researchers by national AIDS control programs and other funders, low wages, and a decline in the quality and availability of higher education in the decades preceding the epidemic (as discussed further below).

AIDS has yet to be firmly established as a field of academic study in many African universities. In the early 1980s, when AIDS first struck the African continent, national AIDS prevention programs drew upon existing expertise within a small pool of researchers who had been trained in tropical disease control. Although this strategy may have been appropriate as a short-term response to the initial outbreak of the epidemic, it is impossible to rely on resources borrowed from other fields over the long term. Now that the nature and magnitude of the epidemic are better understood, there is an urgent need for universities to develop appropriate curricula to train researchers as AIDS specialists. Furthermore, the epidemic led to an immediate need for professionals who were trained in disciplines that were not popular when the epidemic first erupted, such as social anthropology and communication.

As a result of these limitations of indigenous manpower, and given the tremendous pressure on the donor community to respond quickly to the emerging epidemic, donor agencies have preferred to rely on experienced researchers from the United States and Europe. The unintended negative consequences of this and other donor policies that affect capacity building are discussed next.

Unintended Negative Consequences of Donor Policies

Although many donor agencies emphasize the importance of capacity building, the net result of their investments in this area to date has been quite modest (World Bank, 1991; Cohen, 1993; Berg, 1993; Jaycox, 1993). Consequently, the entire modus operandi of donor agencies has come under increasing attack. A recent World Bank report suggests that donors' lack of an overall, consistent, and coherent strategy may have inadvertently contributed to Africa's current shortfall in capacity, of which research capacity would be one element (World Bank, 1991). For example, donor agencies typically design projects on a short (2-year) time-frame that, while appropriate for accomplishing certain program objectives, is insufficient to build a sustainable in-country research capacity. In some instances, donor agencies also "cream off" talented individuals by offering them better pay than they would receive in academia.

Perhaps the most controversial issue in the current literature on capacity building is whether donors employ the right mix of local and foreign workers. In response to weak indigenous research capacity, many donor agencies have favored a model of assistance built around resident foreign consultants as project directors, who are meant to transfer skills to their African counterparts over the life of a project. Many agencies prefer to use expatriate labor, even when local manpower is available. Some African government officials view such donor policies as "biased towards the use of costly external technical assistance with little or no consideration of local capacity building to ensure sustainability of programs" (Msiska, 1994:16). Moreover, persistent reliance on expatriate technical assistance personnel is extremely expensive compared with the cost of hiring local nationals; thus it drives up the cost of conducting research in Africa and leaves fewer resources for other purposes. Furthermore, expatriates often are not skilled in using an apprentice model and often focus too intently on getting the study done at the expense of substantive collaboration or local capacity building (Family Health International, 1992).

Indeed, it is not unusual for the life of a project to take the following course. First, the project identifies a capable African who is designated as the resident consultant's counterpart and local collaborator. Second, as part of the project's activities and with the specific objective of developing local capacity, the counterpart is sent abroad for further graduate studies. Consequently, the counterpart is not on site for half the length of the 2-year project. Third, immediately after the trained counterpart returns, he or she is promoted and reassigned to duties elsewhere. Such scenarios create cynicism and distrust on the part of Africans.

Compounding the above problems is the fact that donor agencies have tended to measure the success of a project in terms of the significance (and quantity) of the scientific publications that result, rather than the number of national staff who have been trained or the extent to which local institutions have been strengthened. Many donor agencies also try to sidestep official bureaucracies, administering programs themselves, as opposed to working with the relevant department in the Ministry of Health or elsewhere. Thus, projects sometimes operate as small, semiautonomous units designed and administered by foreign expatriates. Local personnel for these projects are diverted from other activities, creating a void elsewhere. Sub-Saharan African governments often view such arrangements as the price of financial assistance, rather than as a response to local needs (World Bank, 1991; Ali, 1994). Moreover, once funding for the project has expired, personnel and equipment are dispersed, thus vitiating any lasting impact of the project.

For these and other reasons, it is becoming increasingly evident that the standard model of 2-year development projects with resident foreign advisers has not worked in the area of capacity building. Skills and technologies are not being transferred adequately, local capacity is not being developed, and many projects are being discontinued shortly after expatriate assistance has been withdrawn (World Bank, 1991; Cohen, 1993; Berg, 1993; Jaycox, 1993).

A further problem is that the few African researchers who are currently available are in such high demand that they are often recruited onto projects without any expectation that they will contribute significantly to the projects' goals. Many funding agencies, national research boards, and sub-Saharan African governments require a local element in every international research project, so that most projects are required to list local collaborators as part of the project personnel. An unintended negative consequence of this policy, however, is that it places very heavy demands on a few African researchers. As a result, in far too many instances, Africans are invited to participate in projects without any intention of actually having them integrally involved in the research. The African is paid some (often paltry) consulting wage, and there is no expectation of any work being done. When reinforced over time and over many projects, such a policy creates the expectation among both parties that African collaborators do not function as equal partners in collaborative research projects, which in turn quickly becomes a self-fulfilling prophesy. Thus, there is an urgent need to change work practices and standards on international collaboration research projects and to reestablish a social contract that links pay to productivity.

With the knowledge that AIDS will continue to plague sub-Saharan Africa for many years into the future, it becomes clear that donor agencies would maximize the return on their investment in AIDS research in sub-Saharan Africa by placing greater emphasis on developing an indigenous research capacity relative to utilizing foreign expertise. An important step has been the establishment of the AIDS International Training Research Program in 1989. This program supports the training of foreign scientists in the United States and their home countries, as well as collaborative research between U.S. and foreign scientists. It is the largest global research training program for HIV/AIDS. Between 1989 and 1993, the program provided instruction in the United States for over 200 African health professionals from 18 sub-Saharan African countries. It also supported 65 in-country training courses in 7 sub-Saharan African countries, although only a small number of those trained were in the behavioral and social sciences. Nevertheless, the program has been quite successful, so that a significant proportion of the papers authored or coauthored by African researchers at international AIDS conferences are likely to have been written by former trainees in this program (United States Department of Health and Human Services, 1994).

Inadequate Coordination

Undoubtedly, the major constraints to conducting social and behavioral research in Africa are insufficient money and a lack of capable personnel. However, more could be accomplished with existing funding by eliminating overlap between projects and establishing a system for prioritizing prospective projects. Specific problems include a lack of information on previous and ongoing research efforts, a lack of research-needs assessment and the difficulty of coordinating funding from multiple sources, and a lack of cooperation among donor agencies.

Lack of Information on Previous and Ongoing Research Efforts

Researchers and policy makers in sub-Saharan Africa are often poorly informed about previous research findings. Part of the problem is that the findings of some studies are simply not written up and widely disseminated (e.g., through publication in a major international journal), perhaps because the researchers lacked the necessary time or skill or because an intervention was unsuccessful. This latter reason is particularly disturbing because valuable lessons can often be learned from failed efforts. The other aspect of this problem is that even if the research is written up, it is often difficult to obtain copies of the reports. Often, it is easier to obtain copies of papers from outside the country of the study than from within. Furthermore, English and French are both spoken widely in sub-Saharan Africa, but it is difficult to obtain information about activities in Francophone Africa in English and even more difficult to obtain information about activities in Anglophone Africa in French.

In most sub-Saharan African countries, there is no central repository for research or reports on AIDS-related activities, nor is there a bibliography or database of research efforts. Between August 1988 and February 1989, a team from WHO/GPA conducted a systematic country-by-country inventory of AIDS-related research projects in sub-Saharan Africa. The survey was designed to ascertain what research was being undertaken at the time; to identify the gaps, if any, in the research agenda; and to identify any major duplication of effort (Heymann et al., 1990).[3] Over 50 percent of the 559 studies identified were unknown to the relevant national AIDS control committee. In a small number of countries, such as Uganda and Zimbabwe, there have been recent efforts to develop annotated bibliographies, specifically on published social and behavioral research results (Olowo-Freers and Barton, 1992; Bylmakers, 1992). In Tanza-

[3]A total of 559 AIDS-related research projects were identified in 35 sub-Saharan African countries. Of these, 62 percent were concerned with HIV-1 or HIV-2 seroprevalence among general populations or populations thought to be at risk of infection; 11 percent with knowledge, attitudes, and behavior in response to the AIDS epidemic; 11 percent with perinatal transmission; 9 percent with the association between HIV and other sexually transmitted diseases; 8 percent with the natural history of the infection; 8 percent with the association between HIV and tuberculosis; and 4 percent with rapid field diagnosis of HIV infection (Heymann et al., 1990). The database was updated once in 1991, but insufficient funds forced the cancellation of the project shortly thereafter.

nia, the national AIDS control program recently devoted resources to development of a national database of AIDS research.

Ignorance about other efforts can lead to duplication of research. Moreover, in cases where some duplication or validation of research in a second location would be desirable, the lack of ready access to reports on previous research means that researchers often do not follow the same study design or benefit from the experiences of other researchers. Consequently, "reinvention of the wheel" is a widespread phenomenon. There is an urgent need for more information sharing among AIDS professionals both within and among sub-Saharan African countries. In the absence of an up-to-date inventory of existing research, it is impossible to identify gaps in research relative to any established set of priorities.

Another problem is that because few local outlets exist for publishing research results, researchers rely on international journals for widespread dissemination of their work. Results are withheld until they have been accepted and published, a time-consuming process that can take 2 years or longer. Thus, there is a considerable delay in making study findings available to policy makers and other researchers. Mechanisms are needed to facilitate more rapid dissemination of research results through local conferences and regional journals in which researchers can present and publish interim findings. Information sharing could also be facilitated by donors' sponsoring innovative information exchange activities and mechanisms for communication within and among countries. Such mechanisms might include newsletters; electronic bulletin boards; national or regional clearinghouses for materials, articles, and relevant questionnaires; local, national, or regional HIV-prevention conferences and training workshops; traveling "road shows" that would showcase model programs and experienced program managers; and sending of experienced managers and researchers as consultants to HIV-prevention programs in other countries.

One example of an effort to promote information exchange is ongoing in Zambia, where Morehouse University (Atlanta, Georgia) is planning a workshop to review and disseminate research findings for researchers working there (see Appendix A). This first step is encouraging because to date, there have been no efforts in Zambia to synthesize research findings, and there is no readily accessible bibliography of AIDS-related social and behavioral research.

Lack of Research-Needs Assessment and Difficulty of Coordinating Funding from Multiple Sources

Few African countries have undertaken a needs assessment for social and behavioral research or established research review boards to prioritize and coordinate research proposals. Consequently, the potential for inefficient use of resources and overlap of activities is considerable.

Even if the national AIDS control program or another agency were to achieve a broad consensus on research priorities, the coordination of funding for all priority areas would be difficult. Funds for AIDS-related social and behavioral research come from a variety of sources, many of which have themselves established priorities. Among these sources are (1) national AIDS control programs, which allocate small percentages of their annual budgets to AIDS research (Mann et al., 1992), primarily sentinel surveillance; (2) sub-Saharan African governments that support research through in-kind contributions of manpower and office space; and (3) nongovernmental organizations and international development agencies that fund their own research agendas, as well as support African research institutions through donations of technical equipment and support. In addition, many African researchers collaborate on an ad hoc basis with colleagues from developed countries who have access to research funds.

Lack of Cooperation Among Donor Agencies

AIDS research in sub-Saharan Africa is characterized by an overall lack of cooperation among donor agencies. "Virtually without exception [donors] are reluctant to cooperate and coordinate with each other . . . [resulting in] duplication of activities, while, paradoxically, other critical intervention areas are almost entirely ignored" (Msiska, 1994:16).

The cumulative effect of this lack of cooperation is depressing and contributes to several of the problems discussed earlier in this section: (1) virtually all research projects proposed by outside donors are approved if funding is forthcoming, and local collaborators can be identified; (2) sub-Saharan African governments have been slow to establish their own priorities, and local researchers have no independent means of identifying and mobilizing funds for their projects; and (3) no mechanisms exist for identifying potential duplication of effort in past and current research activities.

Harsh Environment for Social and Behavioral Research

The many constraints inherent in working in developing countries are well known. Overcoming these constraints on a broad scale would require substantial political, economic, social, and technological developments, well beyond the scope of this report. It is important to acknowledge, however, that on a day-to-day basis, researchers working in developing countries must overcome many obstacles that researchers in more developed countries do not have to face.

Unfavorable Political Climate

The overall political climate of a country can be neutral, positive, or negative with regard to AIDS research. Typically, single-party regimes, which historically have been common in sub-Saharan Africa, fall into the last group, tending to favor censorship over open dialogue on the state of the economy and other matters of national interest, including AIDS. Overall, this environment is not conducive to rational decision making on the basis of sound research and policy analysis and results in less-informed debate about policy alternatives (World Bank, 1991). Such political environments also are not supportive of centers that might develop institutional capacity through research and training (World Bank, 1991).

Early in the epidemic, AIDS researchers faced considerable hostility. When AIDS was first discovered, there was a widespread perception that the European and North American press wanted to blame Africa for infecting the world with the disease; this perception caused many African politicians to deny the epidemic's existence (N'Galy et al., 1990). In February 1987, the President of Kenya, perhaps fearing that the presence of the disease would adversely affect international tourism and despite the fact that the Ministry of Health had just launched an anti-AIDS campaign, minimized the extent to which the epidemic had spread through the Kenyan population (Harden, 1987). Furthermore, given the many problems facing sub-Saharan African governments, the problem of AIDS may not appear as immediate as other social issues, a perception that may, in part, explain their attitude toward the disease. In Zaire, the government did not establish a national AIDS control program until 1987 or report AIDS cases to WHO/GPA until 1988, even though a well-known research team in Kinshasa had been presenting papers at international AIDS conferences as early as 1985 that showed hundreds of confirmed cases of AIDS in the country (Mann et al., 1992). Denial and complacency about the epidemic on the part of the general public were equally serious obstacles.

Second, many sub-Saharan African governments have become excessively bureaucratic, in part as a result of social welfare programs that have established governments as the employers of last resort. Researchers petitioning the government, whether for permission to undertake a project, for access to data, or for some other reason, must endure a long and laborious process of obtaining approval.

Third, the existence of corruption is poorly documented but extremely pervasive throughout the region (Kpundeh, 1994). Consequently, sub-Saharan African institutions have experienced serious problems in managing finances and disbursing supplies and equipment. Once widespread corruption and poor work habits had been established at senior levels, they rapidly filtered down through the administrative structure, becoming next-to-impossible to eradicate.

Decline of Higher-Education Systems in Sub-Saharan Africa

Institutes of higher learning in sub-Saharan Africa have not been shielded from the negative consequences of the current economic crisis. In some cases, universities have been viewed as the centers of organized protest against government policies, and as a result some have been closed or starved for resources.

Rapid population growth, coupled with persistently low and, in some cases, negative rates of economic growth, has constrained public expenditures for education. As a result, funds for higher education have declined, enrollment rates have stagnated, and the quality of education has deteriorated substantially.

Since independence, the priority of sub-Saharan African governments has been to expand the number and size of universities without sufficient regard to their quality. Consequently, the growth in the number of university graduates has been spectacular, but the quality of education offered has fallen dramatically (World Bank, 1988). Currently, higher education in sub-Saharan Africa is characterized by (1) a general overproduction of poorly qualified graduates; (2) an overproduction of the wrong types of graduates, that is, an inappropriate mix of outputs; and (3) a high price tag (World Bank, 1989).

The decline in quality at all levels of education, but particularly at the tertiary level, has had severe repercussions for the region's short-term analytical and research capacity. The flight of many top faculty and the rapid deterioration of sub-Saharan African universities have resulted in the loss of high-quality research centers able to supply policy makers with research results and policy analysis for planning purposes. But in the long term, the decline in higher education will result in a much more serious loss: a decline in the quality of these institutions' future graduates.

Inadequate Infrastructure

On a day-to-day operational level, inadequate transportation and communications systems make project implementation infinitely more challenging in sub-Saharan Africa than in developed countries. Inadequate roads make it more difficult for researchers to work in comparatively remote areas; consequently, they are forced to work in more developed areas of the country. Lack of phone systems and electronic communications equipment hinders collaboration and slows the execution of a project. Unstable electrical systems make computer equipment vulnerable to damage and interrupt the project's work plan.

Economic Weakness

AIDS struck the African continent just at a time when it was undergoing its worst financial crisis since independence. The weakness of many African economies contributes to their difficulties in developing an indigenous capacity to conduct research.

In an attempt to stimulate growth and reverse economic declines, many sub-Saharan African governments have been forced to institute structural adjustment programs. A key element of these programs is to bring government budget deficits under control. Despite abundant evidence of overstaffing, most sub-Saharan African governments have found it politically infeasible to reduce the number of government employees and have sought to ease their fiscal burden by allowing inflation to outpace salary increases. In many cases, salaries have fallen below acceptable living standards. A recent survey of eight sub-Saharan African countries found real starting salaries had declined between the early to mid-1970s and 1983 for virtually all grades within the civil service, in some cases by 30 percent or more (Lindauer et al., 1988). In Somalia, salaries in 1985 were only one-twentieth of their real value in 1975 (Robinson, 1990).

The decline in real wages has had disastrous consequences for morale and work efforts throughout the public sector. A report on pay and working conditions in Sudan concluded that:

> . . . the dramatic reduction in real pay has had an equally dramatic effect on performance, motivation and the general level of civil service activities. Attendance at work is unreliable, and performance when at work is low and unsatisfactory for many parts of the civil service . . . it is a matter of some urgency that morale and performance be raised (International Labour Office, 1987:127, 130).

In Uganda, the deterioration of pay and working conditions in the public sector has led to an increase in fraudulent practices such as improper use of allowances, kickbacks on government purchases, illicit payments for not enforcing laws and regulations, diversion of public goods into private hands, and bribes for licenses and permits (Republic of Uganda, 1988, cited in Chew, 1990). The most visible adaptation by civil servants to a reduction in their real wages has been a massive reduction in the number of hours worked. To recover lost wages, many government employees work less than half a normal working day and spend the remainder of the day engaged in small-scale farming or moonlighting in the private sector (Chew, 1990).

Because the majority of sub-Saharan African researchers are employed by public universities, they have experienced declines in real wages comparable to those of other public-sector employees. Not surprisingly, these pay cuts have negatively affected their morale and work performance and made opportunities outside academia more attractive. Many faculty have left. Those who have remained spend much less time than before concentrating on research or other activities necessary to reestablish the university as a center for excellence. Rather, they are forced to spend their time looking for ways to supplement their meager government salaries through consultancies or participation in other business ventures.

Weak Policy Support for the Health Sector

The health sector has not been spared cutbacks as hard times have forced sub-Saharan African governments to implement fiscal austerity measures (Cornia et al., 1987). These measures have seriously impaired the ability of sub-Saharan African health ministries and national AIDS control programs to function efficiently and achieve their objectives. Between 1975 and 1989, the percentage of government expenditures for health fell in 13 of the 22 countries for which time series data are available (World Bank, 1994). In 1985, the average per capita expenditure for health care by sub-Saharan African governments equalled US $5.32, as compared with per capita expenditures of US $1,340 in developed countries and US $323 for the world as a whole (World Bank, 1994).

Low Value Placed on Social and Behavioral Research

An appreciation of the multifaceted cultural, social, and behavioral contexts throughout sub-Saharan Africa and how they are changing in the face of the AIDS epidemic is essential for understanding the spread of the epidemic and for evaluating the potential effect of intervention programs (see Chapter 2). Yet social and behavioral research has been underappreciated and largely neglected. To date, the vast majority of funds for HIV/AIDS research has gone toward clinical research in an attempt to understand the nature of the virus, as a logical starting point for identifying a vaccine or a cure. However, a growing consensus is emerging that while a preventive vaccine and an effective cure remain long-term goals, they will not be achieved soon, and that research on the social and behavioral aspects of the disease—which strongly shape the speed and extent of transmission—has been neglected. Given the social, economic, and cultural diversity in the region, there is an urgent need for more local behavioral and social science knowledge.

A lack of appreciation for the potential contributions of behavioral and social science is not unique to sub-Saharan Africa. In the United States, expert advisory groups similar to this panel have repeatedly demanded more and better behavioral and social science research to increase our understanding of HIV/AIDS and inform policy makers and health planners concerned with slowing the spread of the epidemic (Institute of Medicine [United States], 1986, 1988; Miller et al., 1990; National Commission on AIDS [United States], 1991, 1993; Turner et al., 1989).

Researchers themselves are partly responsible for the lack of appreciation for the role of social and behavioral research in controlling the spread of AIDS. In large part, they have not been successful in working with policy makers to translate their findings into better prevention programs.

RECOMMENDATIONS

In the long run, it is essential to help sub-Saharan African countries develop their own research capacity by strengthening their universities and augmenting the technical skills of their researchers. There is considerable debate and controversy, however, about how best to achieve this goal. Regardless of what the best mechanisms may be, no significant progress is likely to be made until the region's governments understand that they must put AIDS more squarely on their own research and policy agendas. Clearly, a major constraint on the amount of HIV/AIDS research that is undertaken is inadequate funding. Potential sources of funding include communities, private-sector firms, the public sector, and international donors. Because it is unlikely that donors are going to increase significantly their levels of funding in the near future, the governments will have to find additional resources. Given the weak economic position of most sub-Saharan African countries, however, it will be difficult to persuade their governments to pursue more vigorous research agendas in the near future.

There are no easy solutions to the problems discussed in this chapter, but below are several recommendations that could improve the situation marginally in the short run and should be considered in developing any long-term strategies for conducting and using research in Africa.

KEY RECOMMENDATION 5. Linkages between sub-Saharan African institutions and international research centers must be established on a wide range of activities, including teaching, research, and faculty and student exchanges. International donors should seriously consider establishing a sub-Saharan African AIDS research institution with a strong behavioral and social science element.

There is a critical need to strengthen African research institutions in sub-Saharan Africa. Linkages with international organizations, especially if built on an evolving and well-defined research agenda, can help local institutions develop and assist local researchers by providing relatively secure long-term funding, offering support for the preparation of data and manuscripts for publication and dissemination, and providing in-country technical assistance and research training. Experience in a number of settings has demonstrated that such long-term collaboration, in addition to contributing significantly to understanding of the HIV/AIDS epidemic, is mutually beneficial to all institutions involved; it could be very successful in providing highly skilled African researchers with support and the possibility of remaining in their country of origin.

Recommendation 7-1. The number of African scientists well trained to conduct research on HIV and AIDS must be increased.

Research capacity in sub-Saharan Africa cannot be improved without an increase in the number of well-trained local researchers. Many African institutions suffer from a serious shortage of competent professionals, and those that are well staffed have enormous difficulty retaining their best people. The lure of high salaries in the private sector or from international donors is often strong enough to pull many Africans out of local research institutions, including universities. Many others migrate abroad. Furthermore, the rapid emergence of AIDS meant that the only short-run solution to the dearth of AIDS researchers was to borrow from related disciplines. Now that the nature and magnitude of the epidemic are better understood, there is an urgent need for universities to develop appropriate curricula to train researchers as AIDS specialists.

Four possible ways to introduce and keep more researchers in the field are to (1) integrate more graduate students and young professionals into all new AIDS-related research initiatives; (2) establish small grants programs to fund the projects of young researchers; (3) adjust pay scales to attract and retain talented professionals; and (4) provide other incentives for researchers to remain in their home institutions, including small-scale research grants, fewer teaching or administrative responsibilities, and more opportunities for international travel. Providing technical assistance to local researchers is an important priority. Local researchers could benefit from workshops that would help them design research projects, prepare research proposals, identify potential sources of funding, write reports describing interim results, and prepare final manuscripts for submission to peer-reviewed journals.

Recommendation 7-2. Each national AIDS control program should establish a local AIDS-information center that would develop and maintain a database of all AIDS-related research conducted in the country.

These centers should be linked via available technology, such as the Internet. They should also have AIDS databases available on CD-ROM. (CD-ROM equipped computers are available in most national AIDS control program offices.) In addition, national and regional conferences should be held to provide forums at which researchers can discuss their research plans and present their results to a larger group of local researchers than those that attend international conferences.

Recommendation 7-3. There is an urgent need for sub-Saharan African countries to establish and periodically update research priorities at the regional and national levels, providing a basis for discussions with donors on AIDS-related research.

It is important to reduce the proportion of donor-driven research taking place in the region.

Recommendation 7-4. International organizations and donors should utilize existing local resources to the fullest extent possible.

It is paradoxical that donors underutilize existing talent in the region. Utilizing local expertise can strengthen local institutions, generate employment, and create opportunities for talented researchers in sub-Saharan Africa.

Recommendation 7-5. Greater dialogue between researchers and policy makers is necessary.

Not only is there an urgent need to increase indigenous capacity to conduct research, but there is also a need to better synthesize and translate research findings into effective prevention and control programs and policies. Otherwise, prevention programs will be only marginally based on local needs or tailored to local conditions, and research will be even more undervalued and underfunded. Researchers need to do a better job of drawing out the policy implications of their work, and planners and policy makers need to articulate more clearly to researchers what information they need for effective planning and programs (Uganda AIDS Commission, 1992).

Recommendation 7-6. If more effective strategies for AIDS prevention and mitigation are to be developed in the future, better coordination among donors is needed, particularly sharing of information about which prevention and control efforts work and which do not.

The role of the new cosponsored United Nations Programme on AIDS (UNAIDS) will be critical to future work.[4] Success will also require greater political will and commitment on the part of the governments of sub-Saharan Africa and other countries.

---

[4]Announcing Dr. Peter Piot's appointment as the head of the newly formed United Nations Programme on AIDS, Dr. Boutros Boutros-Ghali declared that "faced with a truly global emergency and its multisectoral needs, it is imperative that the UN response is comprehensive and effective. HIV/AIDS will not be controlled unless all of us, acting as a global community, unite our efforts, coordinate our actions, and reduce duplication" (World Health Organization, 1995:1).

References

CHAPTER 1: INTRODUCTION

Ainsworth, M., and A. M. Over

1994a The economic impact of AIDS on Africa. Pp. 559-588 in M. Essex, S. Mboup, P.J. Kanki, and M.R. Kalengayi, eds., *AIDS in Africa*. New York: Raven Press.

1994b AIDS and African development. *World Bank Research Observer* 9(2):203-240.

Barnett, T., and P. Blaikie

1992 *AIDS in Africa: Its Present and Future Impact*. London, UK: Belhaven Press.

Caldwell, J.C.

1995 Understanding the AIDS epidemic and reacting sensibly to it. *Social Science and Medicine* 41(3):299-302.

Caldwell, J.C., and P. Caldwell

1993 The nature and limits of the sub-Saharan Africa AIDS epidemic: Evidence from geographic and other patterns. *Population and Development Review* 19(4):817-848.

Caldwell, J.C., P. Caldwell, E.M. Ankrah, J.K. Anarfi, D.K. Agyeman, K. Awusabo-Asare, and I.O. Orubuloye

1993 African families and AIDS: Context, reactions and potential interventions. *Health Transition Review* 3(Supplement):1-16.

Coates, T.J.

1993 Prevention of HIV-I infection: accomplishments and priorities. *Journal of NIH Research* 5(7):73-76.

Cohen, J.

1993 Jitters jeopardize AIDS vaccine trials. *Science* 262(5136):980-981.

1994a U.S. panel votes to delay real-world vaccine trials. *Science* 264(5167):1839.

1994b Are researchers racing toward success, or crawling? *Science* 265(5177):1373-1375.

Dada, A.J., F. Oyewole, R. Onofowokan, A. Nasidi, B. Harris, A. Levin, L. Diamondstone, T.C. Quinn, and W.A. Blattner

1993 Demographic characteristics of retroviral infections (HIV-1, HIV-2 and HTLV-I) among female professional sex workers in Lagos, Nigeria. *Journal of Acquired Immune Deficiency Syndromes* 6(12):1358-1363.

De Cock, K.M., B. Barrere, L. Diaby, M.F. Lafontaine, E. Gnaore, A. Porter, D. Pantobe, G.C. Lafontant, A. Dagoakribi, M. Ette, K. Odehouri, and W.L. Heyward

1990 AIDS—the leading cause of adult death in the West African city of Abidjan, Ivory Coast. *Science* 249(4970):793-796.

Feachem, R., P. Musgrove, and A.E. Elmendorf

1995 Comment from the World Bank. *AIDS* 9(8):982-983.

Grosskurth, H., F. Mosha, J. Todd, E. Mwijarubi, A. Klokke, K. Senkoro, P. Mayaud, J. Changalucha, A. Nicoll, G. ka-Gina, J. Newell, K. Mugeye, D. Mabey, and R. Hayes

1995 Impact of improved treatment of sexually transmitted diseases on HIV infection in rural Tanzania: randomised controlled trial. *The Lancet* 346(8974):530-536.

Hassig, S.E., J. Perriens, E. Baende, M. Kahotwa, K. Bishagara, N. Kinkela, and B. Kapita

1990 An analysis of the economic impact of HIV infection among patients at Mama Yemo Hospital, Kinshasa, Zaire. *AIDS* 4(9):883-887.

International Ad Hoc Scientific Committee on HIV Vaccines

1994a *HIV Vaccines — Accelerating the Development of Preventive HIV Vaccines for the World. Summary Report and Recommendations of an International Meeting.* March 7-11, 1994. Bellagio, Italy: The Rockefeller Foundation.

1994b *HIV Vaccines — Accelerating the Development of Preventive HIV Vaccines for the World. Summary Report and Recommendations of an International Ad Hoc Scientific Committee.* October 27-28, 1994. Paris, France: The Rockefeller Foundation and the Fondation Mérieux.

Kaijage, F.J.

1994a HIV/AIDS and the orphan crisis in Kagera region: Socio-economic, cultural, and historic dimensions. Unpublished background paper prepared for the USAID/Tanzania AIDS Project's Family Needs Assessment Report, Dar es Salaam, Tanzania. Department of History, University of Dar es Salaam, Tanzania.

1994b HIV/AIDS and the problem of orphans in Arusha region. Unpublished background paper prepared for the USAID/Tanzania AIDS Project's Family Needs Assessment Report, Dar es Salaam, Tanzania. Department of History, University of Dar es Salaam, Tanzania.

Kitange, H.M., D.G. Mclarty, A.B.M. Swai, J. Black, H. Machibya, D. Mtasiwa, G. Masuki, and K.G.M.M. Alberti

1994 HIV disease: The leading cause of adult death in three study areas (urban and rural) in Tanzania. Paper presented to the National Institute for Medical Research's 12th Annual Joint Scientific Conference, 21-25 February, Arusha, Tanzania.

Lamptey, P., T. Coates, P. Piot, and G. Slutkin

1993 HIV prevention: Is it working? Abstract No. PS-02-2, Volume 9(1):9. IXth International Conference on AIDS, June 6-11, Berlin, Germany.

Lurie, P., P. Hintzen, and R.A. Lowe

1995a Socioeconomic obstacles to HIV prevention and treatment in developing countries: the roles of the International Monetary Fund and the World Bank. *AIDS* 9(6):539-546.

1995b Response to the World Bank. *AIDS* 9(8):983-984.

Mann, J., D.J.M. Tarantola, and T.W. Netter, eds.

1992 *AIDS in the World.* Cambridge, MA: Harvard University Press.

McKeown, T.

1979 *The Role of Medicine: Dream, Mirage, or Nemesis?* Princeton, NJ: Princeton University Press.

Mulder, D.W., A.J. Nunn, A. Kamali, and J.F. Kengeya-Kayondo

1995 Decreasing HIV-1 seroprevalence in young adults in a rural Ugandan cohort. *British Medical Journal* 311(7009):833-836.

Mulder, D.W., A.J. Nunn, A. Kamali, J. Nakiyingi, H.U. Wagner, and J.F. Kengeya-Kayondo
1994a Two-year HIV-1-associated mortality in a Ugandan rural population. *The Lancet* 343(8904):1021-1023.

Mulder, D.W., A.J. Nunn, H.U. Wagner, A. Kamali, and J.F. Kengeya-Kayondo
1994b HIV-1 incidence and HIV-1-associated mortality in a rural Ugandan population cohort. *AIDS* 8(1):87-92.

Nelson, A.M., S.E. Hassig, M. Kayembe, L. Okonda, K. Mulanga, C. Brown, K. Kayembe, M.M. Kalengayi, and F.G. Mullick
1991 HIV-1 seropositivity and mortality at University Hospital, Kinshasa, Zaire, 1987. *AIDS* 5(5):583-586.

Nunn, A.J., J.F. Kengeya-Kayondo, S.S. Malamba, J.A. Seeley, and D.W. Mulder
1994 Risk factors for HIV-1 infection in adults in a rural Ugandan community: a population study. *AIDS* 8(1):81-86.

Over, M., and P. Piot
1993 HIV infection and sexually transmitted diseases. Pp. 455-527 in D.T. Jamison, W.H. Mosley, A.R. Measham, and J.L. Bobadilla, eds., *Disease Control Priorities in Developing Countries*. New York: Oxford University Press.

Piot, P., M. Laga, R. Ryder, J. Perriens, M. Temmerman, W. Heyward, and J.W. Curran
1990 The global epidemiology of HIV infection: Continuity, heterogeneity, and change. *Journal of Acquired Immune Deficiency Syndromes* 3(4):403-412.

Potts, M., R. Anderson, and M.C. Boily
1991 Slowing the spread of human immunodeficiency virus in developing countries. *The Lancet* 338(8767):608-613.

Sewankambo, N.K., M.J. Wawer, R.H. Gray, D. Serwadda, C. Li, R.Y. Stallings, S.D. Musgrave, and J. Konde-Lule
1994 Demographic impact of HIV infection in rural Rakai District, Uganda: Results of a population-based cohort study. *AIDS* 8(10):1707-1713.

Stanecki, K.A., L. Heaton, and P. Way
1995 *Sexually Transmitted Diseases in Sub-Saharan Africa and Associated Interactions with HIV*. International Programs Center Staff Paper No. 75. Washington, D.C.: International Programs Center, Population Division, U.S. Bureau of the Census.

Stanecki, K.A. and P. Way
1994 *Review of HIV Spread in Southern Africa*. Washington D.C.: Center for International Research, U.S. Bureau of the Census.

Tembo, G., H. Friesan, G. Asiimwe-Okiror, R. Moser, W. Naamara, N. Bakyaita, and J. Musinguzi
1994 Bed occupancy due to HIV/AIDS in an urban hospital medical ward in Uganda. *AIDS* 8(8):1169-1171.

Turner, C.F., H.G. Miller, and L.E. Moses, eds.
1989 *AIDS: Sexual Behavior and Intravenous Drug Use*. National Research Council. Washington, D.C.: National Academy Press.

U.S. Bureau of the Census
1994 *HIV/AIDS Surveillance Database: Program Diskette, December 1994*. Washington D.C.: Center for International Research, U.S. Bureau of the Census.

Way, P.O., and K.A. Stanecki
1994 *The Impact of HIV/AIDS on World Population*. Washington, D.C.: U.S. Bureau of the Census.

World Bank
1993 *World Development Report, 1993: Investing in Health*. Oxford, UK: Oxford University Press.

World Health Organization
1994 *AIDS: Images of the Epidemic*. Geneva, Switzerland: World Health Organization.

1995 The current global situation of the HIV/AIDS pandemic. *Weekly Epidemiological Record* 70(2):7-8.

CHAPTER 2: SOCIETAL CONTEXT

Anderson, R.M.
1991 The transmission dynamics of sexually transmitted diseases: The behavioral component. Pp. 38-60 in J.N. Wasserheit, S.O. Aral, and K.K. Holmes, eds., *Research Issues in Human Behavior and Sexually Transmitted Diseases in the AIDS Era*. Washington, D.C.: American Society for Microbiology.

Anderson, R.M., and R.M. May
1992 Understanding the AIDS pandemic. *Scientific American* 266(5):58-66.

Andriole, V.T.
1988 Clinical overview of the newer 4-quinolone antibacterial agents. Pp. 155-200 in V.T. Andriole, ed., *The Quinolones*. London, UK: Academic Press.

Antoine, P., and J. Nanitelamio
1991 More single women in African cities: Pikin Abidjan and Brazzaville. *Population: An English Selection* 3:149-169.

Balépa, M., M. Fotso, and B. Barrère
1992 *Enquête Démographique et de Santé: Cameroun, 1991*. Yaoundé, Cameroon: Direction Nationale du Deuxième Recensement Gènèral; Columbia, MD: Macro International.

Barrère, B., J. Schoemaker, M. Barrère, T. Habiyakare, A. Kabagwira, and M. Ngendakumana
1994 *Enquête Démographique et de Santé: Rwanda, 1992*. Kigali, Rwanda: Office National de la Population; Calverton, MD: Macro International.

Bledsoe, C.H. and B. Cohen, eds.
1993 *Social Dynamics of Adolescent Fertility in Sub-Saharan Africa*. Washington, D.C.: National Academy Press.

Bwayo, J.J., A.N. Mutere, M.A. Omari, J.K. Kreiss, W. Jaoko, C. Sekkade-Kigondu, and F.A. Plummer
1991a Long distance truck drivers: 2. Knowledge and attitudes concerning sexually transmitted diseases and sexual behaviour. *East African Medical Journal* 68(9):714-719.

Bwayo, J.J., A.M. Omari, A.N. Mutere, W. Jaoko, C. Sekkade-Kigondo, J. Kreiss, and F.A. Plummer
1991b Long distance truck-drivers: 1. Prevalence of sexually transmitted diseases (STDs). *East African Medical Journal* 68(6):425-429.

Caldwell, J.C.
1995 Understanding the AIDS epidemic and reacting sensibly to it. *Social Science and Medicine* 41(3):299-302.

Caldwell, J.C., and P. Caldwell
1993 The nature and limits of the sub-Saharan Africa AIDS epidemic: Evidence from geographic and other patterns. *Population and Development Review* 19(4):817-848.

Caldwell, J.C., P. Caldwell, and I.O. Orubuloye
1992 The family and sexual networking in sub-Saharan Africa: Historical regional differences and present-day implications. *Population Studies* 46(3):385-410.

Caldwell, J.C., P. Caldwell, and P. Quiggin
1989 The social context of AIDS in sub-Saharan Africa. *Population and Development Review* 15(2):185-234.

Caldwell, J.C., G. Santow, I.O. Orubuloye, P. Caldwell, and J. Anarfi, eds.
1993 *Sexual Networking and HIV/AIDS in West Africa*. Special supplement to *Health Tran-*

sition Review, Volume 3. Canberra: Health Transition Centre, Australian National University.

Carballo, M., and P.I. Kenya
1994 Behavioral issues and AIDS. Pp. 497-512 in M. Essex, S. Mboup, P.J. Kanki, and M.R. Kalengayi, eds., *AIDS in Africa*. New York: Raven Press.

Carswell, J.W., G. Lloyd, and J. Howells
1989 Prevalence of HIV-1 in east African lorry drivers. *AIDS* 3(11):759-761.

Central Statistical Office [Zimbabwe]
1989 *Demographic and Health Survey, 1988*. Harare, Zimbabwe: Central Statistical Office; Columbia, MD: Macro International.

de Zalduondo, B.O., M.H. Avila, and P.U. Zuñiga
1991 Intervention research needs for AIDS prevention among commercial sex workers and their clients. Pp. 165-178 in L.C. Chen, J.S. Amor, and S.J. Segal, eds., *AIDS and Women's Reproductive Health*. New York: Plenum Press.

Denis, F., F. Barin, G. Gershy-Damet, J.L. Rey, M. Lhuillier, M. Mounier, G. Leonard, A. Sangare, A. Goudeau, S. M'Boup, M. Essex, and P. Kanki
1987 Prevalence of human T-lymphotropic retroviruses Type III (HIV) and Type IV in Ivory Coast. *The Lancet* 1(8530):408-411.

Dyson, T., ed.
1992 *Sexual Behaviour and Networking: Anthropological and Socio-Cultural Studies on the Transmission of HIV*. Liège, Belgium: Editions Derouaux-Ordina.

Edmondson, J., M. Wawer, N. Sewankambo, D. Serwadda, and R. Ssengonzi
1993 The rural marketing system as a nexus for HIV transmission in Uganda. Abstract No. PO-D01-3401, Volume 9(2):784. IXth International Conference on AIDS, June 6-11, Berlin, Germany.

Feachem, R., P. Musgrove, and A.E. Elmendorf
1995 Comment from the World Bank. *AIDS* 9(8):982-983.

Federal Office of Statistics [Nigeria]
1992 *Nigeria Demographic and Health Survey, 1990*. Columbia, MD: Institute for Resource Development/Macro International.

Gaisie, K., A.R. Cross, and G. Nsemukila
1993 *Zambia Demographic and Health Survey, 1992*. Lusaka, Zambia: University of Zambia, and Central Statistical Office; Columbia, MD: Macro International.

Gersony, R.
1988 *Summary of Mozambican Refugee Accounts of Principally Conflict-related Experience in Mozambique*. Washington, D.C.: Bureau for Refugee Persons, U.S. Department of State.

Ghana Statistical Service
1989 *Ghana Demographic and Health Survey, 1988*. Columbia, MD: Institute for Resource Development/Macro Systems.

Goldman. N., and A. Pebley
1989 The demography of polygyny in sub-Saharan Africa. Pp. 212-237 in R.J. Lesthaeghe, ed., *Reproduction and Social Organization in Sub-Saharan Africa*. Berkeley, CA: University of California Press.

Guyer, J.I.
1994 Lineal identities and lateral networks: The logic of polyandrous motherhood. Pp. 231-252 in C. Bledsoe and G. Pison, eds., *Nuptiality in Sub-Saharan Africa: Contemporary Anthropological and Demographic Perspectives*. Oxford, UK: Clarendon Press.

Handsfield, H.H.
1991 New macrolides in the treatment of sexually transmitted diseases. Abstract C-20-272.

9th International Meeting of the International Society for STD Research, 6-9 October, Banff, Alberta, Canada.

Handsfield, H.H., W.M. McCormack, E.W. Hook III, J.M. Douglas Jr., J.M. Covino, M.S. Verdon, C.A. Reichart, and J.M. Ehret
1991 A comparison of single-dose cefixime with ceftriaxone as treatment for uncomplicated gonorrhea. The Gonorrhea Treatment Study Group. *New England Journal of Medicine* 325(19):1337-1341.

Heise, L.L., and C. Elias
1995 Transforming AIDS prevention to meet women's needs: a focus on developing countries. *Social Science and Medicine* 40(7):931-943.

Hogsborg, M., and P. Aaby
1992 Sexual relations, use of condoms and perceptions of AIDS in an urban area of Guinea-Bissau with a high prevalence of HIV-2. Pp. 203-231 in T. Dyson, ed., *Sexual Behaviour and Networking: Anthropological and Socio-cultural Studies on the Transmission of HIV*. Liège, Belgium: Editions Derouaux-Ordina.

Hudson, C.P.
1993 Concurrent partners and the results of the Uganda Rakai project. *AIDS* 7(2):286-288.

Hunt, C.W.
1989 Migrant labor and sexually transmitted disease: AIDS in Africa. *Journal of Health and Social Behavior* 30(4):353-373.

Jochleson, K., M. Mothibeli, and J.-P. Leger
1991 Human immunodeficiency virus and migrant labor in South Africa. *International Journal of Health Services* 21(1):157-173.

Jones, R.B., and J.N. Wasserheit
1991 Introduction to the biology and natural history of sexually transmitted diseases. Pp. 11-37 in J.N. Wasserheit, S.O. Aral, and K.K. Holmes, eds., *Research Issues in Human Behavior and Sexually Transmitted Diseases in the AIDS Era*. Washington, D.C.: American Society for Microbiology.

Kaijuka, E.M., E.Z.A. Kaija, A.R. Cross, and E. Loaiza
1989 *Uganda Demographic and Health Survey, 1988/1989*. Entebbe, Uganda: Ministry of Health and Makerere University; Columbia, MD: Macro Systems.

Karanja, W.W.
1987 'Outside wives' and 'inside wives' in Nigeria: A study of changing perceptions in marriage. Pp. 247-261 in D. Parkin and D. Nyamwaya, eds., *Transformations of African Marriage*. Manchester, UK: Manchester University Press.

Katjiuanjo, P., S. Titus, M. Zauana, and J.T. Boerma
1993 *Namibia Demographic and Health Survey, 1992*. Windhoek, Namibia: Ministry of Health and Social Services; Columbia, MD: Macro International.

Konaté, D.L., T. Sinaré, and M. Seroussi
1994 *Enquête Démographique et de Santé: Burkina Faso, 1993*. Ouagadougou, Burkina Faso: Institut National de la Statistique; Calverton, MD: Macro International.

Kourguéni, I.A., B. Garba, and B. Barrère
1993 *Enquête Démographique et de Santé: Niger, 1992*. Niamey, Niger: Direction de la Statistique et des Comptes Nationaux.

Larson, A.
1989 Social context of human immunodeficiency virus transmission in Africa: Historical and cultural bases of east and central African sexual relations. *Review of Infectious Diseases* 11(5):716-731.

Lurie, P., P. Hintzen, and R.A. Lowe
1995 Socioeconomic obstacles to HIV prevention and treatment in developing countries: the roles of the International Monetary Fund and the World Bank. *AIDS* 9(6):539-546.

Mann, J., D.J.M. Tarantola, and T.W. Netter, eds.
1992 *AIDS in the World*. Cambridge, MA: Harvard University Press.

Martin, D.H., T.F. Mroczkowski, Z.A. Dalu, J. McCarty, R.B. Jones, S.J. Hopkins, and R.B. Johnson.
1992 A controlled trial of a single dose of azithomycin for the treatment of chlamydial urethritis and cervicitis. The azithromycin for chlamydial infections study group. *New England Journal of Medicine* 327(13):921-925.

McGinn, T., A. Bamba, and A. Balma
1989 Male knowledge, use and attitudes regarding family planning in Burkina Faso. *International Family Planning Perspectives* 15(3):84-87.

Ministry of Health [Uganda]
1988 *A Guide to Uganda Essential Drug Kits*. Fourth Edition. Kampala, Uganda: Ministry of Health.

Morris, M.W., N. Sewankambo, M. Wawer, D. Serwadda, and B. Lainjo
1995 Concurrent partnerships and HIV transmission in Rakai District, Uganda. Abstract. IXth International Conference on AIDS and STDs in Africa, December 10-14, 1995, Kampala, Uganda.

National Council for Population and Development [Kenya]
1994 *Kenya Demographic and Health Survey, 1993*. Nairobi, Kenya: Central Bureau of Statistics; Calverton, MD: Macro International.

Ndiaye, S., P.D. Diouf, and M. Ayad
1994 *Enquête Démographique et de Santé au Sénégal (EDS-II), 1992/93*. Dakar, Senegal: Ministère de l'Economie; Calverton, MD: Macro International.

Neequaye, A.R., L. Osei, J.A.A. Mingle, G. Ankra-Badu, C. Bentsi, A. Asamoah-Adu, and J.E. Neequaye
1988 Dynamics of human immune deficiency virus (HIV) epidemic the Ghanaian experience. Pp. 9-15 in A.F. Fleming, M. Carballo, D.W. FitzSimons, M.R. Bailey, and J. Mann, eds., *The Global Impact of AIDS*. New York: Alan R. Liss.

Ngallaba, S., S.H. Kapiga, I. Ruyobya, and J.T. Boerma
1993 *Tanzania Demographic and Health Survey, 1991/1992*. Dar es Salaam, Tanzania: Bureau of Statistics; Columbia, MD: Macro International.

Obbo, C.
1993 HIV transmission through social and geographic networks in Uganda. *Social Science & Medicine* 36(7):949-955.

Ogbu, O., and M. Gallagher
1992 Public expenditures and health care in Africa. *Social Science & Medicine* 34(6):615-624.

Okoth-Ogendo, H.W.O.
1991 Africa's migrant millions. *People* 18(4):24-26.

Omara-Otunnu, A.
1987 *Politics and the Military in Uganda 1890-1985*. Basingstoke, Hampshire, UK: Macmillan Press.

Orubuloye, I.O., J.C. Caldwell, and P. Caldwell
1990 *Experimental Research on Sexual Networking in the Ekiti District of Nigeria*. Health Transition Working Paper No. 3. Canberra, Australia: Health Transition Centre, Australian National University.
1991 Sexual networking in the Ekiti district of Nigeria. *Studies in Family Planning* 22(2):61-73.
1992 Diffusion and focus in sexual networking: Identifying partners and partners' partners. *Studies in Family Planning* 23(6):343-351.
1994 *Sexual Networking and AIDS in Sub-Saharan Africa: Behavioural Research and the Social Context*. Canberra: Health Transition Centre, Australian National University.

Orubuloye, I.O., P. Caldwell, and J.C. Caldwell
1993 The role of high-risk occupations in the spread of AIDS: Truck drivers and itinerant market women in Nigeria. *International Family Planning Perspectives* 19(2):43-48.

Oucho, J.O., and W.T.S. Gould
1993 Internal migration, urbanization, and population distribution. Pp. 256-296 in K.A. Foote, K.H. Hill, and L.G. Martin, eds., *Demographic Change in Sub-Saharan Africa*. Washington, D.C.: National Academy Press.

Pebley, A.R., and W. Mbugua
1989 Polygyny and fertility in sub-Saharan Africa. Pp. 338-364 in R.J. Lesthaeghe, ed., *Reproduction and Social Organization in Sub-Saharan Africa*. Berkeley, CA: University of California Press.

Pepin, J., F.A. Plummer, R.C. Brunham, P. Piot, D.W. Cameron, and A.R. Ronald
1989 The interaction of HIV infection and other sexually transmitted diseases: An opportunity for intervention. *AIDS* 3(1):3-9.

Philips, I., A. King, and K. Shannon
1988 In vitro properties of the quinolones. Pp. 83-117 in V.T. Andriole, ed., *The Quinolones*. London, UK: Academic Press.

Piot, P., and R. Tezzo
1990 The epidemiology of HIV and other sexually transmitted infections in the developing world. *Scandinavian Journal of Infectious Diseases Supplementum* 69:89-97.

Plourde, P.J., F.A. Plummer, M. Tyndall, E. Agoki, J. Mobete, L.A. Slaney, L.J. D'Costa, and J.O. Ndinya-Achola
1991 A randomized, open-label study of the efficacy of single dose cefixime vs. single dose ceftriaxone in the treatment of uncomplicated gonorrhoea. Abstract C-20-006. 9th International Meeting of the International Society for STD Research, October 6-9, Banff, Alberta, Canada.

Preston-Whyte, E.
1994 Gender and the lost generation: The dynamics of HIV transmission among black South African teenagers in KwaZulu/Natal. *Health Transition Review* 4(Supplement):241-255.

Quinn, T.C.
1994 Population migration and the spread of types 1 and 2 human immunodeficiency viruses. *Proceedings of the National Academy of Sciences* (USA) 91(7):2407-2414.

Rothenberg, R.B., and J.J. Potterat
1990 Strategies for management of sex partners. Pp. 1081-1086 in K.K. Holmes, P.A. Mardh, and P.F. Sparling, eds., *Sexually Transmitted Diseases*. New York: McGraw-Hill.

Rutenberg, N., A.K. Blanc, and S. Kapiga
1994 Sexual behaviour, social change, and family planning among men and women in Tanzania. *Health Transition Review* 4(Supplement):173-196.

Schoepf, B.G.
1988 Women, AIDS, and the economic crisis in Central Africa. *Canadian Journal of African Studies* 22(3):625-644.
1992 Sex, gender and society in Zaire. Pp. 353-375 in T. Dyson, ed., *Sexual Behaviour and Networking: Anthropological and Socio-cultural Studies on the Transmission of HIV*. Liège, Belgium: Editions Derouaux-Ordina.

Serwadda, D., M.J. Wawer, S.D. Musgrave, N.K. Sewankambo, J.E. Kaplan and R.H. Gray
1992 HIV risk factors in three geographic strata of rural Rakai district, Uganda. *AIDS* 6(9):983-989.

Smallman-Raynor, M.R., and A.D. Cliff
1991 Civil war and the spread of AIDS in central Africa. *Epidemiology and Infection* 107(1):69-80.

Ssengonzi, R., M. Morris, N. Sewankambo, M. Wawer, and D. Serwadda
1995 Economic status and sexual networks in Rakai District, Uganda. Abstract. IXth International Conference on AIDS and STDs in Africa, December 10-14, 1995, Kampala, Uganda.

Stamm, W.E.
1987 Problems in the treatment of bacterial sexually transmitted diseases. *American Journal of Medicine* 82(4A):307-310.

Standing, H., and M.N. Kisekka
1989 *Sexual Behaviour in Sub-Saharan Africa: A Review and Annotated Bibliography*. London, UK: Overseas Development Administration.

Steingrimsson, O., J.H. Olafsson, J. Thorarinsson, R.W. Ryan, R.B. Johnson, and R.C. Tilton
1990 Azithromycin in the treatment of sexually transmitted disease. *Journal of Antimicrobial Chemotherapy* 25(Supplement A):109-114.

United Nations
1991 *World Population Prospects 1990*. New York: Department of International Economic and Social Affairs, United Nations.

United Nations Economic Commission for Africa
1995 *Statistical Compendium on Contraceptive Prevalence and Practice in ECA Member States*. Addis Ababa, Ethiopia: United Nations Economic Commission for Africa.

Wasserheit, J.N.
1992 Epidemiological synergy: Interrelationships between human immunodeficiency virus infection and other sexually transmitted diseases. *Sexually Transmitted Diseases* 19(2):61-77.

Wawer, M.J., D. Serwadda, S.D. Musgrave, J.K. Konde-Lule, M. Musagara, and N.K. Sewankambo
1991 Dynamics of spread of HIV-1 infection in a rural district of Uganda. *British Medical Journal* 303(6813):1303-1306.

Wawer, M.J., L. Gaffikin, V. Ravao, H. Maidouka, and K. Traore
1990 Results of a contraceptive prevalence survey in Niamey, Niger. *International Family Planning Perspectives* 16(3):90-96.

Wood, W.B.
1988 AIDS north and south: Diffusion patterns of a global epidemic and a research agenda for geographers. *Professional Geographer* 40(3):266-279.

CHAPTER 3: EPIDEMIOLOGY OF THE HIV/AIDS EPIDEMIC

Adjorlolo-Johnson, G., K.M. De Cock, E. Ekpini, K.M. Vetter, T. Sibailly, K. Brattegaard, D. Yavo, R. Doorly, J.P. Whitaker, L. Kestens, C.-Y. Ou, J.R. George, and H.D. Gayle
1994 Prospective comparison of mother-to-child transmission of HIV-1, and HIV-2 in Abidjan, Ivory Coast. *Journal of the American Medical Association* 272(6):462-466.

Allen, S., J. Tice, P. Van de Perre, A. Serufilira, E. Hudes, F. Nsengumuremyi, J. Bogaerts, C. Lindan, and S. Hulley
1992 Effect of serotesting with counselling on condom use and seroconversion among HIV discordant couples in Africa *British Medical Journal* 304(6842):1605-1609.

Anderson, R.M., and R.M. May
1988 Epidemiological parameters of HIV transmission. *Nature* 333(6173):514-519.
1992 Understanding the AIDS pandemic. *Scientific American* 266(5):58-66.

Anderson, R.M., R.M. May, M.C. Boily, G.P. Garnett, and J.T. Rowley
1991 The spread of HIV-1 in Africa: Sexual contact patterns and the predicted demographic impact of AIDS. *Nature* 352(6336):581-589.

Aral, S.O., and T.A. Peterman

1993 Defining behavioral methods to prevent sexually transmitted diseases through intervention research. *Infectious Disease Clinics of North America* 7(4):861-873.

Aral, S.O., and J.N. Wasserheit

Forthcoming The hidden epidemic: Are sexually transmitted diseases the key to the control of HIV infection among African-American and Hispanic populations? In M. Antoni, H. Amaro, J. Jemmott, J. Szapocznik, and E.H. Johnson, eds., *African Americans and Hispanics: The Role of Behavioral and Psychosocial Factors*. New York: Praeger.

Arya, O.P., H. Nsanzumuhire, and S.R. Taber

1973 Clinical, cultural and demographic aspects of gonorrhoea in a rural community in Uganda. *Bulletin of the World Health Organization* 49(6):587-595.

Arya, O.P., and S.T. Taber

1975 *Correlates of Venereal Disease and Fertility in Rural Uganda*. Washington, D.C.: World Health Organization.

Ballard, R.C., H.G. Fehler, and P. Piot

1986 Chlamydia infection in the eye and genital tract in developing societies. Pp. 479-486 in J.D. Oriel, G. Ridgway, J. Schachter, D. Taylor-Robinson, and M. Ward, eds., *Chlamydial Infections*. Cambridge, MA: Cambridge University Press.

Barry, M.

1988 Ethical considerations of human investigation in developing countries: The AIDS dilemma. *New England Journal of Medicine* 319(16):1083-1086.

Beauchamp, T.L., and J.F. Childress, eds.

1983 *Principles of Biomedical Ethics*. 2nd edition. Oxford: Oxford University Press.

Behets, F., M. Kashamuka, M. Pappaioanou, T.A. Green, R.W. Ryder, V. Batter, J.R. George, W.H. Hannon, and T.C. Quinn

1992 Stability of human immunodeficiency virus type 1 antibodies in whole blood dried on filter paper and stored under various tropical conditions in Kinshasa, Zaire. *Journal of Clinical Microbiology* 30(5):1179-1182.

Belec, L., S. Lwin, and J. Pillot

1994 Testing for HIV antibody in saliva and HIV-testing centres [letter]. *AIDS* 8(12):1738-1739.

Berger, R.E.

1990 Acute epididymitis. Pp. 641-651 in K.K. Holmes, P-A. Mardh, P.F. Sparling, P.J. Wiesner, W. Cates, S.M. Lemon, and W.E. Stamm, eds., *Sexually Transmitted Diseases*. New York: McGraw Hill.

Berkley, S.F., R. Widy-Wirski, S.I. Okware, R. Downing, M.J. Linnan, K.E. White, and S. Sempala

1989 Risk factors associated with HIV infection in Uganda. *Journal of Infectious Diseases* 160(1):22-30.

Berman, S.M., H.R. Harrison, W.T. Boyce, W.J. Haffner, M. Lewis, and J.B. Arthur

1987 Low birth weight, prematurity and postpartum endometritis: Association with prenatal cervical mycoplasma hominis and chlamydia trachomatis infections. *Journal of the American Medical Association* 257(9):1189-1194.

Berrios, D.C., A.L. Avins, K. Haynes-Sanstad, R. Eversley, and W.J. Woods

1995 Screening for human immunodeficiency virus antibody in urine. *Archives of Pathology and Laboratory Medicine* 119(2):139-141.

Biggar, R.J., S. Pahwa, H. Minkoff, H. Mendes, A. Willoughby, S. Landesman, and J.J. Goedert

1989 Immunosuppression in pregnant women infected with human immunodeficiency virus. *American Journal of Obstetrics and Gynecology* 161(5):1239-1244.

Blanche, S., C. Rouzioux, M.L. Moscato, F. Veber, M.J. Mayaux, C. Jacomet, J. Tricoire, A. Deville, M. Vial, G. Firtion, A. de Crepy, D. Douard, M. Robin, C. Courpotin, N. Ciraru-Vigneron, F. le Deist, C. Griscelli, and the HIV Infection in Newborns French Collaborative Study Group

1989 A prospective study of infants born to women seropositive for human immunodeficiency virus type 1. HIV infection in newborns. *New England Journal of Medicine* 320(25):1643-1648.

Blower, S.M., and A.R. McLean
1994 Prophylactic vaccines, risk behavior change, and the probability of eradicating HIV in San Francisco. *Science* 265(5177):1451-1454.

Bongaarts, J., P. Reining, P. Way, and F. Conant
1989 The relationship between male circumcision and HIV infection in African populations. *AIDS* 3(6):373-377.

Bowie, W.R., S.P. Wang, E.R. Alexander, J. Floyd, P.S. Forsyth, H.M. Pollock, J.S. Lin, T.M. Buchanan, and K.K. Holmes
1977 Etiology of nongonococcal urethritis: Evidence for chlamydia trachomatis and ureaplasma urealyticum. *Journal of Clinical Investigation* 59(5):735-742.

Brokensha, D.
1988 Overview: Social factors in the transmission and control of African AIDS. Pp. 167-173 in N. Miller and R.C. Rockwell, eds., *AIDS in Africa: The Social and Policy Impact.* Lewiston, NY/Queenston, Ontario, Canada: Edwin Mellen Press.

Brunham, R.C., G.P. Garnett, J. Swinton, and R.M. Anderson
1991 Gonococcal infection and human fertility in sub-Saharan Africa. *Proceedings of the Royal Society of London.* Series B: Biological Sciences 246(1316):173-177.

Bulterys M., A. Chao, P. Habimana, A. Dushimimana, P. Nawrocki, and A. Saah
1994 Incident HIV-1 infection in a cohort of young women in Butare, Rwanda. *AIDS* 8(11):1585-1591.

Caldwell, J.C.
1995a Lack of male circumcision and AIDS in sub-Saharan Africa: Resolving the conflict. *Health Transition Review* 5(1):113-117.
1995b Understanding the AIDS epidemic and reacting sensibly to it. *Social Science & Medicine* 41(3):299-302.

Caldwell, J.C., and P. Caldwell
1993 The nature and limits of the sub-Saharan African AIDS epidemic: Evidence from geographic and other patterns. *Population and Development Review* 19(4):817-848.

Caldwell, J.C., G. Santow, I.O. Orubuloye, P. Caldwell, and J. Anarfi, eds.
1993 *Sexual Networking and HIV/AIDS in West Africa.* Special supplement to *Health Transition Review,* Volume 3. Canberra: Health Transition Centre, Australian National University.

Cameron, D.W., J.N. Simonsen, L.J. D'Costa, A.R. Ronald, G.M. Maitha, M.N. Gakinya, M. Cheang, J.O. Ndinya-Achola, P. Piot, R.C. Brunham, and F.A. Plummer
1989 Female to male transmission of human immunodeficiency virus type 1: Risk factors for seroconversion in men. *The Lancet* 2(8660):403-407.

Cao, Y., A.E. Friedman-Kien, J.V. Chuba, M. Mirabile, and B. Hosein
1988 IgG antibodies to HIV-1 in urine of HIV-1 seropositive individuals. *The Lancet* 1(8589):831-832.

Cates, W., T.M. Farley, and P.J. Rowe
1985 Worldwide patterns of infertility: Is Africa different? *The Lancet* 2(8455):596-598.

Cates, W., and A.R. Hinman
1991 Sexually transmitted diseases in the 1990's. *New England Journal of Medicine* 325(19):1368-1370.

Chernesky, M.A., H. Lee, J. Schachter, J.D. Burczak, W.E. Stamm, W.M. McCormack, and T.C. Quinn
1994 Diagnosis of Chlamydia trachomatis urethral infection in symptomatic and

asymptomatic men by testing first-void urine in a ligase chain reaction assay. *Journal of Infectious Diseases* 170(5):1308-1311.

Chin, J.
1990 Current and future dimensions of the HIV/AIDS pandemic in women and children. *The Lancet* 336(8709):221-224.

Choto, R.G.
1990 Breastfeeding: Breast milk banks and human immunodeficiency virus. *Central African Journal of Medicine* 36(12):296-300.

Christakis, N.A.
1988 The ethical design of an AIDS vaccine trial in Africa. *Hastings Center Report* June/July:31-37. New York: The Hastings Center.

Clavel, F., M. Guyader, D. Guetard, M. Salle, L. Montagnier, and M. Alizon
1986 Molecular cloning and polymorphism of the human immune deficiency virus type 2. *Nature* 324(6098):691-695.

Cooper-Poole, B.
1986 Prevalence of syphilis in Mbeya, Tanzania: The validity of the VDRL as a screening test. *East African Medical Journal* 63(10):646-650.

Cotch, M.F., and J.K. Pastorek
1991 Effect of Trichomonas vaginalis (Tv) carriage on pregnancy outcome. Abstract C-04-150. Paper presented at the 9th International Meeting of the International Society for STD Research, October 6-9, Banff, Alberta, Canada.

Council for International Organizations of Medical Sciences and World Health Organization
1992 *Ethics and Research on Human Subjects: International Guidebook.* Proceedings of the XXVIth CIOMS Conference, 5-7 February, 1992, Geneva, Switzerland. Geneva: CIOMS.

Dada, A.J., F. Oyewole, R. Onofowokan, A. Nasidi, B. Harris, A. Levin, L. Diamondstone, T.C. Quinn, and W.A. Blattner
1993 Demographic characteristics of retroviral infections (HIV-1, HIV-2 and HTLV-I) among female professional sex workers in Lagos, Nigeria. *Journal of Acquired Immune Deficiency Syndromes* 6(12):1358-1363.

Daly, C.C., G.E. Helling-Giese, J.K. Mati, and D.J. Hunter
1994 Contraceptive methods and the transmission of HIV: Implications for family planning. *Genitourinary Medicine* 70(2):110-117.

Damiba, A.E., S.H. Vermund, and K.F. Kelly
1990 The trend of reported gonorrhoea and urethritis incidence in Burkina Faso from 1978-1983. *Transactions of the Royal Society of Tropical Medicine & Hygiene* 84(1):132-135.

de Bruyn, M.
1992 Women and AIDS in developing countries. *Social Science & Medicine* 34(3):249-262.

De Cock, K.M., and F. Brun-Vezinet
1989 Epidemiology of HIV-2 infection. *AIDS* 3(Supplement 1):S89-S95.

Decosas, J., F. Kane, J.K. Anarfi, K.D.R. Sodji, and H.U. Wagner
1995 Migration and AIDS. *The Lancet* 346(8978):826-828.

Decosas, J., and V. Pedneault
1992 Women and AIDS in Africa: Demographic implications for health promotion. *Health Policy & Planning* 7(3):227-233.

De Schryver, A., and A. Meheus
1990 Epidemiology of sexually transmitted diseases: The global picture. *Bulletin of the World Health Organization* 68(5):639-654.

de Vincenzi, I., for the European Study Group on Heterosexual Transmission of HIV

1994 A longitudinal study of human immunodeficiency virus transmission by heterosexual partners. *New England Journal of Medicine* 331(6):341-346.

Dunn, D.T., M.L. Newell, A.E. Ades, and C.S. Peckham

1992 Risk of human immunodeficiency virus type 1 transmission through breastfeeding. *The Lancet* 340(8819):585-588.

Dyson, T., ed.

1992 *Sexual Behaviour and Networking: Anthropological and Socio-Cultural Studies on the Transmission of HIV*. Liège, Belgium: Editions Derouaux-Ordina.

Eschenbach, D.A.

1993 History and review of bacterial vaginosis. *American Journal of Obstetrics & Gynecology* 169(2 Part 2):441-445.

European Collaborative Study

1991 Children born to women with HIV-1 infection: Natural history and risk of transmission. *The Lancet* 337(8736):253-260.

Frank, O.

1983 Infertility in sub-Saharan Africa: Estimates and implication. *Population and Development Review* 9(1):137-144.

Frerichs, R.R., N. Eskes, and M.T. Htoon

1994 Validity of three assays for HIV-I antibodies in saliva. *Journal of Acquired Immune Deficiency Syndromes* 7(5):522-525.

Frost, E., M. Collet, J. Raniers, A. Leclerc, B. Ivanoff, and A. Meheus.

1987 Importance of chlamydial antibodies in acute salpingitis in central Africa. *Genitourinary Medicine* 63(3):176-178.

Garner, P., T. Tan Torres, and P. Alonso

1994 Trial design in developing countries. *British Medical Journal* 309(6958):825-826.

Gibbs, R.S.

1993 Chorioamnionitis and bacterial vaginosis. *American Journal of Obstetrics & Gynecology* 169(2 Part 2):460-462.

Greenberg, A.E., P. Nguyen-Dinh, J.M. Mann, N. Kabote, R.L. Colebunders, H. Francis, T.C. Quinn, P. Baudoux, B. Lyamba, F. Davachi, J.M. Roberts, N. Kabeya, J.W. Curran, and C.C. Campbell

1988 The association between malaria, blood transfusions, and HIV seropositivity in a pediatric population in Kinshasa, Zaire. *Journal of the American Medical Association* 259(4):545-549.

Grosskurth, H., F. Mosha, J. Todd, E. Mwijarubi, A. Klokke, K. Senkoro, P. Mayaud, J. Changalucha, A. Nicoll, G. ka-Gina, J. Newell, K. Mugeye, D. Mabey, and R. Hayes

1995 Impact of improved treatment of sexually transmitted diseases on HIV infection in rural Tanzania: randomised controlled trial. *The Lancet* 346(8974):530-536.

Guyader, M., M. Emerman, P. Sonigo, F. Clavel, L. Montagnier, and M. Alizon

1987 Genome organization and transactivation of the human immunodeficiency virus type 2. *Nature* 326(6114):662-669.

Hammerschlag, M.R.

1991 STDs and pregnancy outcome: Chlamydia, GC and syphilis. Abstract C-04-268. Paper presented at the 9th International Meeting of the International Society for STD Research, October 6-9, Banff, Alberta, Canada.

Hardy, L.M., ed.

1991 *HIV Screening of Pregnant Women and Newborns*. Washington, D.C.: National Academy Press.

Haverkos, H.W., and T.C. Quinn

1995 The third wave: HIV infection among heterosexuals in the United States and Europe. *International Journal of STDs & AIDS* 6(June/August):227-232.

Henig, R.M.

1993 *A Dancing Matrix: Now Science Confronts Emerging Viruses*. New York: Vintage Books.

Hillier, S.L.

1993 Diagnostic microbiology of bacterial vaginosis. *American Journal of Obstetrics and Gynecology* 169(2 Part 2):455-459.

Hillier, S.L., M.A. Krohn, R.P. Nugent, and R.S. Gibbs

1992 Characteristics of three vaginal flora patterns assessed by Gram Stain among pregnant women. Vaginal Infections and Prematurity Study Group. *American Journal of Obstetrics and Gynecology* 166(3):938-44.

Hillier, S.L., M.A. Krohn, L.K. Rabe, S.J. Klebanoff, and D.A. Eschenbach

1993 The normal vaginal flora, H_2O_2-producing lactobacilli, and bacterial vaginosis in pregnant women. *Clinical Infectious Diseases* 16(Supplement 4):S273-S281.

Hira, S.K., G.J. Bhat, D.M. Chikamata, B. Nkowane, G. Tembo, P.L. Perine, and A. Meheus

1990 Syphilis intervention in pregnancy: Zambia demonstration project. *Genitourinary Medicine* 66(3):159-164.

Hira, S.K., J. Kamanga, G.J. Bhat, C. Mwale, G. Tembo, N. Luo, and P.L. Perine

1989 Perinatal transmission of HIV-1 in Zambia. *British Medical Journal* 299(6710):1250-1252.

Hira, S., and R. Sunkutu

1993 Zambian National STD Control Program: A model program. Abstract No. WS-C22-6, Volume 9(1):103. IXth International Conference on AIDS, June 6-11, Berlin, Germany.

Horsburgh, C.R., Jr., and S.D. Holmberg

1988 The global distribution of human immunodeficiency virus type 2 (HIV-2) infection. *Transfusion* 28(2):192-195.

Hu, D.J., W.L. Heyward, R.H. Byers Jr., B.M. Nkowane, M.J. Oxtoby, S.E. Holck, and D.L. Heymann

1992 HIV infection and breast-feeding: Policy implications through a decision analysis model. *AIDS* 6(12):1505-1513.

Hudson, C.P.

1993 Concurrent partners and the results of the Uganda Rakai project. *AIDS* 7(2):286-8.

Johnson, P.D., S.R. Graves, L. Stewart, R. Warren, B. Dwyer, and C.R. Lucas

1991 Specific syphilis serological tests may become negative in HIV infection. *AIDS* 5(4):419-423.

Kaheru, Z.,

1989 Remarks made at a press conference at the International Conference Center, Kampala, Uganda. November 30, 1989.

Kanki, P.J.

1991 Biologic features of HIV-2: An update. *AIDS Clinical Review* 17-38.

1994 Simian retroviruses in Africa. Pp. 97-107 in M. Essex, S. Mboup, P.J. Kanki, and M.R. Kalengayi, eds., *AIDS in Africa*. New York: Raven Press.

Kanki, P., S. M'Boup, R. Marlink, K. Travers, C.C. Hsieh, A. Gueye, C. Boye, J.-L. Sankalé, C. Donnelly, W. Leisenring, T. Siby, I. Thior, M. Dia, E.-H. Gueye, I. N'Doye, and M. Essex

1992 Prevalence and risk determinants of human immunodeficiency virus type 2 (HIV-2) and human immunodeficiency virus type 1 (HIV-1) in West African female prostitutes. *American Journal of Epidemiology* 136(7):895-907.

Kanki, P.J., K.U. Travers, S. MBoup [sic.], C.C. Hsieh, R.G. Marlink, A. Gueye-NDiaye, T. Siby, I. Thior, M. Hernandez-Avila, J.-L. Sankalé, I. NDoye [sic], and M.E. Essex

1994 Slower heterosexual spread of HIV-2 than HIV-1. *The Lancet* 343(8903):943-946.

Kennedy, K.I., J.A. Fortney, M.G. Bonhomme, M. Potts, P. Lamptey, and W. Carswell
1990 Do the benefits of breastfeeding outweigh the risk of postnatal transmission of HIV via breastmilk? *Tropical Doctor* 20(1):25-29.

Killewo, J., K. Nyamurayekunge, A. Sandstrom, U. Bredberg-Raden, S. Wall, F. Mhalu, and G. Biberfeld
1990 Prevalence of HIV-1 infection in the Kagera region of Tanzania: A population-based study. *AIDS* 4(11):1081-1085.

Konde-Lule, J.K., S.F. Berkley, and R. Downing
1989 Knowledge, attitudes and practices concerning AIDS in Ugandans. *AIDS* 3(8):513-518.

Kreiss, J.K., R. Coombs, F. Plummer, K.K. Holmes, B. Nikora, W. Cameron, E. Ngugi, J.O. Ndinya Achola, and L. Corey
1989 Isolation of human immunodeficiency virus from genital ulcers in Nairobi prostitutes. *Journal of Infectious Diseases* 160(3):380-384.

Kreiss, J.K, D.M. Willerford, M. Hensel, W. Emonyi, F. Plummer, J. Ndinya-Achola, P.L. Roberts, J. Hoskyn, S. Hillier, and N. Kiviat
1994 Association between cervical inflammation and cervical shedding of human immunodeficiency virus DNA. *Journal of Infectious Diseases* 170(6):1597-1601.

Kretzschmar, M., and M. Morris
Forthcoming Measures of concurrency in sexual networks and the spread of STDs. *Mathematical Biosciences.*

Laga, M., M. Alary, N. Nzila, A.T. Manoka, M. Tuliza, F. Behets, J. Goeman, M. St. Louis, and P. Piot
1994 Condom promotion, sexually transmitted diseases treatment, and declining incidence of HIV-1 infection in female Zairian sex workers. *The Lancet* 344(8917):246-248.

Laga, M., A. Manoka, M. Kivuvu, B. Malele, M. Tuliza, N. Nzila, J. Goeman, F. Behets, V. Batter, M. Alary, W.L. Heyaward, R.W. Ryder, and P. Piot
1993 Non-ulcerative sexually transmitted diseases as risk factors for HIV-1 transmission in women: Results from a cohort study. *AIDS* 7(1):95-102.

Laga, M., F.A. Plummer, H. Nzanze, W. Namaara, R.C. Brunham, J.O. Ndinya-Achola, G. Maitha, A.R. Ronald, L.J. D'Costa, V.B. Bhullar, J.K. Mati, L. Fransen, M. Cheang, and P. Piot
1986 Epidemiology of ophthalmia neonatorum in Kenya. *The Lancet* 2(8516):1145-1148.

Lallemant, M., S. Lallemant-Le Coeur, D. Cheynier, S. Nzingoula, G. Jourdain, M. Sinet, M.C. Dazza, S. Blanche, C. Griscelli, and B. Larouze
1989 Mother-child transmission of HIV-1 and infant survival in Brazzaville, Congo. *AIDS* 3(10):643-646.

Larsen, U.
1994 Sterility in sub-Saharan Africa. *Population Studies* 48(3):459-474.

Latif, A.S.
1989 Epidemiology and control of chancroid. Abstract No. 66. VIIIth International Society for Sexually Transmitted Diseases Research, September 10-13, Copenhagen, Denmark.

Leclerc, A., E. Frost, M. Collet, J. Goeman, and L. Bedjabaga
1988 Urogenital chlamydia trachomatis in Gabon: An unrecognised epidemic. *Genitourinary Medicine* 64(5):308-311.

Lee, H.H., M.A. Chernesky, J. Schachter, J.D. Burczak, W.W. Andrews, S. Muldoon, G. Leckie, and W.E. Stamm
1995 Diagnosis of Chlamydia trachomatis genitourinary infection in women by ligase chain reaction assay of urine. *The Lancet* 345(8944):213-216.

Lepage, P., P. Van de Perre, M. Carael, F. Nsengumuremyi, J. Nkurunziza, J.P. Butzler, and S. Sprecher
1987 Postnatal transmission of HIV from mother to child. *The Lancet* 2(8555):400.

Mabey, D.C., N.E. Lloyd-Evans, S. Conteh, and T. Forsey
1984 Sexually transmitted diseases among randomly selected attenders at an antenatal clinic in The Gambia. *British Journal of Venereal Diseases* 60(5):331-336.

Mabey, D.C., G. Ogbaselassie, J.N. Robertson, J.E. Heckels, and M.E. Ward
1985 Tubal infertility in The Gambia: Chlamydial and gonococcal serology in women with tubal occlusion compared with pregnant controls. *Bulletin of the World Health Organization* 63(6):1107-1113.

Mabey, D.C., R.A. Wall, and C.S. Bello
1987 Aetiology of genital ulceration in the Gambia. *Genitourinary Medicine* 63(5):312-315.

Mabey, D.C., and H.C. Whittle
1982 Genital and neonatal chlamydial infection in a trachoma endemic area. *The Lancet* 2(8293):300-301.

MacDonald, K.S., D.W. Cameron, L. D'Costa, J.O. Ndinya-Achola, F.A. Plummer, and A.R. Ronald
1989 Evaluation of fleroxacin (RO23-6240) as single-oral-dose therapy of culture-proven chancroid in Nairobi, Kenya. *Antimicrobial Agents and Chemotherapy* 33(5):612-614.

Mann, J.M., H. Francis, F. Davachi, P. Baudoux, T.C. Quinn, N. Nzilambi, N. Bosenge, R.L. Colebunders, P. Piot, N. Kabote, P.K. Asila, M. Malonga, and J.W. Curran
1986a Risk factors for human immunodeficiency virus seropositivity among children 1-24 months old in Kinshasa, Zaire. *The Lancet* 2(8508):654-657.

Mann, J.M., H. Francis, F. Davachi, P. Baudoux, T.C. Quinn, N. Nzilambi, R.L. Colebunders, N. Kabote, and P. Piot
1986b Human immunodeficiency virus seroprevalence in pediatric patients 2 to 14 years of age at Mama Yemo Hospital, Kinshasa, Zaire. *Pediatrics* 78(4):673-677.

Mann, J.M., H. Francis, T.C. Quinn, K. Bila, P.K. Asila, N. Bosenge, N. Nzilambi, L. Jansegers, P. Piot, K. Ruti, and J.W. Curran
1986c HIV seroprevalence among hospital workers in Kinshasa, Zaire: Lack of association with occupational exposure. *Journal of the American Medical Association* 256 (22):3099-3102.

Markovitz, D.M.
1993 Infection with the human immunodeficiency virus type 2. *Annals of Internal Medicine* 118(3):211-218.

Marlink, R.
1994 The biology and epidemiology of HIV-2. Pp. 47-65 in M. Essex, S. Mboup, P.J. Kanki, and M.R. Kalengayi, eds., *AIDS in Africa*. New York: Raven Press.

Mason, P.R., D.A. Katzenstein, T.H. Chimbira, and L. Mtimavalye
1989 Microbial flora of the lower genital tract of women in labour at Harare Maternity Hospital. The Puerperal Sepsis Study Group. *Central African Journal of Medicine* 35(3):337-344.

Mastro, T.D., G.A. Satten, T. Nopkesorn, S. Sangkharomya, and I.M. Longini
1994 Probability of female-to-male transmission of HIV-1 in Thailand. *The Lancet* 343 (8891):204-207.

Matheron, S., C. Courpotin, F. Simon, H. Di Maria, H. Balloul, S. Bartzack, D. Dormont, F. Brun Vezinet, A.G. Saimon, and J.P. Coulaud
1990 Vertical transmission of HIV-2. *The Lancet* 335(8697):1103-1104.

McDonald, H.M., J.A. O'Loughlin, P. Jolley, R. Vigneswaran, and P.J. McDonald
1991 Vaginal infection and preterm labour. *British Journal of Obstetrics and Gynaecology* 98(5):427-435.

McGregor, J.A., J.I. French, and K. Seo
1993 Premature rupture of membranes and bacterial vaginosis. *American Journal of Obstetrics and Gynecology* 169(2 Part 2):463-466.

Meheus, A., K.F. Schulz, and W. Cates
1990 Development of prevention and control programs for sexually transmitted diseases in developing countries. Pp. 1041-1046 in K.K. Holmes, P.A. Mardh, F.P. Sparling, and P.J. Wiesner, eds., *Sexually Transmitted Diseases*. New York: McGraw-Hill.

Mertens, T.E., R.J. Hayes, and P.G. Smith
1990 Epidemiological methods to study the interaction between HIV infection and other sexually transmitted diseases. *AIDS* 4(1):57-65.

Mhalu, F., V. Bredberg-Raden, E. Mbena, K. Pallangyo, J. Kiango, R. Mbise, K. Nyamuryekunge, and G. Biberfeld
1987 Prevalence of HIV infection in healthy subjects and groups of patients in Tanzania. *AIDS* 1(4):217-221.

Mhalu, F., and R.W. Ryder
1988 Blood transfusion and AIDS in the tropics. *Baillieres Clinical Tropical Medicine and Communicable Diseases* 3(1):157-166.

Miles, S.A., E. Balden, L. Magpantay, L. Wei, A. Leiblein, D. Hofheinz, G. Toedter, E.R. Stiehm, and Y. Bryson
1993 Rapid serologic testing with immune-complex-dissociated HIV p24 antigen for early detection of HIV infection in neonates. Southern California Pediatric AIDS Consortium. *New England Journal of Medicine* 328(5):297-302.

Ministry of Health [Uganda]
1989 *Report of the National Serosurvey of Human Immunodeficiency Virus in Uganda.* Entebbe, Uganda: Ministry of Health.

Miotti, P.G., G. Dallabetta, E. Ndovi, G. Liomba, A.J. Saah, and J. Chiphangwi
1990 HIV-1 and pregnant women: Associated factors, prevalence, estimate of incidence and role in fetal wastage in central Africa. *AIDS* 4(8):733-736.

Morris, M., and M. Kretzchmar
Forthcoming Concurrent partnerships and transmission dynamics in networks. *Social Networks.*

Moss, G.B., D. Clemetson, L. D'Costa, F.A. Plummer, J.O. Ndinya-Achola, M. Reilly, K.K. Holmes, P. Piot, G.M. Maitha, S.L. Hillier, N.C. Kiviat, C.W. Cameron, I.A. Wamola, and J.K. Kreiss
1991 Association of cervical ectopy with heterosexual transmission of human immunodeficiency virus: Results of a study of couples in Nairobi, Kenya. *Journal of Infectious Diseases* 164(3):588-591.

Mputo, L., M. Wolomby, and K. Mahekele
1986 La contribution de la composante masculine dans l'infertilité du couple à Kinshasa (Zaire). *Journal of Gynecology and Obstetrics in Biological Reproduction* 15(1):51-58.

Muir, D.G., and M.A. Belsey
1980 Pelvic inflammatory disease and its consequences in the developing world. *American Journal of Obstetrics and Gynecology* 138(7 Part 2):913-928.

Mulder, D.W.
1993 Health seeking behavior and the problem of delayed treatment for women. Pp. 1-3 in *MRC/ODA Programme on AIDS in Uganda*. Entebbe: Uganda Virus Research Institute.

Mulder, D.W., A.J. Nunn, A. Kamali, J. Nakiyingi, H.U. Wagner, and J.F. Kengeya-Kayondo
1994a Two-year HIV-1-associated mortality in a Ugandan rural population. *The Lancet* 343(8904):1021-1023.

Mulder, D.W., J.F. Kengeya-Kayonda, S.D.K. Sempala, and A.J. Nunn
1994b *MRC/ODA/UVRI Programme, Annual Report, 1993.* Entebbe, Uganda: Uganda Virus Research Institute.

Myers, G.

1994 Tenth anniversary perspectives on AIDS. HIV: Between past and future. *AIDS Research & Human Retroviruses* 10(11):1317-1324.

Nasah, B.T., R. Nquematcha, M. Eyong, and S. Godwin

1980 Gonorrhea, trichomonas and candida among gravid and nongravid women in Cameroon. *International Journal of Gynecology and Obstetrics* 18(1):48-52.

Naucler, A., P. Albino, A.P. da Silva, P.A. Andreasson, S. Andersson, and G. Biberfeld

1991 HIV-2 infection in hospitalized patients in Bissau, Guinea-Bissau. *AIDS* 5(3):301-304.

N'Galy, B., R.W. Ryder, K. Bila, K. Mwandagalirwa, R.L. Colebunders, H. Francis, J.M. Mann, and T.C. Quinn

1988 Human immunodeficiency virus infection among employees in an African hospital. *New England Journal of Medicine* 319(17):1123-1127.

Nicoll, A., J.Z. Killewo, and C. Mgone

1990 HIV and infant feeding practices: Epidemiological implications for sub-Saharan African countries. *AIDS* 4(7):661-665.

Nsubuga, P.S., W.L. Roseberry, F. Judson, D. Hu, S. Kalibbala, E. Van Dyck, Baingana-Baingi, F. Mirembe, E.K. Mbidde, and B. Nkowane

1994 Rapid assessment of STD prevalence: The validity of STD rapid indicators in Uganda. Abstract No. 135. *Sexually Transmitted Diseases* 21(2 Supplement):S143.

Ntozi, J.P.M., and M. Lubega

1990 Patterns of sexual behavior and the spread of AIDS in Uganda. Paper presented at the International Union for the Scientific Study of Population Seminar on Anthropological Studies Relevant to the Sexual Transmission of HIV, November 19-22, Sonderborg, Denmark.

Nugent, R.P., M.A. Krohn, and S.L. Hillier

1991 Reliability of diagnosing bacterial vaginosis is improved by a standardized method of gram stain interpretation. *Journal of Clinical Microbiology* 29(2):297-301.

Nyambi, P.N., K. Fransen, H. De Beenhouwer, E.N. Chomba, M. Temmerman, J.O. Ndinya-Achola, P. Piot, and G. van der Groen

1994 Detection of human immunodeficiency virus type 1 (HIV-1) in heel prick blood on filter paper from children born to HIV-1 seropositive mothers. *Journal of Clinical Microbiology* 32(11):2858-2860.

Nzilambi, N., K.M. De Cock, D.N. Forthal, H. Francis, R.W. Ryder, I. Malebe, J. Getchell, M. Laga, P. Piot, and J.B. McCormick

1988 The prevalence of infection with human immunodeficiency virus over a 10-year period in rural Zaire. *New England Journal of Medicine* 318(5):276-279.

Oakley A., D. Fullerton, and J. Holland

1995 Behavioural interventions for HIV/AIDS prevention. *AIDS* 9(5):479-486.

Obbo, C.

1993 HIV transmission through social and geographic networks in Uganda. *Social Science & Medicine* 36(7):949-955.

Olaleye, O.D., L. Bernstein, C.C. Ekweozor, Z. Sheng, S.A. Ormilabu, X.-Y. Li, J. Sullivan-Halley, and S. Rasheed

1993 Prevalence of human immunodeficiency virus types 1 and 2 infections in Nigeria. *Journal of Infectious Diseases* 167(3):710-714.

Orubuloye, I.O., J.C. Caldwell, and P. Caldwell

1990 *Experimental Research on Sexual Networking in the Ekiti District of Nigeria.* Health Transition Centre Working Paper No. 3. Canberra, Australia: Health Transition Centre, Australian National University.

1994 *Sexual Networking and AIDS in Sub-Saharan Africa: Behavioural Research and the Social Context.* Canberra: Health Transition Centre, Australian National University.

Oxtoby, M.J.
1990 Perinatally acquired human immunodeficiency virus infection. *Pediatric Infectious Disease Journal* 9(9):609-619.

Pappaioanou, M., M. Kashamuka, F. Behets, S. Mbala, K. Biyela, F. Davachi, J.R. George, T.A. Green, T.J. Dondero, W.L. Heyward, and R.W. Ryder
1993 Accurate detection of maternal antibodies to HIV in newborn whole blood dried on filter paper. *AIDS* 7(4):483-488.

Parkin, D., and D. Nyamwaya
1987 *Transformations of African Marriage*. Manchester: Manchester University Press.

Pepin, J., D. Dunn, I. Gaye, P. Alonso, A. Egboga, R. Tedder, P. Piot, N. Berry, D. Schellenberg, H. Whittle, and A. Wilkins
1991 HIV-2 infection among prostitutes working in The Gambia: Association with serological evidence of genital ulcer diseases and with generalized lymphadenopathy. *AIDS* 5(1):69-75.

Pepin, J., F.A. Plummer, R.C. Brunham, P. Piot, D.W. Cameron, and A.R. Ronald
1989 The interaction of HIV infection and other sexually transmitted diseases: An opportunity for intervention. *AIDS* 3(1):3-9.

Pickering, H., J. Todd, D. Dunn, J. Pepin, and A. Wilkins
1992 Prostitutes and their clients: A Gambian survey. *Social Science & Medicine* 34(1):75-88.

Piot, P., J. Goeman, and M. Laga
1994 The epidemiology of HIV and AIDS in Africa. Pp. 157-171 in M. Essex, S. Mboup, P.J. Kanki, and M.R. Kalengayi, eds., *AIDS in Africa*. New York: Raven Press.

Piot, P., and M. Laga
1989 Genital ulcers, other sexually transmitted diseases, and the sexual transmission of HIV. *British Medical Journal* 298(6674):623-624.

Piot, P., M. Laga, R. Ryder, J. Perriens, M. Temmerman, W. Heyward, and J.W. Curran
1990 The global epidemiology of HIV infection: Continuity, heterogeneity, and change. *Journal of Acquired Immune Deficiency Syndromes* 3(4):403-412.

Piot, P., F.A. Plummer, F.S. Mhalu, J.-L. Lamboray, J. Chin, and J.M. Mann
1988 AIDS: An international perspective. *Science* 239(4840):573-579.

Piot, P., F.A. Plummer, M.A. Rey, E.N. Ngugi, C. Rouzioux, J.O. Ndinya-Achola, G. Veracauteren, L.J. D'Costa, M. Laga, H. Nsanze, L. Fransen, D. Haase, G. Van der Groen, R.C. Brunham, A.R. Ronald, and F. Brun-Vezinet
1987 Retrospective seroepidemiology of AIDS virus infection in Nairobi populations. *Journal of Infectious Diseases* 155(6):1108-1112.

Piot, P., T.C. Quinn, H. Taelman, F.M. Feinsod, K.B. Minlangu, O. Wobin, N. Mbendi, P. Mazebo, K. Ndangi, W. Stevens, K. Kalambayi, S. Mitchell, C. Bridts, and J.B. McCormick
1984 Acquired immunodeficiency syndrome in a heterosexual population in Zaire. *The Lancet* 2(8394):65-69.

Piot, P., and R. Tezzo
1990 The epidemiology of HIV and other sexually transmitted infections in the developing world. *Scandinavian Journal of Infectious Diseases Supplementum* 69:89-97.

Pison, G.
1989 La nuptialité en Afrique au Sud du Sahara: Changements en cours et impact sur la fécondité. *Population* 44(4-5):949-959.

Pison, G., B. Le Guenno, E. Lagarde, C. Enel, and C. Seck
1993 Seasonal migration: A risk factor for HIV infection in rural Senegal. *Journal of Acquired Immune Deficiency Syndromes* 6(2):196-200.

Plummer, F.A., M. Laga, R.C. Brunham, P. Piot, A.R. Ronald, V. Bhullar, J.Y. Mati, J.O. Ndinya-Achola, M. Cheang, and H. Nsanze

1987 Postpartum upper genital tract infections in Nairobi, Kenya: Epidemiology, etiology and risk factors. *Journal of Infectious Diseases* 156(1):92-98.

Plummer, F.A., J.N. Simonsen, D.W. Cameron, J.O. Ndinya-Achola, J.K. Kreiss, M.N. Gakinya, P. Waiyaki, M. Cheang, P. Piot, A.R. Ronald, and E.N. Ngugi

1991 Cofactors in male-female sexual transmission of human immunodeficiency virus type 1. *Journal of Infectious Diseases* 163(2):233-239.

Plummer, F.A., J.N. Simonsen, H. Chubb, L. Slaney, J. Kimata, M. Bosire, J.O. Ndinya-Achola, and E.N. Ngugi

1989 Epidemiological evidence for the development of serovar-specific immunity after gonococcal infection. *Journal of Clinical Investigation* 83(5):1472-1476.

Poulsen, A.G., P. Aaby, A. Gottschau, B.B. Kvinesdal, F. Dias, K. Molbak, and E. Lauritzen

1993 HIV-2 infection in Bissau, West Africa, 1987-1989: Incidence, prevalences, and routes of transmission. *Journal of Acquired Immune Deficiency Syndromes* 6(8):941-948.

Poulsen, A.G., B.B. Kvinesdal, P. Aaby, I.M. Lisse, A. Gottschau, K. Molbak, F. Dias, and E. Lauritzen

1992 Lack of evidence of vertical transmission of human immunodeficiency virus type 2 in a sample of the general population in Bissau. *Journal of Acquired Immune Deficiency Syndromes* 5(1):25-30.

Preble, E.A.

1990 Impact of HIV/AIDS on African children. *Social Science & Medicine* 31(6):671-680.

Quinn, T.C.

1991 AIDS in Africa. *AIDS Updates* 4(6):1-16.

1994 Population migration and the spread of types 1 and 2 human immunodeficiency viruses. *Proceedings of the National Academy of Sciences* (USA) 91(7):2407-2414.

Quinn, T.C., A. Ruff, and N. Halsey

1994 Special considerations for developing nations. Pp. 31-49 in P.A. Pizzo and C.M. Wilfert, eds., *Pediatric AIDS: The Challenge of HIV Infection in Infants, Children, and Adolescents*. Baltimore, MD: Williams & Wilkins.

Ratman, A.V., S.N. Din, S.K. Hira, G.J. Bhat, D.S.O. Wacha, A. Rukmini, and R.C. Mulenga

1982 Syphilis in pregnant women in Zambia. *British Journal of Venereal Diseases* 58(6):355-358.

Read, J.S., and M.A. Klebanoff

1993 Sexual intercourse during pregnancy and preterm delivery: Effects of vaginal microorganisms. The Vaginal Infections and Prematurity Study Group. *American Journal of Obstetrics & Gynecology* 168(2):514-519.

Riduan, J.M., S.L. Hillier, B. Utomo, G. Wiknjosastro, M. Linnan, and N. Kandun

1993 Bacterial vaginosis and prematurity in Indonesia: Association in early and late pregnancy. *American Journal of Obstetrics & Gynecology* 169(1):175-178.

Rogers, M.F., C.Y. Ou, M. Rayfield, P.A. Thomas, E.E. Schoenbaum, E. Abrams, K. Krasinski, P.A. Selwyn, J. Moore, A. Kaul, K.T. Grimm, M. Banji, G. Schochetman, The New York City Collaborative Study of Maternal HIV Transmission and Montefiore Medical Center HIV Perinatal Transmission Study Group

1989 Use of the polymerase chain reaction for early detection of the proviral sequences of human immunodeficiency virus in infants born to seropositive mothers. *New England Journal of Medicine* 320(25):1649-1654.

Rowley, J.T., R.M. Anderson, and T.W. Ng

1990 Reducing the spread of HIV infection in sub-Saharan Africa: Some demographic and economic implications. *AIDS* 4(1):47-56.

Rwandan HIV Seroprevalence Study Group
1989 Nationwide community-based serological survey of HIV-1 and other human retrovirus infections in a central African country. *The Lancet* 1(8644):941-943.

Ryder, R.W., and S.E. Hassig
1988 The epidemiology of perinatal transmission of HIV. *AIDS* 2(Supplement 1):S83-S89.

Ryder, R.W., T. Manzila, E. Baende, U. Kabagabo, F. Behets, V. Batter, E. Paquot, E. Binyingo, and W.L. Heyward
1991 Evidence from Zaire that breast-feeding by HIV-1 seropositive mothers is not a major route for perinatal HIV-1 transmission but does decrease morbidity. *AIDS* 5(6):709-714.

Ryder R.W., W. Nsa, S.E. Hassig, F. Behets, M. Rayfield, B. Ekungola, A.M. Nelson, U. Mulenda, H. Francis, K. Mwandagalirwa, F. Davachi, M. Rogers, N. Nzilambi, A. Greenberg, J. Mann, T.C. Quinn, P. Piot, and J.W. Curran
1989 Perinatal transmission of the human immunodeficiency virus type 1 to infants of seropositive women in Zaire. *New England Journal of Medicine* 320(25):1637-1642.

St. Louis, M.E., M. Kamenga, C. Brown, A.M. Nelson, T. Manzila, V. Batter, F. Behets, U. Kabagabo, R.W. Ryder, M. Oxtoby, T.C. Quinn, and W.L. Heyward
1993 Risk for perinatal HIV-1 transmission according to maternal immunologic, virologic, and placental factors. *Journal of the American Medical Association* 269(22):2853-2859.

Schoepf, B.G.
1990 Sex, gender and society in Zaire. Paper presented at the International Union for the Scientific Study of Population Seminar on Anthropological Studies Relevant to the Sexual Transmission of HIV, November 19-22, Sonderborg, Denmark.

Schmutzhard, E., D. Fuchs, P. Hengster, A. Hausen, J. Hofbauer, P. Pohl, J. Rainer, G. Reibnegger, D. Tibyampansha, E.R. Werner, M.P. Dierich, F. Gerstenbrand, and H. Wachter
1989 Retroviral infections (HIV-1, HIV-2, and HTLV-I) in rural northwestern Tanzania: Clinical findings, epidemiology, and association with infections common in Africa. *American Journal of Epidemiology* 130(2):309-318.

Semba, R.D., P.G. Miotti, J.D. Chiphangwi, A.J. Saah, J.K. Canner, G.A. Dallabetta, and D.R. Hoover
1994 Maternal vitamin A deficiency and mother-to-child transmission of HIV-1. *The Lancet* 343(8913):1593-1597.

Serwadda, D., R.H. Gray, M.J. Wawer, R.Y. Stallings, N.K. Sewankambo, J.K. Konde-Lule, B. Lainjo, and R. Kelly
1995 The social dynamics of HIV transmission as reflected through discordant couples in rural Uganda. *AIDS* 9(7):745-750.

Serwadda, D., R.D. Mugerwa, N.K. Sewankambo, A. Lwegaba, J.W. Carswell, G.B. Kirya, A.C. Bayley, R.G. Downing, R.S. Tedder, S.A. Clayden, R.A. Weiss, and A.G. Dalgleish
1985 Slim disease, a new disease in Uganda and its association with HTLV-III infection. *The Lancet* 2(8460):849-852.

Serwadda, D., M.J. Wawer, S.D. Musgrave, N.K. Sewankambo, J.E. Kaplan and R.H. Gray
1992 HIV risk factors in three geographic strata of rural Rakai district, Uganda. *AIDS* 6(9):983-989.

Sewankambo, N.K., M.J. Wawer, R.H. Gray, D. Serwadda, C. Li, R.Y. Stallings, S.D. Musgrave, and J. Konde-Lule
1994 Demographic impact of HIV infection in rural Rakai district, Uganda: Results of a population-based cohort study. *AIDS* 8(12):1707-1713.

Shulz, K.F., W. Cates Jr., and P.R. O'Mara
1987 Pregnancy loss, infant death and suffering: Legacy of syphilis and gonorrhoea in Africa. *Genitourinary Medicine* 63(5):320-325.

Simonsen, J.N., F.A. Plummer, E.N. Ngugi, C. Black, J.K. Kreiss, M.N. Gakinya, P. Waiyaki, L.J. D'Costa, J.O. Ndinya-Achola, P. Piot, and A. Ronald

1990 HIV infection among lower socioeconomic strata prostitutes in Nairobi. *AIDS* 4(2):139-144.

Smith, K.R., S. Ching, H. Lee, Y. Ohhashi, H.Y. Hu, H.C. Fisher, III, and E.W. Hook, III

1995 Evaluation of ligase chain reaction for use with urine for identification of Neisseria honorrhoeae in females attending a sexually transmitted disease clinic. *Journal of Clinical Microbiology* 33(2):455-457.

Spiegel, C.A., R. Amsel, and K.K. Holmes

1983 Diagnosis of bacterial vaginosis by direct gram stain of vaginal fluid. *Journal of Clinical Microbiology* 18(1):170-177.

Sweet, R.L., D.V. Landers, C. Walker, and J. Schachter

1987 Chlamydia trachomatis infection and pregnancy outcome. *American Journal of Obstetrics and Gynecology* 156(4):824-833.

Taha, T.E.T., G.A. Dallabetta, J.K. Canner, J.D. Chiphangwi, G. Liomba, D.R. Hoover, and P.G. Miotti

Forthcoming The effect of human immunodeficiency virus infection on birthweight and infant and child mortality in urban Malawi. *International Journal of Epidemiology* 24(4).

Temmerman, M., J. Ndinya-Achola, J. Ambani, and P. Piot

1995 The right not to know HIV-test results. *The Lancet* 345(8955):969-970.

Travers, K., S. Mboup, R. Marlink, A. Guèye-Ndiaye, T. Siby, I. Thior, I. Traore, A. Dieng-Sarr, J. Sankalé, C. Mullins, I. Ndoye, C. Hsieh, M. Essex, and P. Kanki

1995 Natural protection against HIV-1 infection provided by HIV-2. *Science* 268(5217): 1612-1615.

Udvardy, M.

1990 Taking social and cultural factors into account: Dimensions of sexuality and reproduction relevant to HIV/AIDS in Africa. Pp. 73-90 in F. Staugard, ed., *The Role of Women in Health Development*. Stockholm, Sweden: The Nordic School of Public Health and the World Health Organization.

United Nations

1993 *The Sex and Age Distribution of the World Populations: The 1992 Revision*. New York: Department of Economic and Social Development, United Nations.

U.S. Bureau of the Census

1994a *HIV/AIDS Surveillance Database: Program Diskette, December 1994*. Washington, D.C.: Center for International Research, U.S. Bureau of the Census.

1994b *Recent HIV Seroprevalence Levels by Country: December 1994*. Research Note No. 15. Washington, D.C.: Health Studies Branch, Center for International Research, U.S. Bureau of the Census.

1994c *Trends and Patterns of HIV/AIDS Infection in Selected Developing Countries: Country Profiles: June 1994*. Research Note No. 14. Washington, D.C.: Health Studies Branch, Center for International Research, U.S. Bureau of the Census.

Valleroy, L.A., J.R. Harris, and P.O. Way

1990 The impact of HIV-1 infection on child survival in the developing world. *AIDS* 4(7): 667-672.

Van de Perre, P., D. Rouvroy, P. Lepage, J. Bogaarts, P. Kestelyn, J. Kayihigi, A.C. Hekker, J.P. Butzler, and N. Clumek

1984 Acquired Immunodeficiency Syndrome in Rwanda. *The Lancet* 2(8394):62-65.

Van de Perre, P., A. Simonon, P. Msellati, D.G. Hitimana, D. Vaira, A. Bazubagira, C. Van Goethem, A.M. Stevens, E. Karita, D. Sondag-Thull, F. Dabis, and P. Lepage

1991 Postnatal transmission of human immunodeficiency virus type 1 from mother to infant:

A prospective cohort study in Kigali, Rwanda. *New England Journal of Medicine* 325(9):593-598.

Wabwire-Mangen, F.
1995 *Maternal and Placental Risk Factors for Vertical Transmission of the Human Immunodeficiency Virus in Uganda.* Unpublished PhD Dissertation. Baltimore, MD: Department of Epidemiology, School of Hygiene and Public Health, Johns Hopkins University.

Wagner H-U., A. Kamali, A.J. Nunn, J.F. Kengeya-Kayondo, and D.W. Mulder
1993 General and HIV-1-associated morbidity in a rural Ugandan community. *AIDS* 7(11):1 461-1467.

Wasserheit, J.N.
1992 Epidemiological synergy: Interrelationships between human immunodeficiency virus infection and other sexually transmitted diseases. *Sexually Transmitted Diseases* 19(2): 61-77.

Wasserheit, J.N., and K.K. Holmes
1992 Reproductive tract infection: Challenges for international health policy, program and research, Pp. 7-33 in A. Germain, K.K. Holmes, P. Piot, and J.N. Wasserheit, eds., *Reproductive Tract Infections: Global Impact and Priorities for Women's Reproductive Health.* New York: Plenum Press.

Watson, P.A.
1985 The use of screening tests for sexually transmitted diseases in a third world community: A feasibility study in Malawi. *European Journal of Sexually Transmitted Diseases* 2(2):63-65.

Wawer, M.J., D. McNairn, F. Wabwire-Mangen, L. Paxton, R.H. Gray, and N. Kiwanuka
1995a Self administered vaginal swabs for population-based assessment of Trichomonas vaginalis prevalence [letter]. *The Lancet* 345(8942):131-132.

Wawer, M.J., D. Serwadda, S.D. Musgrave, J.K. Konde-Lule, M. Musagara, and N.K. Sewankambo
1991 Dynamics of spread of HIV-1 infection in a rural district of Uganda. *British Medical Journal* 303(6813):1303-1306.

Wawer, M.J., N.K. Sewankambo, S. Berkley, and D. Serwadda
1994a Incidence of HIV-1 infection in a rural region of Uganda. *British Medical Journal* 308(6922):171-173.
1994b Trends in crude prevalence may not reflect incidence in communities with mature epidemics. Abstract No. 289C, Volume 10(1):84. Xth International Conference on AIDS, August 7-12, Yokohama, Japan.

Wawer, M.J., R.H. Gray, T.C. Quinn, N.K. Sewankambo, F. Wabwire-Mangen, D. Serwadda, and L. Paxton
1995b Design and feasibility of population-based mass STD treatment, rural Rakai district, Uganda. Abstract 079, XIth Meeting of the International Society for STD Research, August 27-30, 1995, New Orleans, LA.

Welgemoed, N.C., A. Mahaffey, and J. Van den Ende
1986 Prevalence of neisseria gonorrhoeae infection in patients attending an antenatal clinic. *South African Medical Journal* 69(1):32-34.

Widy-Wirsky, R.R., and L.J. D'Costa
1989 Prévalence des maladies transmisés par voie sexuelle dans la population des femmes enceités en milieu urbain en Centrafrique. Pp. 655-660 in *13ieme Conference Technique: Rapport Final.* Yaoundé, Cameroon: OSEAC.

World Bank
1995 *World Development Report 1995.* Oxford: Oxford University Press.

World Health Organization
1992 Consensus statement from the WHO/UNICEF consultation on HIV transmission and breast-feeding. *Weekly Epidemiological Record* 67(24):177-179.
1993 Profile of the HIV/AIDS epidemic, Cameroon. *Weekly Epidemiological Record* 68(11):74-77.
1994 *AIDS: Images of the Epidemic.* Geneva, Switzerland: World Health Organization.
1995a The current global situation of the HIV/AIDS pandemic. *Weekly Epidemiological Record* 70(2):7-8.
1995b WHO calls on policy-makers to reduce women's growing vulnerability to HIV/AIDS. Press Release WHO/11. Geneva, Switzerland: Office of Information, World Health Organization.
Forthcoming *Recommendations from the Meeting on Mother-to-Infant Transmission of HIV by Use of Antiretrovirals.* Geneva 23-25 June, 1994. Geneva: World Health Organization.

World Health Organization Expert Committee on Venereal Diseases and Treponematoses
1986 *6th Report*, Technical Report Series No. 736. Geneva, Switzerland: World Health Organization.

World Health Organization Scientific Group on the Epidemiology of Infertility
1975 *The Epidemiology of Infertility.* Report of a WHO Scientific Group, Technical Report Series 582. Geneva, Switzerland: World Health Organization.

CHAPTER 4: SEXUAL BEHAVIOR AND HIV/AIDS

Agounké, A., M. Assogba, and K. Anipah
1989 *Enquête Démographique et de Santé au Togo, 1988.* Lomé, Togo: Unité de Recherche Démographique, Direction de la Statistique; Columbia, MD: Institute for Resource Development/Westinghouse.

Ahmed, S.A., and A.H.H.M. Kheir
1992 Sudanese sexual behaviour, socio-cultural norms and the transmission of HIV. Pp. 303-314 in T. Dyson, ed., *Sexual Behaviour and networking: Anthropological and Socio-Cultural Studies on the Transmission of HIV.* Liège, Belgium: Editions Derouaux-Ordina.

Anarfi, J.K.
1993 Sexuality, migration and AIDS in Ghana—a socio-behavioural study. *Health Transition Review* 3(Supplement):45-67.

Anarfi, J.K., and K. Awusabo-Asare
1993 Experimental research on sexual networking in some selected areas of Ghana. *Health Transition Review* 3(Supplement):29-43.

Awusabo-Asare, K., J.K. Anarfi, and D.K. Agyeman
1993 Women's control over their sexuality and the spread of STDs and HIV/AIDS in Ghana. *Health Transition Review* 3(Supplement):69-84.

Baingana, G., K. Choi, D.C. Barrett, R. Byansi, and N. Hearst
1995 Female partners of AIDS patients in Uganda: Reported knowledge, perceptions and plans. *AIDS* 9(Supplement 1):S15-S19.

Balépa, M., M. Fotso, and B. Barrère
1992 *Enquête Démographique et de Santé: Cameroun, 1991.* Yaoundé, Cameroon: Direction Nationale du Deuxième Recensement Gènèral; Columbia, MD: Macro International.

Barrère, B., J. Schoemaker, M. Barrère, T. Habiyakare, A. Kabagwira, and M. Ngendakumana
1994 *Enquête Démographique et de Santé: Rwanda, 1992.* Kigali, Rwanda: Office National de la Population; Calverton, MD: Macro International.

Bledsoe, C.
1990 Transformations in sub-Saharan African marriage and fertility. *Annals of the American Academy of Political and Social Science* 510(July):115-125.

Bleek, W.
1987 Lying informants: A fieldwork experience from Ghana. *Population and Development Review* 13(2):314-322.

Bongaarts, J., P. Reining, P. Way, and F. Conant
1989 The relationship between male circumcision and HIV infection in African populations. *AIDS* 3(6):373-377.

Brown, J.E., O.B. Ayowa, and R.C. Brown
1993 Dry and tight: Sexual practices and potential AIDS risk in Zaire. *Social Science & Medicine* 37(8):989-994.

Caldwell, J.C., and P. Caldwell
1993 The nature and limits of the sub-Saharan African AIDS epidemic: Evidence from geographic and other patterns. *Population and Development Review* 19(4):817-848.

Caldwell, J.C., P. Caldwell, and P. Quiggin
1989 The social context of AIDS in sub-Saharan Africa. *Population and Development Review* 15(2):185-234.

Caldwell, J.C., P. Caldwell, E.M. Ankrah, J.K. Anarfi, D.K. Agyeman, K. Awusabo-Asare, and I.O. Orubuloye
1993 African families and AIDS: Context, reactions and potential interventions. *Health Transition Review* 3(Supplement):1-16.

Caraël, M.
1995 Sexual behaviour. Pp. 75-123 in J. Cleland and B. Ferry, eds., *Sexual Behaviour and AIDS in the Developing World*. London. Taylor and Francis.

Caraël, M., T.E. Mertens, T. Burton, and P. Sato
1994 *Bright Lights, Red Lights, and Sex*. Paper presented at the International Union for the Scientific Study of Population seminar on Sexual Sub-Cultures, Migration, and AIDS/ STDs, February 27-March 3, Bangkok, Thailand.

Central Bureau of Statistics [Ghana]
1983 *Ghana Fertility Survey 1979-1980, First Report, Volume 1: Background, Methodology and Findings*. Accra, Ghana: Central Bureau of Statistics (Ghana) in collaboration with the World Fertility Survey.

Central Statistical Office [Zimbabwe]
1989 *Demographic and Health Survey, 1988*. Harare, Zimbabwe: Central Statistical Office; Columbia, MD: Macro International.
1995 *Demographic and Health Survey, 1994*. Harare, Zimbabwe: Central Statistical Office; Columbia, MD: Macro International.

Chesney, M.A., P. Lurie, and T.J. Coates
1995 Strategies for addressing the social and behavioral challenges of prophylactic HIV vaccine trials. *Journal of Acquired Immune Deficiency Syndromes and Human Retrovirology* 9(1):30-35.

Cleland, J.G.
1995 Risk perception and behavioural change. Pp. 157-192 in J.G. Cleland and B. Ferry, eds., *Sexual Behaviour and AIDS in the Developing World*. London, UK: Taylor & Francis.

Cleland, J.G., and B. Ferry, eds.
1995 *Sexual Behaviour and AIDS in the Developing World*. London, UK: Taylor & Francis.

Conant, F.P.
1995 Regional HIV prevalence and ritual circumcision in Africa. *Health Transition Review* 5(1):108-112.

Cook, L.S., L.A. Koutsky, and K.K. Holmes
1994 Circumcision and sexually transmitted diseases. *American Journal of Public Health* 84(2):197-201.

Dallabetta, G.A., P.G. Miotti, J.D. Chiphangwi, G. Liomba, J.K Canner, and A.J. Saah
1995 Traditional vaginal agents: use and association with HIV infection in Malawian Women. *AIDS* 9(3):293-297.

Dare, O.O., and J.G. Cleland
1994 Reliability and validity of survey data on sexual behaviour. *Health Transition Review* 4(Supplement):93-110.

de Vincenzi, I., and T. Mertens
1994 Male circumcision: a role in HIV prevention? *AIDS* 8(2):153-160.

Enel, C., E. Lagarde, and G. Pison
1994 The evaluation of surveys of sexual behaviour: A study of couples in rural Senegal. *Health Transition Review* 4(Supplement):111-124.

Federal Office of Statistics [Nigeria]
1992 *Nigeria Demographic and Health Survey, 1990.* Columbia, MD: Institute for Resource Development/Macro International.

Ferry, B., with J.C. Deheneffe, M. Mamdani, and R. Ingham
1995a Characteristics of Surveys and Data Quality. Pp. 10-42 in J. Cleland and B. Ferry, eds., *Sexual Behaviour and AIDS in the Developing World.* London: Taylor & Francis.

Ferry, B.
1995b Risk factors related to HIV transmission: Sexually transmitted diseases, alcohol consumption and medically-related injections. Pp. 193-207 in J. Cleland and B. Ferry, eds., *Sexual Behaviour and AIDS in the Developing World.* London: Taylor and Francis.

Gaisie, K., A.R. Cross, and G. Nsemukila
1993 *Zambia Demographic and Health Survey, 1992.* Lusaka, Zambia: University of Zambia, and Central Statistical Office; Columbia, MD: Macro International.

Ghana Statistical Service
1989 *Ghana Demographic and Health Survey, 1988.* Columbia, MD: Institute for Resource Development/Macro Systems.
1994 *Ghana Demographic and Health Survey, 1993.* Calverton, MD: Demographic and Health Surveys, Macro International.

Guyer, J.I.
1994 Lineal identities and lateral networks: The logic of polyandrous motherhood. Pp. 231-252 in C. Bledsoe and G. Pison, eds., *Nuptiality in Sub-Saharan Africa: Contemporary Anthropological and Demographic Perspectives.* Oxford, UK: Clarendon Press.

Hogsborg, M., and P. Aaby
1992 Sexual relations, use of condoms and perceptions of AIDS in an urban area of Guinea-Bissau with a high prevalence of HIV-2. Pp. 203-231 in T. Dyson, ed., *Sexual Behaviour and Networking: Anthropological and Socio-cultural Studies on the Transmission of HIV.* Liège, Belgium: Editions Derouaux-Ordina.

Hunter, D.J., B.N. Maggwa, J.K.G. Mati, P.M. Tukei, and S. Mbugua
1994 Sexual behavior, sexually transmitted diseases, male circumcision and risk of HIV infection among women in Nairobi, Kenya. *AIDS* 8(1):93-99.

Ingham, R.
1995 AIDS: Knowledge, Awareness and Attitudes. Pp. 43-74 in J.G. Cleland and B. Ferry, eds., *Sexual Behaviour and AIDS in the Developing World.* London, UK: Taylor & Francis.

IRESCO
1992 *Pratiques Sexuelles et Maladies Sexuellement Transmissibles dans les Milleux de la Prostitution de la Ville de Douala.* Yaoundé, Cameroon: Institut de Recherche et des Études de Comportements (IRESCO).

1994 *Evaluation du Projet de Prevention de la Transmission du SIDA par Voie Sexuelle auprès des Populations à Risque.* Yaoundé, Cameroon: Institut de Recherche et des Études de Comportements (IRESCO).

1995 *Barriers to the Prevention and Treatment of STDS/AIDS in Cameroon.* Yaoundé, Cameroon: Institut de Recherche et des Études de Comportements (IRESCO).

Irwin, K., J. Bertrand, N. Mibandumba, K. Mbuyi, C. Muremeri, M. Mukoka, K. Munkolenkole, N. Nzilambi, N. Bosenge, and R. Ryder

1991 Knowledge, attitudes and beliefs about HIV infection and AIDS among healthy factory workers and their wives, Kinshasa, Zaire. *Social Science & Medicine* 32(8):917-930.

Kaijage, F.J.

1994a HIV/AIDS and the orphan crisis in Kagera region: Socio-economic, cultural, and historic dimensions. Unpublished background paper prepared for the USAID/Tanzania AIDS Project's Family Needs Assessment Report, Dar es Salaam, Tanzania. Department of History, University of Dar es Salaam, Tanzania.

1994b HIV/AIDS and the problem of orphans in Arusha region. Unpublished background paper prepared for the USAID/Tanzania AIDS Project's Family Needs Assessment Report, Dar es Salaam, Tanzania. Department of History, University of Dar es Salaam, Tanzania.

Kaijuka, E.M., E.Z.A. Kaija, A.R. Cross, and E. Loaiza

1989 *Uganda Demographic and Health Survey, 1988/1989.* Entebbe, Uganda: Ministry of Health and Makerere University; Columbia, MD: Macro Systems.

Katjiuanjo, P., S. Titus, M. Zauana, and J.T. Boerma

1993 *Namibia Demographic and Health Survey, 1992.* Windhoek, Namibia: Ministry of Health and Social Services; Columbia, MD: Macro International.

Kisekka, M.

No date *Socio-Cultural Beliefs and Practices Related to Condom Acceptability Among Hausa in Nigeria and Baganda in Uganda.* Zaria, Nigeria: Centre for Social and Economic Research, Ahmadu Bello University.

Kivumbi, G.W.

1993 Experience with HIV prevention campaigns in Uganda: A case study of Rakai district. Paper presented at the International Union for the Scientific Study of Population seminar on AIDS Impact and Intervention in the Developing World: The Contribution of Demography and The Social Sciences, December 5-9, Annecy, France.

Konaté, D.L., T. Sinaré, and M. Seroussi

1994 *Enquête Démographique et de Santé: Burkina Faso, 1993.* Ouagadougou, Burkina Faso: Institut National de la Statistique; Calverton, MD: Macro International.

Konde-Lule, J.K.

1993 Focus group interviews about AIDS in Rakai district of Uganda. *Social Science & Medicine* 37(5):679-684.

Konings, E., W.A. Blattner, A. Levin, G. Brubaker, Z. Siso, J. Shao, J.J. Goedert, and R.M. Anderson

1994 Sexual behaviour survey in a rural area of northwest Tanzania. *AIDS* 8(7):987-993.

Kouba, L.J., and J. Muasher

1985 Female circumcision in Africa: An overview. *African Studies Review* 28(1):95-110.

Kourguéni, I.A., B. Garba, and B. Barrère

1993 *Enquête Démographique et de Santé: Niger, 1992.* Niamey, Niger: Direction de la Statistique et des Comptes Nationaux.

Larson, A.

1989 *The Social Context of HIV Transmission in Africa.* Health Transition Centre Working Paper No. 1. Canberra, Australia: Health Transition Centre, Australian National University.

Lesthaeghe, R.J.
1989 Production and reproducation in sub-Saharan Africa: An overview of organizing principles. Pp. 13-59 in R.J. Lesthaeghe, ed., *Reproduction and Social Organization in Sub-Saharan Africa*. Berkeley, CA: University of California Press.
Lindan, C., S. Allen, M. Caraël, F. Nsengumuremyi, P. Van de Perre, A. Serufilira, J. Tice, D. Black, T. Coates, and S. Hulley
1991 Knowledge, attitudes, and perceived risk of AIDS among urban Rwandan women: Relationship to HIV infection and behavior change. *AIDS* 5(8):993-1002.
Lurie, P., M. Bishaw, M.A. Chesney, M. Cooke, M.E.L. Fernandes, N. Hearst, E. Katongole-Mbidde, S. Koetsawang, C.P. Lindan, J. Mandel, M. Mhloyi, and T.J. Coates
1994 Ethical, behavioral, and social aspects of HIV vaccine trials in developing countries. *Journal of the American Medical Association* 271(4):295-301.
Meekers, D.
1992 The process of marriage in African societies: A multiple indicator approach. *Population and Development Review* 18(1):61-78.
1994 Sexual initiation and premarital childbearing in sub-Saharan Africa. *Population Studies* 48(1):47-64.
Mehryar, A.
1995 Condoms: Awareness, attitudes, and use. Pp. 124-156 in J. Cleland and B. Ferry, eds., *Sexual Behaviour and AIDS in the Developing World*. London. Taylor & Francis.
Mertens, T.E., and M. Caraël
1995 Sexually transmitted diseases, genital hygiene, and male circumcision may be associated: a working hypothesis for HIV prevention. *Health Transition Review* 5(1):104-108.
Messersmith, L.J., T.T. Kane, A.I. Odebiyi, and A.A. Adewuyi
1994 Patterns of sexual behaviour and condom use in Ile-Ife, Nigeria: Implications for AIDS/STD prevention and control. *Health Transition Review* 4(Supplement):197-216.
Meursing, K., T. Vos, O. Coutinho, M. Moyo, S. Mpofu, O. Oneko, V. Mundy, S. Dubc, T. Mahlangu, and F. Sibindi
Forthcoming Child sexual abuse in Matabeleland, Zimbabwe. *Social Science & Medicine*.
Moses, S., J.A. Bradley, N.J.D. Nagelkerke, A.R. Ronald, J.O. Ndinya-Achola, and F.A. Plummer
1990 Geographical patterns of male circumcision practices in Africa: association with HIV seroprevalence. *International Journal of Epidemiology* 19(3):693-697.
Moses, S., F.A. Plummer, J.E. Bradley, J.O. Ndinya-Achola, N.J.D. Nagelkerke, and A.R. Ronald
1995 Male circumcision and the AIDS epidemic in Africa. *Health Transition Review* 5(1):100-103.
National Council for Population and Development [Kenya]
1994 *Kenya Demographic and Health Survey, 1993*. Nairobi, Kenya: Central Bureau of Statistics; Calverton, MD: Macro International.
Ndiaye, S., P.D. Diouf, and M. Ayad
1994 *Enquête Démographique et de Santé au Sénégal (EDS-II), 1992/93*. Dakar, Senegal: Ministère de l'Economie; Calverton, MD: Macro International.
Ngallaba, S., S.H. Kapiga, I. Ruyobya, and J.T. Boerma
1993 *Tanzania Demographic and Health Survey, 1991/1992*. Dar es Salaam, Tanzania: Bureau of Statistics; Columbia, MD: Macro International.
O'Toole Erwin, J.
1993 Reproductive tract infections among women in Ado-Ekiti, Nigeria: Symptoms recognition, perceived causes and treatment choices. *Health Transition Review* 3(Supplement):135-149.

Obbo, C.

1993a HIV transmission: Men are the solution. *Population and Environment* 14(3):211-243.

1993b HIV transmission through social and geographical networks in Uganda. *Social Science & Medicine* 36(7):949-955.

Ogbuagu, S.C., and J.O. Charles

1993 Survey of sexual networking in Calabar. *Health Transition Review* 3(Supplement):105-119.

Okie, S.

1993 Mutilation and rape 'normal' for girls. *Toronto Star*, April 7, A15.

Olowo-Freers, B.P.A., and T.G. Barton

1992 *In Pursuit of Fulfillment: Studies of Cultural Diversity and Sexual Behaviour in Uganda*. Kampala, Uganda: UNICEF.

Omorodion, F.I.

1993 Sexual networking among market women in Benin City, Bendel State, Nigeria. *Health Transition Review* 3(Supplement):159-169.

Orubuloye, I.O., J.C. Caldwell, and P. Caldwell

1990 Experimental Research on Sexual Networking in the Ekiti District of Nigeria. Health Transition Working Paper No. 3., 1990. Canberra, Australia: Health Transition Centre, Australian National University.

1991 Sexual networking in the Ekiti district of Nigeria. *Studies in Family Planning* 22(2):61-73.

1992 Diffusion and focus in sexual networking: Identifying partners and partners' partners. *Studies in Family Planning* 23(6):343-351.

1993 African women's control over their sexuality in an era of AIDS: A study of the Yoruba of Nigeria. *Social Science & Medicine* 37(7):859-872.

Oyeneye, O.Y., and S. Kawonise

1993 Sexual networking in Ijebu-Ode, Nigeria: An exploratory study. *Health Transition Review* 3(Supplement):171-183.

Phits'ane, K.

1994 AIDS soars in Lesotho. *Southern African Political and Economic Monthly* 7(9):10-11.

Pickering, H., J. Todd, D. Dunn, J. Pepin, and A. Wilkins

1992 Prostitutes and their clients: A Gambian survey. *Social Science & Medicine* 34(1):75-88.

Pickering H., and H.A. Wilkins

1993 Do unmarried women in African towns have to sell sex, or is it a matter of choice? *Health Transition Review* 3(Supplement):17-27.

Preston-Whyte, E.

1994 Gender and the lost generation: The dynamics of HIV transmission among black South African teenagers in KwaZulu Natal. *Health Transition Review* 4(Supplement):241-255.

Rutenberg, N., A.K. Blanc, and S. Kapiga

1994 Sexual behaviour, social change, and family planning among men and women in Tanzania. *Health Transition Review* 4(Supplement):173-196.

Sandala, L., P. Lurie, M.R. Sunkutu, E.M. Chani, E.S. Hudes, and N. Hearst

1995 'Dry sex' and HIV infection among women attending a sexually transmitted diseases clinic in Lusaka, Zambia. *AIDS* 9(supplement 1):S61-S68.

Schopper, D., S. Doussantousse, and J. Orav

1993 Sexual behaviors relevant to HIV transmission in a rural African population. *Social Science & Medicine* 37(3):401-412.

Segamba, L., V. Ndikumasabo, C. Makinson, and M. Ayad
1988 *Enquête Démographique et de Santé au Burundi, 1987.* Gitega, Burundi: Ministère de l'Intérieur; Columbia, MD: Institute for Resource Development/Westinghouse.

Serwadda, D., M.J. Wawer, S.D. Musgrave, N.K. Sewankambo, J.E. Kaplan, and R.H. Gray
1992 HIV risk factors in three geographic strata of rural Rakai district, Uganda. *AIDS* 6(9):983-989.

Standing, H., and M.N. Kisekka
1989 *Sexual Behaviour in Sub-Saharan Africa: A Review and Annotated Bibliography.* London, UK: Overseas Development Administration.

Stone, L., and J.G. Campbell
1984 The use and misuse of surveys in international development: An experiment from Nepal. *Human Organization* 43(1):27-37.

Ulin, P.R.
1992 African women and AIDS: Negotiating behavioral change. *Social Science & Medicine* 34(1):63-73.

van de Walle, E.
1993 Recent trends in marriage ages. Pp. 117-152 in K.A. Foote, K.H. Hill, and L.G. Martin, eds., *Demographic Change in Sub-Saharan Africa.* Washington, D.C.: National Academy Press.

van de Walle, E., and F. van de Walle
1991 Breastfeeding and popular aetiology in the Sahel. *Health Transition Review* 1(1):69-81.

Vos, T.
1994 Attitudes to sex and sexual behaviour in rural Matabeleland, Zimbabwe. *AIDS Care* 6(2):193-203.

Wilson, D., R. Greenspan, and C. Wilson
1989 Knowledge about AIDS and self-reported behaviour among Zimbabwean secondary school pupils. *Social Science & Medicine* 28(9):957-961.

CHAPTER 5: PRIMARY HIV-PREVENTION STRATEGIES

Allen, S., A. Serufilira, J. Bongaarts, P. Van de Perre, F. Nsengumuremyi, C. Lindan, M. Carael, W. Wolf, T. Coates, and S. Hulley
1992a Confidential HIV testing and condom promotion in Africa: Impact on HIV and gonorrhea rates. *Journal of the American Medical Association* 268(23):3338-3343.

Allen, S., J. Tice, P. Van de Perre, A. Serufilira, E. Hudes, F. Nsengumuremyi, J. Bogaarts, C. Lindan, and S. Hully
1992b Effect of serotesting with counselling on condom use and seroconversion among HIV discordant couples in Africa. *British Medical Journal.* 304(6842):1605-1609.

Ankomah, B.
1994 AIDS: More revelations. *New African* 319(May):9-11.

Ankrah, E.M.
1994 Empowering women may help retard HIV. *Network* 15(12):20-21. Research Triangle Park, NC: Family Health International.

Asamoah-Adu, A., S. Weir, M. Pappoe, N. Kanlisi, A. Neequaye, and P. Lamptey
1994 Evaluation of a targeted AIDS prevention intervention to increase condom use among prostitutes in Ghana. *AIDS* 8(2):239-246.

Barton, T.
1993 *The District Speak-Out: A Preliminary Community Planning Workshop in Uganda.* Kampala, Uganda: UNICEF.

Beaton, G.H., R. Martorell, K.J. Aronson, B. Edmonston, G. McCabe, A.C. Ross, and B. Harvey
1993 *Effectiveness of Vitamin A Supplementation in the Control of Young Child Morbidity and Mortality in Developing Countries.* United Nations Administrative Committee on Coordination/SubCommittee on Nutrition State-of-the-Art Series Nutrition Policy Discussion Paper No. 13. Toronto, Ontario, Canada: University of Toronto.

Bulterys, M., A. Chao, P. Habimana, A. Dushimimana, P. Nawrocki, and A. Saah
1994 Incident HIV-1 infection in a cohort of young women in Butare, Rwanda. *AIDS* 8(11):1585-1591.

Caravano, K.
1991 More than mothers and whores: redefining the AIDS preemption needs of women. *International Journal of Health Services* 21(1):131-142.

Cates, W. and A.R. Hinman
1992 AIDS and absolutism—the demand for perfection in prevention. *The New England Journal of Medicine* 327(7):492-494.

Centers for Disease Control
1994 Zidovudine for the prevention of HIV transmission from mother to infant. *Morbidity and Mortality Weekly Report* 43(16):285-287.

Choi, K.H., and T.J. Coates
1994 Prevention of HIV infection. *AIDS* 8(10):1371-1389.

Cleland, J., J.F. Phillips, S. Amin, and G.M. Kamal
1994 *The Determinants of Reproductive Change in Bangladesh: Success in a Challenging Environment.* Washington, D.C.: World Bank.

Coates, T.
1993 Prevention of HIV-1 Infection: accomplishments and priorities. *Journal of NIH Research* 5(7):73-76.

Cohen, J.
1995 Bringing AZT to poor countries. *Science* 269(5224):624-626.

Coutsoudis, A., R.A. Bobat, H.M. Coovadia, L. Kuhn, W.Y. Tsai, and Z.A. Stein
1995 The effects of vitamin A supplementation on the morbidity of children born to HIV-infected women. *American Journal of Public Health* 85(8):1076-1081.

Coyle, S.L., R.F. Boruch, and C.F. Turner, eds.
1991 *Evaluating AIDS Prevention Programs, Expanded Edition.* Panel on the Evaluation of AIDS Interventions, Committee on AIDS Research and the Behavioral, Social, and Statistical Sciences, Commission on Behavioral and Social Sciences and Education, National Research Council. Washington, D.C.: National Academy Press.

Crump, S.
1995 *The Quality of Evaluation Research on HIV Prevention Strategies in Sub-Saharan Africa.* Unpublished Master's thesis. Atlanta, GA: School of Public Health, Emory University.

Delehanty, D.
1993 AIDS: Providing a coping mechanism. *Trickle Up Continent Report (Asia, 1993)*:9. New York: Trickle Up Program.

De Zoysa, I., K. Phillips, M.C. Kamenga, K. O'Reilly, M. Sweat, R. White, O. Grinstead, and T. Coates
1995 Role of HIV counselling and testing in changing risk behavior in developing countries. *AIDS* 9(Supplement A):S95-S101.

du Guerny, J., and E. Sjöberg
1993 Inter-relationship between gender relations and the HIV/AIDS epidemic: some possible considerations for policies and programmes. *AIDS* 7(8):1027-1034.

Elias, C.J., and L.L. Heise
1994 Challenges for the development of female-controlled vaginal microbicides. *AIDS* 8(1):1-9.

Faden, R.R., G. Geller, and M. Powers, eds.
1991 *AIDS, Women and the Next Generation: Towards a Morally Acceptable Public Policy for HIV Testing of Pregnant Women and Newborns.* New York: Oxford University Press.

Family Health International/AIDSCAP Project
1992 *USAID HIV/AIDS Database Report.* Arlington, VA: Family Health International.
1994 *AIDSCAP Project Annual Report.* Arlington, VA: Family Health International.
1995 *AIDSCAP Behavioral Change and Communication Theoretical Framework.* Arlington, VA: Family Health International.

Ford, N., A. Ankomah, A.F. D'Auriol, E. Davies, and E. Mathie
1992 *Review of Literature on the Health and Behavioural Outcomes of Population and Family Planning Education Programmes in School Settings in Developing Countries.* Unpublished review commissioned by the World Health Organization Global Programme on AIDS. Geneva: World Health Organization.

Gebru, A., Y. Workeneh, D. Flanagan, and A. Kebret
1990 A pilot project for AIDS/STD education in Ethiopian schools. *Ethiopian Journal of Health Development* 4(2):231-237.

Grosskurth, H., F. Mosha, J. Todd, E. Mwijarubi, A. Klokke, K. Senkoro, P. Mayaud, J. Changalucha, A. Nicoll, G. ka-Gina, J. Newell, K. Mugeye, D. Mabey, and R. Hayes
1995 Impact of improved treatment of sexually transmitted diseases on HIV infection in rural Tanzania: Randomised controlled trial. *The Lancet* 346(8974):530-536.

Grunseit, A., and S. Kippax
1993 *Effects of Sex Education on Young People's Sexual Behavior.* Geneva, Switzerland: World Health Organization Global Programme on AIDS.

Gupta, G.R., and E. Weiss
1993 Women's lives and sex: Implications for AIDS prevention. *Culture, Medicine and Psychiatry* 17(4):399-412.

Hanenberg, R.S., W. Rojanapithayakorn, P. Kunasol, and D.C. Sokal
1994 Impact on Thailand's HIV-control programme as indicated by the decline of sexually transmitted diseases. *The Lancet* 344(8917):243-245.

Hankins, C.A., and M.A. Handley
1992 HIV disease and AIDS in women: Current knowledge and a research agenda. *Journal of Acquired Immune Deficiency Syndromes* 5(10):957-971.

Heise, L.L., and C. Elias
1995 Transforming AIDS prevention to meet women's needs: A focus on developing countries. *Social Science & Medicine* 40(7):931-943.

Herdt, G., and A.M. Boxer
1991 Ethnographic issues in the study of AIDS. *Journal of Sex Research* 28(2):171-187.

Hess, L.L.
1993 Prevention is still the best medicine: Condom social marketing campaign changes attitudes and actions in Guinea. *Front Lines* 33(8):6-7. Washington, DC: U.S. Agency for International Development.

Higgins, D.L., C. Galavotti, K.R. O'Reilly, D.J. Schnell, M. Moore, D.L. Rugg, and R. Johnson
1991 Evidence for the effects of HIV antibody counseling and testing on risk behaviors. *Journal of the American Medical Association* 266(17):2419-2429.

Holland, J., C. Ramazanoglu, S. Scott, S. Sharpe, and R. Thomson
1994 Methodological issues in researching young women's sexuality. Pp. 219-239 in M. Boulton, ed., *Challenge and Innovation: Methodological Advances in Social Research on HIV/AIDS.* London, UK: Taylor & Francis.

Kagimu, M., E. Marum, and D. Serwadda
1995 Planning and evaluating strategies for AIDS Health Education Interventions in the Muslim community in Uganda. *AIDS Education and Prevention* 7(1):10-21.

Kamenga, M., R.W. Ryder, M. Jingu, N. Mbuyi, L. Mbu, F. Behets, C. Brown, and W.L. Heyward
1991 Evidence of marked sexual behavior change associated with low HIV-1 seroconversion in 149 married couples with discordant HIV-1 serostatus: experience at an HIV counselling center in Zaire. *AIDS* 5(1):61-67.

Katende, M., and R. Bunnell
1993 Involving communities through feedback on evaluation. *AIDS Health Promotion Exchange* 4:4-5. Amsterdam, The Netherlands: Royal Tropical Institute (KIT).

Kirby, D., L. Short, J. Collins, D. Rugg, L. Kolbe, M. Howard, B. Miller, F. Sonenstein, and L.S. Zabin
1994 School-based programs to reduce sexual risk behaviors: A review of effectiveness. *Public Health Reports* 109(3):339-360.

Klepp, K.I., S.S. Ndeki, A.M. Seha, P. Hannan, B.A. Lyimo., M.H. Msuya, M.N. Irema, and A. Schreiner
1994 AIDS education for primary school children in Tanzania: An evaluation study. *AIDS* 8(8):1157-1162.

Konde-Lule, J.K., M.J. Wawer, and B. Lainjo
1994 Condom Use in Young Adults in Rural Uganda. Abstract No. PC0505, Volume 10(2):282. Xth International Conference on AIDS, August 7-12, Yokohama, Japan.

Kreiss, J.K., D. Koech, F.A. Plummer, K.K. Holmes, M. Lightfoote, P. Piot, A.R. Ronald, J.O. Ndinya-Achola, L.J. D'Costa, P. Roberts, E.N. Ngugi, and T.C. Quinn
1986 AIDS virus infection in Nairobi prostitutes: Spread of the epidemic to East Africa. *New England Journal of Medicine* 314(7).414-418.

Krynen, P.
1994 Rethinking AIDS: Africa's Answer to Western Controlled Health Programmes. Unpublished paper. Victoria Programme, Partage, Tanzania.

Laga, M., M. Alary, N. Nzila, A.T. Manoka, M. Tuliza, F. Behets, J. Goeman, M. St. Louis, and P. Piot
1994 Condom promotion, sexually transmitted diseases treatment, and declining incidence of HIV-1 infection in female Zairian sex workers. *The Lancet* 344(8917):246-248.

Laga, M., N. Nzila, and J. Goeman
1991 The interrelationship of sexually transmitted diseases and HIV infection: implications for the control of both epidemics in Africa. *AIDS* 5(Supplement):S55-S63.

Lamptey, P.
1994 Slowing AIDS: Lessons from a decade of prevention efforts. *AIDSCaptions* August:2-4. Arlington, VA: Family Health International/AIDSCAP.

Lamptey, P., and T.J. Coates
1994 Community-Based AIDS Interventions in Africa. Pp. 513-531 in M. Essex, S. Mboup, P.J. Kanki, and M. Kalengayi, eds., *AIDS in Africa*. New York: Raven Press.

Lamptey, P., T. Coates, G. Slutkin, and P. Piot
1993 HIV prevention: Is it working? Plenary address to IXth International Conference on AIDS/IVth STD World Congress, Berlin, Germany. June 7-11.

Lamptey, P., and M. Potts
1990 Targeting prevention programs in Africa. Pp. 144-180 in P. Lamptey and P. Piot, eds. *The Handbook for AIDS Prevention in Africa*. Research Triangle Park, NC: Family Health International.

Leonard, A.
1994 *Community-Based AIDS Prevention and Care in Africa: Building on Local Initiatives. Case Studies from Five African Countries*. New York: The Population Council.

Levine, C.
1991 AIDS and the ethics of human subjects research. Pp. 77-104 in F.G. Reamer, ed., *AIDS and Ethics*. New York: Columbia University Press.
Liskin, L., C. Wharton, and R. Blackburn
1990 Condoms: Now more than ever. *Population Reports* 23(3)(Series H., No. 8):1-36.
Loodts, P., and P. Van de Perre
1989 STD/HIV prevention, education and promotion of condom use among military recruits in Rwanda. Kigale, Rwanda: National AIDS Control Programme, Ministry of Defense.
Mann, J., D.J.M. Tarantola, T.W. Netter, eds.
1992 *AIDS in the World: The Global AIDS Policy Coalition*. Cambridge, MA: Harvard University Press.
May, J., N. Mukamanzi, and M. Vekemans
1990 Family planning in Rwanda: Status and prospects. *Studies in Family Planning* 21(1):20-32.
McCombie, S., and R. Hornik
1992 *Evaluation of a Workplace-Based Peer Education Program Designed to Prevent AIDS in Uganda*. Working paper #1011. Philadelphia, PA.: Annenberg School of Communications/Center for International Health and Development Communication.
Mercer, M.A., C.E. Mariel, and S.J. Scott
1993 Lessons and Legacies: The Final Report of a Grants Program for HIV/AIDS Prevention in Africa. Institute of International Programs, School of Hygiene and Public Health, The Johns Hopkins University, Baltimore, MD.
Minkoff, H.L., and A. Duerr
1994 Obstetric issues—relevance to women and children. Pp. 773-784 in P.A. Pizzo and C.M. Wilfert, eds., *Pediatric AIDS: The Challenge of HIV Infection in Infants, Children and Adolescents*. Baltimore, MD: Williams & Wilkins.
Moore, M., E. Tukwasiibwe, E. Marum, C. Taremwa, K. O'Reilly, and L. Rosner
1993 Impact of HIV counselling and testing (CT) in Uganda. Abstract No. WS-C-16-4, Volume 9(1):97. IXth International Conference on AIDS, June, 6-11, Berlin, Germany.
Mouli, V.C.
1992 *All Against AIDS: The Copperbelt Health Education Project, Zambia*. London, UK: ACTIONAID, AMREF, CHRISTIAN AID.
Mwizarubi, B., U. Laukamm-Josten, C. Maijonga, G. Lwihula, A. Outwater, and D. Nyamwaga
1992 HIV/AIDS education and condom promotion for truck drivers, their assistants and sex partners in Tanzania. Abstract No. W.D. 4017, Volume 7(2):392. VIIIth International Conference on AIDS, June 16-21, Geneva, Switzerland.
Nature
1993 New-style abuse of press freedom. *Nature* 366(6455):493-494.
Ndyetabura, E.F., and M. Paalman
1994 *The People in Kagera Do Not Believe the Misinformation on AIDS by the Krynens*. Report of the visit to Partage Project in Kagera. Dar es Salaam, Tanzania: Ministry of Health.
Ngugi, E.N., J.N. Simonsen, M. Bosire, A.R. Ronald, F.A. Plummer, D.W. Cameron, P. Waiyaki, and J.O. Ndinya-Achola
1988 Prevention of transmission of human immunodeficiency virus in Africa: Effectiveness of condom promotion and health education among prostitutes. *The Lancet* 2(8616):887-890.
Norr, K.F., B.J. McElmurry, M. Moeti, and S.D. Tlou
1992 AIDS prevention for women. *Nursing Outlook* 40(6):250-256.
Oakley, A., D. Fullerton, and J. Holland
1995 Behavioural interventions for HIV/AIDS prevention. *AIDS* 9(5):479-486.

Over, M., and P. Piot
1993 HIV infection and sexually transmitted diseases. Pp. 455-527 in D.T. Jamison, W.H. Mosley, A.R. Measham, and J.L. Bobadilla, eds., *Disease Control Priorities in Developing Countries*. New York: Oxford University Press.

Population Council
1995 *Community-Based AIDS Prevention and Care in Africa: Building on Local Initiatives. Case Studies from Five African Countries*. New York, New York: The Population Council.

Population Services International
1992 *The Zaire Mass Media Project: A Model AIDS Prevention Communications and Motivation Project*. PSI Special Reports No. 1. Washington, D.C.: Population Services International.
1994a *PSI 1993/1994 Annual Report*. Washington, D.C.: Population Services International.
1994b Social marketing for AIDS prevention in post-apartheid South Africa. *PSI Profile*, April. Washington, D.C.: Population Services International.
1994c *The 1993 Year-end Sales Report*. Washington, D.C.: Population Services International.
1994d Zambia social marketing project has maximum impact on war against AIDS. *PSI Profile*, February. Washington, D.C.: Population Services International.
1995 *December 1994 and Year-end Sales Reports*. Washington, D.C: Population Services International.

Robey, B., S.O. Rutstein, and L. Morris
1992 The reproductive revolution: New survey findings. *Population Reports* 20(4)(Series M, No. 11):1-43.

Seeley, J., U. Wagner, J. Mulemwa, J. Kengeya-Kayondo, and D. Mulder
1991 The development of a community-based HIV/AIDS counselling service in a rural area in Uganda. *AIDS Care* 3(2):207-217.

Semba, R.D., P.G. Miotti, J.D. Chiphangwi, A.J. Saah, J.K. Canner, G.A. Dallabetta, and D.R. Hoover
1994 Maternal vitamin A deficiency and mother-to-child transmission of HIV-1. *The Lancet* 343(8913):1593-1597.

Sokal, D., S. Seitz, B. Auvert, W. Namaara, J. Stover, and R. Bernstein
1991 *Simulation Modeling of Single and Combined Interventions to Control a Heterosexual HIV Epidemic: Preliminary Results*. Research Triangle Park, NC: Family Health International.

Stanecki, K., and P.O. Way
1994 *Review of HIV Spread in Southern Africa*. Washington D.C.: Center for International Research, U.S. Bureau of the Census.

Stryker, J., T.J. Coates, P. DeCarlo, K. Haynes-Sanstad, M. Shriver, and H.J. Makadon
1995 Prevention of HIV infection: Looking back, looking ahead. *Journal of the American Medical Association* 273(14):1143-1148.

Tlou, S.
1995 AIDS prevention for women: A community-based approach in Botswana. Paper presented at the World Health Organization Global Programme on AIDS Meeting on Effective Approaches for the Prevention of HIV/AIDS in Women, February 8-11, Geneva, Switzerland.

Turner, C.F., H.G. Miller, and L.E. Moses, eds.
1989 *AIDS: Sexual Behavior and Intravenous Drug Use*. Committee on AIDS Research and the Behavioral, Social, and Statistical Sciences, Commission on Behavioral and Social Sciences and Education, National Research Council. Washington, D.C.: National Academy Press.

Ulin, P.R.
1992 African women and AIDS: Negotiating behavioral change. *Social Science & Medicine* 34(1):63-73.

UNICEF
1995 Annex 7: Evaluations and studies: Their findings and recommendations. Pp. 36-58 in *A Review of UNICEF Support to AIDS Control and Prevention in Uganda and Zimbabwe*. New York: UNICEF Health Promotion Unit, UNICEF.

U.S. Bureau of the Census
1994a *Recent HIV Seroprevalence Levels by Country: December 1994*. Research Note No. 15. Washington, D.C.: Health Studies Branch, Center for International Research, U.S. Bureau of the Census.
1994b *Trends and Patterns of HIV/AIDS Infection in Selected Developing Countries: Country Profiles: June 1994*. Research Note No. 14. Washington, D.C.: Health Studies Branch, Center for International Research, U.S. Bureau of the Census.

Van de Perre, P., N. Clumeck, M. Carael, E. Nzabihimana, M. Robert-Guroff, P. De Mol, P. Freyens, J.P. Butzler, R.C. Gallo, and J.B. Kanyamupira
1985 Female prostitutes: A risk group for infection with human T-cell lymphotrophic virus type III. *The Lancet* 2(8454):524-526.

Visrutaratna, S., C.P. Lindan, A. Sirhorachai, and J.S. Mandel
1995 'Superstar' and 'model brothel': developing and evaluating a condom promotion program for sex establishments in Chiang Mai, Thailand. *AIDS* 9(Supplement 1):S69-S75.

Williams, E., N. Lamson, S. Efem, S. Weir, and P. Lamptey
1992 Implementation of an AIDS prevention program among prostitutes in the Cross River State of Nigeria. *AIDS* 6(2):229-230.

Williams, G., and S. Ray
1993 *Work Against AIDS: Workplace-based AIDS Initiatives in Zimbabwe*. London, UK: ACTIONAID.

Wilson, D., B. Myathi, and M. Whariwa
1992 *A Community-level AIDS Prevention Program Among Sexually Vulnerable Groups and the General Population in Bulawayo, Zimbabwe*. Harare, Zimbabwe: University of Zimbabwe.

World Bank
1993 *Education in Sub-Saharan Africa: Policies for Adjustment, Revitalization, and Expansion*. Washington, D.C.: World Bank.

World Health Organization
1986 *Young People's Health—A Challenge for Society: Report of a WHO Study Group on Young People and "Health for All by the Year 2000."* WHO Technical Report Series 731. Geneva, Switzerland: World Health Organization.
1992a Consensus statement from the WHO/UNICEF consultation on HIV transmission and breast-feeding. *Weekly Epidemiological Record* 67(24):177-179.
1992b *Current and Future Dimensions of the HIV/AIDS Pandemic: A Capsule*. Geneva, Switzerland: World Health Organization Global Programme on AIDS.
1992c *Effective Approaches to AIDS Prevention: Report of the Meeting, May 26-29*. Geneva, Switzerland: World Health Organization Global Programme on AIDS.
1994a *AIDS: Images of the Epidemic*. Geneva, Switzerland: World Health Organization.
1994b *WHO/UNESCO Pilot Projects on School-Based AIDS Education: A Summary*. Geneva, Switzerland: World Health Organization.
1995 The current global situation of the HIV/AIDS pandemic. *Weekly Epidemiological Record* 70(2):7-8.

Wynendaele, B., W. Bomba, W. M'Manga, S. Bhart, and L. Fransen
1995 Impact of counselling on safer sex and STD occurrence among STD patients in Malawi. *International Journal of STD & AIDS* 6(2):105-109.

CHAPTER 6: MITIGATING THE IMPACT OF THE EPIDEMIC

Ainsworth, M., and M. Over
1994a AIDS and African development. *World Bank Research Observer* 9(2):203-240.
1994b The economic impact of AIDS on Africa. Pp. 559-588 in M. Essex, S. Mboup, P.J. Kanki, and M.R. Kalengayi, eds., *AIDS in Africa*. New York: Raven Press.

Ainsworth, M., and A.A. Rwegarulira
1992 *Coping with the AIDS Epidemic in Tanzania: Survivor Assistance*. Technical Working Paper No. 6. Washington, D.C.: Africa Technical Department, Population, Health and Nutrition Division, The World Bank.

Awusabo-Asare, K., and D.K. Agyeman
1993 Social science research and the challenge of the AIDS epidemic. Pp. 357-368 in *International Union for the Scientific Study of Population Conference, Montreal, 1993*. Volume 4. Liège, Belgium: International Union for the Scientific Study of Population.

Baggaley, R., P. Godfrey-Faussett, R. Msiska, D. Chilangwa, E. Chitu, J. Porter, and M. Kelly
1994 *Impact of HIV infection on Zambian businesses*. *British Medical Journal* 309(6968): 1549-1550.

Barnett, T.
1994 *The Effects of HIV/AIDS on Farming Systems and Rural Livelihoods in Uganda, Tanzania, and Zambia*. Unpublished report prepared for the Food and Agriculture Organization. Norwich, UK: Overseas Development Group, University of East Anglia.

Barnett, T., and P. Blaikie
1992 *AIDS in Africa: Its Present and Future Impact*. London, UK: Guilford Press.

Biggar, R.J.
1993 When ideals meet reality: The global challenge of HIV/AIDS. *American Journal of Public Health* 83(10):1383-1384.

Bledsoe, C., and U. Isiugo-Abanihe
1989 Strategies of child-fosterage among Mende Grannies in Sierra Leone. Pp. 442-474 in R.J. Lesthaeghe, ed., *Reproduction and Social Organization in Sub-Saharan Africa*. Berkeley, CA: University of California Press.

Bongaarts, J.
1994 Projection of the mortality impact of AIDS in Africa. Pp. 187-205 in W. Lutz, ed., *The Future Population of the World: What Can We Assume Today*. London, UK: Earthscan Publications.

Bongaarts, J., and P. Way
1989 *Geographic Variation in the HIV Epidemic and Mortality Impact of AIDS in Africa*. Research Division Working Paper No. 1. New York: Population Council.

Bos, E., and R.A. Bulatao
1992 The demographic impact of AIDS in sub-Saharan Africa: short and long-term projections. *International Journal of Forecasting* 8(3):367-384.

Brugha, R.
1994 HIV counseling and care programmes at the district level in Ghana. *AIDS Care* 6(2): 129-137.

Buvé, A., S.D. Foaster [sic.], C. Mbwili, E. Mungo, N. Tollenare, and M. Zeko

1994 Mortality among female nurses in the face of the AIDS epidemic: A pilot study in Zambia. *AIDS* 8(3):396.

Caldwell, J.C., P. Caldwell, E.M. Ankrah, J.K. Anarfi, D.K. Agyeman, K. Awusabo-Asare, and I.O. Orubuloye

1993 African families and AIDS: Context, reactions, and potential interventions. *Health Transition Review* 3(Supplement):1-16.

Caldwell, J.C., I.O. Orubuloye, and P. Caldwell

1994 Underreaction to AIDS in sub-Saharan Africa. Pp. 217-234 in I.O. Orubuloye, J.C. Caldwell, P. Caldwell, and G. Santow, eds., *Sexual Networking and AIDS in Sub-Saharan Africa: Behavioral Research and the Social Context.* Canberra, Australia: Health Transition Centre, Australian National University.

Caraël, M., J. Cleland, and R. Ingham

1994 Extramarital sex: Implications of survey results for STD/HIV Transmission. *Health Transition Review* 4(Supplement):153-172.

Castle, C.S.

1994 The (re)negotiation of illness diagnoses and responsibility for child death in rural Mali. *Medical Anthropology Quarterly* 8(3):314-335.

Chela, C.M., R. Malska, T. Chava, A. Martin, A. Mwanza, B. Yamba, and E. van Prang

1994 Costing and evaluating home based care in Zambia. Abstract No. 099B/D, Volume 10(1):31. IXth International Conference on AIDS, August 7-12, Yokohama, Japan.

Chela, C.M., and Z.C. Siankanga

1991 Home and community care: The Zambian experience. *AIDS* 5(Supplement):S157-S161.

Chin, J.

1990 Current and future dimensions of the HIV/AIDS pandemic in women and children. *The Lancet* 336(8709):221-224.

Colebunders, R.L., and B. Kapita

1994 Treatments of HIV infection. Pp. 423-437 in M. Essex, S. Mboup, P.J. Kanki, and M.R. Kalengayi, eds., *AIDS in Africa.* New York: Raven Press.

Cuddington, J.T.

1993 Modelling the macroeconomic effects of AIDS with an application to Tanzania. *World Bank Economic Review* 7(2):173-189.

Cuddington, J.T., and J.D. Hancock

1994 Assessing the impact of AIDS on the growth path of the Malawian economy. *Journal of Development Economics* 43(2):363-368.

Danziger, R.

1994 The social impact of HIV/AIDS in developing countries. *Social Science & Medicine* 39(7):905-917.

De Cock, K.M., B. Barrere, L. Diaby, M.F. Lafontaine, E. Gnaore, A. Porter, D. Pantobe, G.C. Lafontant, A. Dagoakribi, M. Ette, K. Odehouri, and W.L. Heyward

1990 AIDS—the leading cause of adult death in the West African city of Abidjan, Ivory Coast. *Science* 249(4970):793-796.

De Cock, K.M., S.B. Lucas, S. Lucas, J. Agness, A. Kadio, and H.D. Gayle

1993 Clinical research, prophylaxis, therapy, and care for HIV disease in Africa. *American Journal of Public Health* 83(10):1385-1389.

Foster, S.

1993 *Cost and Burden of AIDS on the Zambian Health Care System: Policies to Mitigate the Impact on Health Services.* Unpublished report. London, UK.: Department of Public Health and Policy, London School of Hygiene and Tropical Medicine.

1994 HIV/AIDS in Africa. *American Journal of Public Health* 8(7):1178.

Gillespie, S.
1989 Potential impact of AIDS on farming systems: A case study from Rwanda. *Land Use Policy* 6(4):301-312.

Hassig, S.E., J. Perriëns, E. Baende, M. Kahotwa, K. Bishagara, N. Kinkela, and B. Kapita
1990 An analysis of the economic impact of HIV infection among patients at Mama Yemo Hospital, Kinshasa, Zaire. *AIDS* 4(9):883-887.

IRESCO
1995 *Social and Psychological Impact of HIV and AIDS in Sub-Saharan Africa.* Yaoundé, Cameroon: Institut de Recherche et des Études de Comportements (IRESCO).

Kaijage, F.J.
1994a *HIV/AIDS and the Orphan Crisis in Kagera Region: Socio-economic, Cultural, and Historical Dimensions.* Unpublished report. Dar es Salaam, Tanzania: Department of History, University of Dar es Salaam.
1994b *HIV/AIDS and the Problem of Orphans in Arusha Region.* Unpublished report. Dar es Salaam, Tanzania: Department of History, University of Dar es Salaam.

Katabira, E.T., and K.R. Wabitsch
1991 Management issues for patients with HIV infection in Africa. *AIDS* 5(Supplement): S149-S155.

Kitange, H.M., D.G. Mclarty, A.B.M. Swai, J. Black, H. Machibya, D. Mtasiwa, G. Masuki, and K.G.M.M. Alberti
1994 HIV disease: The leading cause of adult death in three study areas (urban and rural) in Tanzania. Paper presented to the National Institute for Medical Research's 12th Annual Joint Scientific Conference, 21-25 February, Arusha, Tanzania.

Lwihula, G., L. Dahlgren, J. Killewo, and A. Sanstrom
1993 AIDS epidemic in Kagera region, Tanzania the experiences of local people. *AIDS Care* 5(3):347-358.

Lwihula, G., and M. Over
1993 Impact of adult deaths from AIDS and other fatal illnesses on the cultural practices of local people in the Kagera Area, Tanzania. Paper presented at the International Union for the Scientific Study of Population seminar on AIDS Impact and Intervention in the Developing World: The Contribution of Demography and the Social Sciences, December 5-9, Annecy, France.

Mann, J.M., H. Francis, T.C. Quinn, B. Kapita, P.K. Asilo, N. Bosenge, N. Nzilambi, L. Jansegers, P. Piot, K. Ruti, and J.W. Curran
1986 HIV seroprevalence among hospital workers in Kinshasa, Zaire: Lack of association with occupational exposure. *Journal of the American Medical Association* 256(22): 3099-3102.

Metrikin, A.S., M. Zwarenstein, M.H. Steinberg, E. Van Der Vyver, G. Maartens, and R. Wood
1995 Is HIV/AIDS a primary-care disease? Appropriate levels of outpatient care for patients with HIV/AIDS. *AIDS* 9(6):619-623.

Ministry of Health [Zambia]
1994 *Report of the Workshop on the Effects of HIV/AIDS on Agricultural Production Systems.* Lusaka, Zambia: Ministry of Health.

M'Pelé, P., S. Lallemant-Le Coeur, and M.J. Lallemant
1994 AIDS counseling in Africa. Pp. 463-472 in M. Essex, S. Mboup, P.J. Kanki, and M.R. Kalengayi, eds., *AIDS in Africa.* New York: Raven Press.

Mulder, D.W., A.J. Nunn, H.U. Wagner, N. Kamali, and J.F. Kengeya-Kayondo
1994a HIV-1 incidence and HIV-1-associated mortality in a rural Ugandan population cohort. *AIDS* 8(1):87-92.

Mulder, D.W., A.J. Nunn, A. Kamali, J. Nakiyingi, H.U. Wagner, and J.F. Kengeya-Kayondo
1994b Two-year HIV-1-associated mortality in a Ugandan rural population. *The Lancet* 343(8904):1021-1023.

National AIDS Control Programme [Kenya]
no date *AIDS in Kenya: Background, Projections, Impact, Interventions.* Nairobi, Kenya: National AIDS Control Programme.

Nelson, A.M., S.E. Hassig, M. Kayembe, L. Okonda, K. Mulanga, C. Brown, K. Kayembe, M.M. Kalengayi, and F.G. Mullick
1991 HIV-1 seropositivity and mortality at University Hospital, Kinshasa, Zaire, 1987. *AIDS* 5(5):583-586.

Norse, D.
1991 Socio-economic impact of AIDS on food production in East Africa. Abstract No. TU.D.57, Volume 7(1):71. VIIth International Conference on AIDS, June 16-21, Florence, Italy.

Obbo, C.A.
1993 Reflections on the AIDS orphans problem in Uganda. Pp. 108-109 in M. Berer and S. Ray, eds., *Women and HIV/AIDS: An International Resource Book.* London, UK: Pandora Press.

Over, M.
1992 *The Macroeconomic Impact of AIDS in Sub-Saharan Africa.* Technical Working Paper No. 3. Population Health and Nutrition Division, African Technical Department, The World Bank. Washington, D.C.: The World Bank.

Over, M., S. Bertozzi. J. Chin, B. N'Galy, and K. Nyamuryekung'e
1988 The direct and indirect cost of HIV infection in developing countries: The cases of Zaire and Tanzania. Pp. 123-125 in A. Fleming, M. Carbalo, D.W. FitzSimmons, M.R. Bailey, and J. Mann, eds., *The Global Impact of AIDS.* New York: Alan R. Liss.

Over, M., and P. Mujinja
1993 Expenditure on health care and use of medical services prior to death. Pp. 41-46 in *The Economic Impact of Fatal Adult Illness in Sub-Saharan Africa: Proceedings of a Workshop.* Washington, D.C.: The World Bank.

Over, M., and P. Piot
1993 HIV infection and sexually transmitted diseases. Pp. 455-527 in D.T. Jamison and H. Mosley, eds., *Disease Control Priorities in Developing Countries.* New York: Oxford University Press.

Page, H.J.
1989 Childrearing versus childbearing: Coresidence of mother and child in sub-Saharan Africa. Pp. 401-441 in R.J. Lesthaeghe, ed., *Reproduction and Social Organization in Sub-Saharan Africa.* Berkeley, CA: University of California Press.

Porter, R.W.
1994 AIDS in Ghana: Priorities and policies. Pp. 90-106 in D.A. Feldman, ed., *Global AIDS Policy.* Westport, CT: Bergin and Garvey.

Preble, E.A.
1990 Impact of HIV/AIDS on African children. *Social Science & Medicine* 31(6):671-680.

Quinn, T.C., P. Piot, J.B. McCormick, F.M. Feinsod, H. Taelman, B. Kapita, W. Stevens, and A.S. Fauci
1987 Serologic and immunologic studies in patients with AIDS in North America and Africa: The potential role of infectious agents as cofactors in human immunodeficiency virus infection. *Journal of the American Medical Association* 257(19):2617-2621.

Ryder, R.W., M. Kamenga, M. Nkusu, V. Batter, and W.L. Heyward
1994 AIDS orphans in Kinshasa, Zaire: Incidence and socioeconomic consequences. *AIDS* 8(5):673-679.

Ryder, R.W., and R.D. Mugerwa
1994 The clinical definition and diagnosis of AIDS in African adults. Pp. 269-281 in M. Essex, S. Mboup, P.J. Kanki, and M.R. Kalengayi, eds., *AIDS in Africa*. New York: Raven Press.

Schietinger, H., C. Almedal, B.N. Marianne, R.K. Jacqueline, and B.L. Ravn
1993 Teaching Rwandan families to care for people with AIDS at home. *The Hospice Journal* 9(1):33-53.

Schoepf, B.G.
1988 Women, AIDS, and economic crisis in Central Africa. *Canadian Journal of African Studies* 22(3):625-644.

Schopper, D., and J. Walley
1992 Care for AIDS patients in developing countries: A review. *AIDS Care* 4(1):89-102.

Seitz, S.
1991 *IWGAIDS User's Manual, Version 3.0*. Urbana/Champaign, IL: Merriam Laboratory for Analytic Political Science, Department of Political Science, University of Illinois.

Sewankambo, N.K., M.J. Wawer, R.H. Gray, D. Serwadda, C. Li, R.Y. Stallings, S.D. Musgrave, and J. Konde-Lule
1994 Demographic impact of HIV infection in rural Rakai District, Uganda: Results of a population-based cohort study. *AIDS* 8(10):1707-1713.

Shepard, D.S.
1991 *Costs of Care for Persons with AIDS in Rwanda*. Cambridge, MA: Harvard Institute for International Development, Harvard University.

Social Policy Research Group
1993 *Orphans, Widows, and Widowers in Zambia: A Situation Analysis and Options for HIV/AIDS Survival Assistance*. Lusaka, Zambia: Institute for African Studies, University of Zambia.

Stanley, E.A., S.T. Seitz, P.O. Way, P.D. Johnson, and T.F. Curry
1989 The United States interagency working group approach: The IWG model for the heterosexual spread of HIV and the demographic impact of the AIDS epidemic. Pp. 119-136 in *The AIDS Epidemic and Its Demographic Consequences: Proceedings of the United Nations/World Health Organization Workshop on Modelling the Demographic Impact of the AIDS Epidemic in Pattern II Countries: Progress to Date and Policies for the Future*. New York: United Nations/World Health Organization.

Stover, J.
1993 *The Impact of HIV/AIDS on Population Growth in Africa*. Washington, D.C.: African Population Advisory Committee.
1994 The impact of HIV/AIDS on adult and child mortality in the developing world. *Health Transition Review* 4(Supplement):47-63.

Tanzania AIDS Project
1994 *National Assessment of Families and Children Affected by AIDS*. Dar es Salaam, Tanzania: Tanzania AIDS Project.

U.S. Bureau of the Census
1994 *Recent HIV Seroprevalence Levels by Country: December 1994*. Research Note No. 15. Washington, D.C.: Health Studies Branch, Center for International Research, U.S. Bureau of the Census.

Wasserheit, J.N.
1989 The significance and scope of reproductive tract infections among Third World women. *International Journal of Gynecology and Obstetrics* 3(Supplement):145-168.

Way, P., and K. Stanecki
1993 How bad will it be? Modelling the AIDS epidemic in Eastern Africa. *Population and Environment* 14(3):265-278.

1994 The Demographic Impact of an AIDS Epidemic on an African Country: Application of the IWGAIDS Model. CIR Staff Paper No. 58, Center for International Research. Washington, D.C.: U.S. Bureau of the Census.

World Bank

1992a *Tanzania: AIDS Assessment and Planning Study*. Washington, D.C.: The World Bank.

1992b *World Development Report*. New York: Oxford University Press.

1993 *World Development Report*. New York: Oxford University Press.

World Health Organization

1991 *Review of Six HIV/AIDS Home Care Programmes in Uganda and Zambia*. Geneva, Switzerland: World Health Organization.

1993 *AIDS Home Care Handbook*. Geneva, Switzerland: World Health Organization.

1994 *AIDS: Images of the Epidemic*. Geneva, Switzerland: World Health Organization.

CHAPTER 7: BUILDING CAPACITY FOR AIDS-RELATED RESEARCH

Ali, M.M.

1994 Capacity building and donor coordination in sub-Saharan Africa. Paper presented at the African Studies Association Meetings, November 3-6, Toronto, Ontario, Canada.

Berg, E.J.

1993 *Rethinking Technical Cooperation: Reforms for Capacity Building in Africa*. New York: United Nations Development Programme.

Bylmakers, L.

1992 *Directory of Socio-Behavioural Research on HIV Infection and AIDS in Zimbabwe*. Harare: UNICEF.

Chew, D.C.E.

1990 Internal adjustments to falling civil service salaries: Insights from Uganda. *World Development* 18(7):1003-1014.

Cohen, J.M.

1993 *Building Sustainable Public Sector Managerial, Professional, and Technical Capacity: A Framework for Analysis and Intervention*. Development Discussion Paper No. 473. Cambridge, MA: Harvard Institute for International Development, Harvard University.

Cornia, G.A., R. Jolly, and F. Stewart, eds.

1987 *Adjustment with a Human Face*. Oxford, UK: Clarendon Press.

Elford, J., R. Bor, and P. Summers

1991 Research into HIV and AIDS between 1981 and 1990: The epidemic curve. *AIDS* 5(12):1515-1519.

Family Health International

1992 *AIDSTECH Final Report*. Volume 1, September 16, 1987-September 15, 1992: Cooperative Agreement. Durham, NC: Family Health International.

Harden, B.

1987 Africans recognize AIDS problem; nations begin public health drives, but resent publicity. *The Washington Post*, February 20, 1987. Section A, p. A21. Washington D.C.: The Washington Post.

Heymann, D.L., P. Bres, M. Karam, R. Biritwum, B. Nkowane, A. Sow, P. Kenya, E.G. Beausoleil, R. Widdus, and J.M. Mann

1990 AIDS-related research in sub-Saharan Africa [letter]. *AIDS* 4(5):469-470.

Institute of Medicine [United States]

1986 *Confronting AIDS: Directions for Public Health, Health Care, and Research*. Washington, D.C.: National Academy Press.

1988 *Confronting AIDS: Update 1988.* Washington, D.C.: National Academy Press.

International Labour Office

1987 *Employment and Economic Reform: Toward a Strategy for The Sudan.* Geneva, Switzerland: International Labour Office.

Jaycox, E.V.K.

1993 Capacity building: The missing link in African development. Paper presented at the African American Institute Conference on Capacity Building, May 20, Reston, Virginia.

Kpundeh, S.J.

1994 Limiting administrative corruption in Sierra Leone. *Journal of Modern African Studies* 32(1):139-157.

Lindauer, D.L., O. Meesook, and P. Suebsaeng

1988 Government wage policy in Africa: Some findings and policy issues. *World Bank Research Observer* 3(1):1-25.

Mann, J.M., and D.J.M. Tarantola, eds.

Forthcoming *AIDS in the World*, Volume 2. New York: Oxford University Press.

Mann, J.M., D.J.M. Tarantola, and T.W. Netter, eds.

1992 *AIDS in the World.* Cambridge, MA: Harvard University Press.

Miller, H.G., C.F. Turner, and L.E. Moses, eds.

1990 *AIDS: The Second Decade.* Washington, D.C.: National Academy Press.

Msiska, R.

1994 Building an effective response: International cooperation. *Integration* 42(December):16-17.

N'Galy B., S. Bertozzi, and R.W. Ryder

1990 Obstacles to the optimal management of HIV infection/AIDS in Africa. *Journal of Acquired Immune Deficiency Syndromes* 3(4):430-437.

National Commission on Acquired Immune Deficiency Syndrome [United States]

1991 *Executive Summary: America Living with AIDS.* Washington, D.C.: National Commission on AIDS.

1993 *Behavioral and Social Sciences and the HIV/AIDS Epidemic.* Washington, D.C.: National Commission on AIDS.

Olowo-Freers, B.P., and T.G. Barton

1992 *In Pursuit of Fulfillment: Studies of Cultural Diversity and Sexual Behaviour in Uganda.* Kampala, Uganda: UNICEF.

Robinson, D.

1990 *Civil Service Pay in Africa.* Geneva, Switzerland: International Labour Office.

Serwadda, D., and E. Katongole-Mbidde

1990 AIDS in Africa: Problems for research and researchers. *The Lancet* 335(8693):842-843.

Turner, C.F., H.G. Miller, and L.E. Moses, eds.

1989 *AIDS: Sexual Behavior and Intravenous Drug Use.* National Research Council. Washington, D.C.: National Academy Press.

Uganda AIDS Commission

1992 *Research Needs Assessment.* Kampala, Uganda: Uganda AIDS Commission and Child Health and Development Centre, Makerere University.

United Republic of Tanzania

1991 *Research Priorities on Human Immunodeficiency Virus Infection and AIDS in Tanzania.* Dar es Salaam, Tanzania: National AIDS Control Programme.

United States Department of Health and Human Services

1994 *AIDS International Training and Research Programs: Fifth Year Progress Report and Cumulative Report for the First Five Years.* Washington, D.C.: National Institutes of Health.

World Bank

1988 *Education in Sub-Saharan Africa: Policies for Adjustment, Revitalization, and Expansion.* Washington, D.C.: The World Bank.

1989 *Sub-Saharan Africa: From Crisis to Sustainable Growth: A Long-Term Perspective Study.* Washington, D.C.: The World Bank.

1991 *The African Capacity Building Initiative: Toward Improved Policy Analysis and Development Management.* Washington, D.C.: The World Bank.

1994 *Better Health in Africa: Experience and Lessons Learned.* Washington, D.C.: The World Bank.

World Health Organization

1994 *AIDS: Images of the Epidemic.* Geneva, Switzerland: World Health Organization.

1995 Peter Piot to head new joint UN programme. *Global AIDS News* 1:1.

APPENDIX A
Panel Visits to Three African Countries January 20-February 12, 1995

INTRODUCTION

During January 20-February 12, 1995, a subset of the panel visited three African countries to observe first-hand the state of the response to the HIV/AIDS epidemic. The purpose of these visits was to (1) learn more about the current prevention and mitigation efforts taking place in these sub-Saharan African countries; (2) brief key African researchers on the efforts of the National Research Council with respect to HIV/AIDS; and (3) gather information to help the panel carry out its mission of identifying the research and data priorities, particularly in the social and behavioral arena, for HIV/AIDS prevention and mitigation in sub-Saharan Africa over the next 5 to 7 years.

Given time and financial constraints, it was impossible to visit more than three countries. The countries were selected to maximize the panel's exposure to countries undergoing different stages of the epidemic, with differing responses and with differing social and behavioral research capacities, while at the same time minimizing the overlap in knowledge reflected in the panel members' considerable expertise. The countries thus selected were Zambia, Tanzania, and Cameroon.

Zambia is a country with a mature epidemic that is being countered with a coordinated response from a strong Ministry of Health, including innovative workplace and traditional healer prevention programs. In comparison with other countries in the region, relatively little HIV-related research focusing on the social and behavioral aspects of the disease is being conducted in Zambia. Tanzania is a second country with a mature epidemic, but one that is being countered by a fragmented response, mainly through nongovernmental organizations. On the other hand, some interesting and important social and behavioral research has been conducted in Tanzania. The AIDS epidemic in Cameroon is not as far advanced as in Zambia or Tanzania, and is characterized by a relatively low level of response. Although the country enjoys some limited social and behavioral research capacity, no prioritization of research needs has yet been conducted.

The visiting team included Deborah Rugg (Centers for Disease Control and Prevention), Carl Kendall (Tulane University), and Peter Way (U.S. Bureau of the Census), together with Barney Cohen (National Research Council). A fourth member of the panel, Dr. Eustace Muhondwa, joined the team in Dar es Salaam, and Peter Way left the team there for a brief visit to learn more about the situation in Kenya. Additionally, Dr. Tom Barton (UNICEF and Makerere University) was invited to join the team for 2 days in Dar es Salaam so he could brief them on the research needs assessment he had conducted for the Uganda AIDS Commission in October 1992.

The team met with the national AIDS control program managers in each of the three countries, as well as many other government officials, social and behavioral scientists, donors, university researchers, policy makers, caregivers, and employees of national and international nongovernmental organizations.

This appendix presents findings from the team's visits to Zambia, Tanzania, and Cameroon.[1] For each, it presents an overview of the current HIV/AIDS situation, summarizes the history of AIDS-prevention efforts, describes ongoing prevention and mitigation initiatives, and reviews the state of social and behavioral research. The final section presents overall themes emerging from the visits to the three countries.

ZAMBIA
JANUARY 23-27, 1995

Overview of Current HIV/AIDS Situation

In Zambia, the AIDS epidemic is already at an advanced stage and has become a major health crisis for the government. The first AIDS cases in Zambia were reported in 1984 and 1985. By 1986, the disease had been recognized as a major public health problem. Over the last 10 years, the number of AIDS cases has risen dramatically. Although exact figures are unreliable, the magnitude of the problem is enormous. Data are available from selected sentinel surveillance sites around the country for 1992, and preliminary data are available for 1993. These data indicate that HIV prevalence among sexually active adults in urban areas ranges from 15 to 37 percent in urban areas, with an average figure of

[1]A list of the people contacted by the team can be found at the end of this appendix.

around 25 percent. In rural areas, where approximately 58 percent of the population resides, HIV prevalence among sexually active adults ranges from 7 to 15 percent, with an estimated average figure of 10 percent. Rural areas close to truck routes, military bases, or mines are likely to have higher rates. In sum, these data indicate that over 600,000 Zambian sexually active adults are HIV-positive and will, sometime in the future, develop AIDS.

History of AIDS-Prevention Efforts

Early efforts at HIV/AIDS prevention in Zambia followed quite closely the typical sub-Saharan African pattern. In 1986, the Government of Zambia set up a National AIDS Surveillance Committee and an Intersectoral AIDS Health Education Committee to coordinate all activities of AIDS prevention and control. With the assistance of WHO, the National AIDS Surveillance Committee implemented an emergency Short-Term Plan to deal with the immediate problem of ensuring a safe blood supply. Under this plan, two laboratories at the University Teaching Hospital in Lusaka and the Tropical Diseases Research Centre in Ndola were designated as national reference centers, with the task of supervising the 31 blood screening centers that were set up subsequently throughout the country. A mass media campaign was launched to create public awareness about HIV infection and AIDS.

In July 1987, the Ministry of Health, recognizing the long-term implications of AIDS, formulated a 5-year Medium-Term Plan covering the period 1988 to 1992, with technical assistance from WHO. This plan identified several priority areas for interventions. It was adopted in September 1988, with a financial outlay of US $12 million over the 5-year period. At a donor meeting in Lusaka in March 1989, a total of US $4.9 million was pledged—$1.9 million more than the amount required for the first fiscal year of the plan. Over the life of the plan, seven functional units evolved: Programme Management; Information, Education, and Communication (IEC); Laboratory Support; Epidemiology and Research; Counseling; Home-Based Care; and STD and Clinical Care. A key turning point in AIDS awareness for Zambians came in 1989 with the untimely death of the former president's son as a result of AIDS.

Over the period of the Medium-Term Plan, the Zambian National AIDS Programme received approximately US $10 million through the WHO Trust Fund. In addition, the Government of Zambia receives assistance for AIDS prevention and control from most of the major donor countries, including the United States, the United Kingdom, Canada, The Netherlands, France, Japan, Norway, and Sweden, in the form of bilateral agreements. Each donor organization has its own readily identifiable AIDS prevention or control activities, but these are integrated reasonably well into the overall national strategy. In addition, a large number of national and international nongovernmental organizations operate throughout the country.

In 1992, three major external reviews were conducted—by the World Bank, WHO, and the Swedish International Development Authority (SIDA)—which revealed that, although each of the above seven functional units had achieved major success, their combined efforts had failed to slow the spread of the epidemic. In effect, increased knowledge among the general population about the dangers of HIV/AIDS and its modes of transmission had not translated into safer sexual behavior. There was a growing realization that all prevention and control efforts were too medically focused, and that there was an urgent need to develop a multisectoral response to the epidemic. At the same time, there was also the need to improve condom distribution and make STD services more accessible.

In response to these reviews, the government, recognizing the need for a broad participatory approach, organized a 3-day consensus workshop in May 1993 in Livingstone as a basis for preparing the second Medium-Term Plan. To ensure the broadest possible base for consensus, the Ministry of Health invited to the workshop over 60 participants from other government ministries and departments, local and international nongovernmental organizations and parastatal organizations operating in Zambia, and representatives from bilateral and multilateral donors. The consensus workshop was followed by technical workshops in the areas of youth, women, the workplace, defense, management, and behavioral change.

The planning process for the second Medium-Term Plan coincided with a change in political structure and ongoing health reform. The Ministry of Health has now moved toward a decentralized model, with responsibility for decision making transferred to the district level.

In 1994, the National AIDS/STD/TB & Leprosy Programme produced its strategic plan for 1994-1998 and launched its enhanced prevention strategies and mitigation/care efforts. Currently, the National AIDS Programme is part of the National AIDS/STD/TB & Leprosy Programme. It is situated in the Ministry of Health, and the program manager reports to the Deputy Director of Medical Services (Primary Health Care). The onset of the AIDS epidemic has coincided with a period of general economic malaise in the country, so that resources for health education and prevention have become even scarcer than usual. Consequently, the National AIDS Programme has been forced to rely heavily on the generosity of the international community. Foreign donors fund virtually all of Zambia's HIV/AIDS prevention and mitigation activities. For example, a large share of prevention activities is implemented through a 3-year, US $8.24 million Morehouse University School of Medicine project funded by the U.S. Agency for International Development (USAID). At the same time, Overseas Development Aid (ODA) is developing a model of home-based care for people with AIDS, and UNICEF is working with orphans. An immediate and important constraint for the National AIDS Programme is a lack of condoms for free distribution.

Ongoing Prevention and Mitigation Initiatives

It would be impossible to review all the worthy HIV/AIDS prevention and mitigation initiatives that are currently taking place in Zambia. Three of the more innovative programs are discussed below.

Workplace Peer Education and Counseling

The Morehouse project, together with the Institute of African Studies of the University of Zambia, has designed and started implementing a workplace peer education and counseling model intended to reach 30,000 workers at approximately 300 sites over 3 years. The project has been designed to provide a mechanism whereby Zambian public- and private-sector employers can assume responsibility for, and institutionalize, a continuing peer education program that will increase STD/AIDS awareness, promote safer sexual behavior, and reduce STD/HIV transmission among their employees. The project includes the training of peer educators and the development of health communication activities within the work site, the provision of assistance to workplaces in designing effective prevention policies, and ultimately the use of workers and management to reach the larger communities affected by the workplace. The project has encouraged interested employers to develop their own HIV/AIDS prevention and counseling programs and has developed a workshop for training peer educators, for which it has designed accompanying manuals and materials.

The project is currently working at 22 worksites in two areas: Lusaka and the Copperbelt. Among the first sites where the project was implemented were Standard Bank and Chibote Farms in Lusaka Province; the Ministries of Tourism, Information, and Agriculture and the Pamodzi Hotel in Lusaka City; and Indeni Petroleum in the Copperbelt Region. These sites represent a variety of work environments, with different kinds of staffing, and each accordingly has a specially designed program. At each site, approximately 1 of every 40 workers is nominated to serve as a peer educator. Approximately 600 workers attended workshops in 1994. The strategy for curriculum development is participatory, with workers playing an active role.

Obviously, one of the goals of the project is to induce major behavioral change. Although the project has been established for only a relatively short period of time, and STD/HIV trends have not been formally tracked, recent evaluation revealed that the project may be having some impact on those trends. The Chiboti Meat Corporation reported that STD cases among its employees had declined by about one-half, and the company's drug procurement costs dropped significantly between May-June at the outset of the project and July-August 1994.

Traditional Healer Component

Traditional healers have always played a major role in the provision of health care in Zambia and have been well organized for over 30 years. Registration of traditional healers in Zambia began in the mid-1960s. A major challenge to STD/HIV prevention in Zambia is that many people seek treatment for STDs from traditional healers, rather than from doctors who use western medicine. Although healers tend to express great faith in their prescribed treatments for STDs, these treatments are usually considered nonefficacious from a biomedical perspective. There is considerable confusion among traditional healers about some of the facts pertaining to the epidemic, for example, the difference between HIV and AIDS, and many traditional healers are reluctant to tell patients that AIDS is a fatal disease. In fact, some healers identify AIDS with the symptoms of "kalyonde-onde," which is thought to be curable.

Against this background, it was decided that any HIV-prevention program in Zambia should include a traditional healer component. Currently, this component is conducting workshops to prepare healers to play the role of community educators, individual counselors, and condom distributors. A series of 20 workshops trained approximately 400 traditional healers in 1994. In addition, routine monthly meetings of healers are used to review topics not well understood; cover additional topics; provide support to the healers in their communities; and identify needed changes in the materials and presentations, incorporating the healers' own suggestions. The strategy for curriculum development is also participatory, with healers playing an active role.

The project is still in its initial stages. Thus it has yet to be formally evaluated, which will be a challenge. However, initial indications are very positive: healers representing the national organization appear quite willing to promote biomedical models of disease transmission, refer clients to hospitals if they suspect AIDS, and promote greater use of condoms and partner reduction among their clients. Additionally, some healers counsel patients whom they believe to be seropositive that repeated unsafe sex will make them sicker. These preliminary findings about the project encourage further exploration of the potential role of traditional healers in HIV prevention and care.

Programs for Orphans

Currently, there are two government initiatives to help orphans and children in need. The Ministry of Community Development and Social Welfare has introduced a Public Welfare Assistance Scheme that is accessible in all districts through the Social Welfare Department offices. It assists the poor and vulnerable by providing money for medical fees, house rentals, educational fees, and material goods. Each district has its own District Welfare Assistance Committee. The other initiative is the Child Care and Adoption Society of Zambia, which is operating in Lusaka and Ndola. This society is promoting fostering (for varying lengths of time) and adoption of children.

In response to the emerging orphan crisis, UNICEF, in collaboration with other nongovernmental organizations, has set up a Children in Need Secretariat, whose mandate is to strengthen family and community capacities to protect and promote the welfare of children. Note that one has to be careful in defining an "orphan" in Zambia. Because of the system of inheritance and property grabbing, the loss of one's father is much more damaging than that of one's mother. Consequently, in a recent Ministry of Health study, 24 percent of "orphans" had lost both parents, 25 percent had lost only their mothers, and 51 percent had lost only their fathers. In all, the study found that 4 out of every 10 households had one or more orphans under their care (Social Policy Research Group, 1993).

The State of Social and Behavioral Research

In general, AIDS-related research activities have been largely uncoordinated in Zambia. Currently, multiple research activities are being carried out, but as far as the team could ascertain, they are not being coordinated by the National AIDS/STD/TB & Leprosy Control Programme or by any other organization. Most research appears to be driven by donors rather than the government of Zambia. The government has not conducted a research-needs assessment or a prioritization exercise to develop a national plan of action for research on AIDS in Zambia. There appears to have been no effort to synthesize research findings for Zambia, and there is no readily accessible bibliography of AIDS-related research either completed or currently in progress. However, in an effort to promote information exchange, Morehouse is sponsoring a one-day research workshop to review and disseminate research findings. Despite the obvious potential for overlap and duplication of effort, the team found no evidence that a serious duplication of effort is taking place.

With regard to social and behavioral research, a number of important initiatives are currently under way in Zambia. For example, research is taking place on the socioeconomic impact of AIDS. As part of the ongoing process of integrating AIDS activities into sectors of the economy outside the health sector, the government of Zambia has commissioned a series of studies to evaluate the social and economic impact of the disease. Each study will assess the impact of HIV/AIDS on one sector of the economy, including, among others, agricultural production systems, transport, mining, and hotels. Some of these reports are still in preparation, but the report on the effects of HIV/AIDS on agricultural production systems has been completed; according to its findings, most labor farming systems are not immediately vulnerable to the epidemic (Barnett, 1994). However, case studies from two rural communities, Teta and Chipese, indicate that in these two communities at least, the epidemic is already affecting quite large numbers of households. Furthermore, large-scale agricultural schemes or the "estate" sector is feeling the impact of the epidemic at all levels of the workforce, particularly among migrant workers and among the more-skilled and more-educated members of the workforce, although in economic and financial terms the impact is not very serious (Barnett, 1994).

UNICEF is currently sponsoring research to develop a better understanding of the trends and the magnitude of the orphan problem in Zambia. A recent Ministry of Health study found that 25 percent of urban orphans and 40 percent of rural orphans quit school because their guardians could not pay uniform and school fees. Furthermore, the majority of orphans did not go to health facilities when ill because of the expense.

Given the advanced state of the epidemic, the enormous number of people suffering, and the limited financial and human resources the public sector can provide, there is an urgent need to develop appropriate models of home-based and community care. With this in mind, ODA is supporting health systems research on costing and evaluation of home-based care in Zambia. The goal of the research is to develop alternative models of home-based care to alleviate the burden of hospitals and to extend the quantity and quality of care available. Initial research on this topic was carried out by Chela et al. (1994), who found that hospital-initiated home-based care cost approximately three times more than community-initiated home care. The largest cost item in hospital-initiated home care was the cost of transportation for caregivers. There was also considerable variation found in the type of service provided, as indicated by the statistic that the average duration per visit was 30 minutes for the hospital-initiated home care, as compared with 120 minutes for the community-initiated home care.

With regard to AIDS prevention, there has been little major research apart from a few studies conducted in communities restricted to urban areas and the Copperbelt. Studies on the social aspects of HIV/AIDS are being carried out by a few institutions, including the University of Zambia, the Commonwealth Youth Program, Family Health Trust, the Churches Medical Association of Zambia, and the Copperbelt Health Education Project. Under the University of Zambia, the Institute for African Studies has been particularly active. Each of these institutions has a library in which it keeps records of work done.

A good number of individuals in Zambia have conducted research related to HIV/AIDS. Most have at least masters degrees in the social sciences from universities abroad, coupled with relevant experience at various levels of governmental or nongovernmental organizations. A directory of Zambian consultants working in the HIV/AIDS field was published in 1993.

TANZANIA
JANUARY 30-FEBRUARY 3, 1995

Overview of Current HIV/AIDS Situation

The first three cases of AIDS in Tanzania were clinically diagnosed in Bukoba regional hospital in Kagera in 1983. From 1983 on, the number of people infected with HIV increased exponentially, mainly through heterosexual contact. AIDS cases were increasingly diagnosed throughout the country, using the Bangui criteria of two major and one minor clinical sign or symptom, and by 1986 were found throughout Tanzania. Although some seroprevalence studies have been conducted in Kagera and elsewhere, it is difficult to know precisely the seroprevalence for Tanzania. The World Bank estimates that 400,000 new infections occur in Tanzania each year and projects a cumulative total of 1.6 million cases by 2010. AIDS kills between 20,000 and 30,000 people every year in Tanzania. It is believed to be the leading cause of death among adults and is likely to be the leading cause of death among children in the very near future (World Bank, 1992). An estimated 130,000 children have lost a parent to AIDS, and by the year 2000 there could be 750,000 AIDS orphans in Tanzania. In Dar es Salaam, HIV infection levels among antenatal care attenders have almost doubled, from 8.9 percent in 1989 to 16.1 percent in 1993.

The extent of the epidemic varies widely by region, with some parts of the country much more affected than others. The levels of infection are highest in Kagera, Iringa, Mwanza, and Rukwa regions, ranging from 12 to 21 percent among pregnant women attending antenatal clinics. In other regions, levels range from 2.9 to 9 percent. Whether seroprevalence levels in these latter regions will ultimately reach levels similar to those recorded in Kagera and other more heavily affected regions will depend crucially on what happens to patterns of sexual behavior. Regardless of whether behavior changes or not, however, there is no doubt that AIDS will be a major health problem in Tanzania for many years to come.

History of AIDS-Prevention Efforts

In 1985, the first institutionalized efforts were initiated with the formation of the AIDS Task Force, later named the Technical Advisory Committee on AIDS. Efforts to control the pandemic in Tanzania began with small-scale studies among selected population groups in 1986 and a population-based study in Kagera in 1987. In 1988, the Technical Advisory Committee assisted in the creation of the Tanzanian national AIDS control program, which is now in its second 5-year Medium-Term Plan.

Ongoing Prevention and Mitigation Initiatives

Although many HIV/AIDS prevention and mitigation activities have been undertaken in Tanzania, there is relatively little coordination through the national AIDS control program or consensus on the best approaches, nor is there much integration of the various programs. Each donor has its own interventions. For example, USAID focuses on condom social marketing, while other donors focus on STDs or family planning. Ideally, there should be more donor coordination to meet national needs and use resources optimally. Instead, donor programs are offered on a "take it or leave it" basis. Little Tanzanian national funding for HIV/AIDS prevention and mitigation has been forthcoming. The presence of international donors, especially the bilateral donors, has permitted the country to invest national financial resources in other areas; however, this has made the national AIDS control program almost completely dependent on international donors and their priorities. (See the discussion of these issues in Chapter 7.) This problem has also existed for the multilaterals, but the new reorganization of United Nations services may resolve the problem for those programs.

There is a general feeling within the national AIDS control program that the choice of interventions and strategies to be adopted is imposed on the basis of international or individual nongovernmental organization agendas, rather than being based on research on what works in Tanzania. This leads to some obvious tensions and conflicts of interest. For example, the national AIDS control program would like to see a behavior-change focus and more emphasis placed on improved materials. However, donors have identified commodities, such as condoms and STD therapy, as the focus of their intervention programs.

The Tanzania AIDS Project, funded by USAID, is the largest single AIDS-prevention effort in Tanzania. The main purpose of the project is to support nongovernmental organizations in complementing the government's efforts through the national AIDS control program.

Components of the Tanzania AIDS Project

The Tanzania AIDS Project has five main components:

- *Social Marketing of Condoms*: The project provides the national AIDS control program with technical assistance in condom logistics for the public sector, while also managing the Population Services International social marketing campaign. Last year, 3 million condoms had been sold at 20 Tanzanian schillings each. Social marketing has been so successful that people would now rather buy a condom than get one for free.
- *Behavior-Change Communication and Information, Education, and Communication (IEC)*: The project has supported the presentation of AIDS-related messages in both electronic and print media. These have included radio spots,

since many Tanzanians listen to the radio at some point in a given day or week, even if they do not own one. The project also borrowed the idea of a newspaper for schoolchildren ("Straight Talk") that has been so successful in Uganda. Videos have been supported, as well as a film entitled "More Time."

- *STD Control:* The project is working with the private sector to facilitate training in STD diagnosis among health-care providers.
- *Nongovernmental Organization Support*: The project has facilitated the establishment of coalitions or "clusters" of nongovernmental organizations in nine regions. Operating through a designated "anchor" organization in each region, the project conducts training of nongovernmental organization staff in management skills, leadership skills, and financial management and provides technical assistance as needed. A nongovernmental organization workplace project started as a demonstration project in 1990 and supports 22 organizations. This project has yet to be formally evaluated. Peer educators have generally noted that knowledge of the modes of transmission and means to prevent AIDS has greatly increased in the last 2 years, but they are uncertain whether this has translated into behavior change. Consequently, despite the successes experienced by the nongovernmental organizations involved, this effort has not been scaled up.
- *Workplace Education*: The project supports the African Medical Research Foundation (AMREF) in its truck driver/truck stop project, which trains peer educators, distributes condoms, and now offers STD treatment near the truck stop sites. AMREF also works with the women's clubs that have sprung up along the trucking routes. The problem is that these naturally occurring community-based groups have proved difficult to sustain because the women die or move on down the truck route.

The Nongovernmental Organization Strategy

Tanzania is unusual among the countries visited by the team in that USAID-funded interventions are channeled exclusively through nongovernmental organizations. This strategy arose from concerns on the part of the USAID mission that there was a divergence between the mission goals and the GPA-linked national AIDS control program. There was also concern about the effectiveness of the utilization of funds in the public sector. (For example, a recent condom audit uncovered a substantial divergence between warehouse records and condoms on hand in a warehouse.)

Not surprisingly, a policy of funding only nongovernmental organizations leads to obvious questions surrounding the capacity of those organizations. Although there are many excellent examples of nongovernmental organizations doing AIDS-related work in Tanzania, many require substantial technical assistance, as envisioned in the Tanzania AIDS Project. Although a nongovernmental organization strategy, at its best, promises local control and ownership, great commitment, and popular support to build investment in the organization for sustainability, not all nongovernmental organizations are local, legitimate, or grass-roots. Furthermore, the sustainability of these organizations needs to be explored. Finally, there is the danger that this investment simply frees nongovernmental organization funding for other activities, such as religious proselytizing. For example, according to the assessment document, one recipient of funding, the Lutheran Church, believes that condom promotion leads to promiscuity (even though scientific evidence contradicts this assertion) and provides condoms only to discordant couples.

From the perspective of the nongovernmental organizations, the major constraints to their effective operation are (1) basic infrastructure issues, including a lack of transport, facilities, office supplies, equipment, and training; (2) difficulties in knowing how to evaluate their efforts; and (3) their dependence on single foreign donors, which they regard as a vulnerability.

In sum, it remains to be seen whether this investment in nongovernmental organizations is effective, either in delivering appropriate services or in building sustainable programs.

Social and Economic Mitigation of AIDS

In addition to all the conventional components of USAID-funded AIDS Control and Prevention (AIDSCAP) projects, the Tanzania AIDS Project attempts to address directly the issue of social and economic mitigation of the impact of the epidemic, focusing especially on women and children. The project has benefited from a national assessment of families and children affected by AIDS, conducted in collaboration with the Tanzanian Ministry of Labor and Youth Development and Muhimbili University College of the Health Sciences. This report highlights the following:

- Issues of vulnerability associated with widows and orphans and how these difficulties are exacerbated by high levels of general poverty and unemployment;
- Costs associated with prolonged illness and death and special costs associated with HIV disease;
- The inability of the traditional marriage, inheritance, and fosterage system to protect individual women and children; and
- Inappropriate local behavioral responses to the epidemic.

Just as prevention programs have been reluctant to address care issues because of the enormous potential costs involved, they have been reluctant to address mitigation issues. Mitigation issues cannot easily be separated from general socioeconomic development issues, and many of the hardest-hit areas are economically too fragile to respond adequately. However, there are issues related to the protection of widows and orphans, the education of children and others, and similar concerns that can and should be addressed.

Overall, efforts to address mitigation issues involve complex intervention issues, necessitating close cooperation across ministries in the government sector; cooperation from professionals such as healers, ministers, and teachers; and local participation. These efforts are unlikely to resemble traditional programs in the health sector.

The State of Social and Behavioral Research

A repeated theme throughout the team's meetings in Tanzania was that research agendas are set outside Tanzania, rather than collaboratively with the Tanzanians (a theme raised also in our visit to Zambia, as discussed earlier). Domestic research priorities are funded either inadequately or not at all. Moreover, funded research does not follow the priorities established by the national AIDS control program in 1991. (Although the program acknowledges that these priorities are somewhat dated, it still believes they have relevance in many areas.) The problem is highlighted by a table compiled by Dr. Susan Hunter, USAID (see Table 6-1). This table lists 12 research priorities and 7 data collection priorities and reviews the agendas of AIDS experts in Washington, the national AIDS control program, and the Tanzania AIDS Project. There is no agreement on any of the 12 research priorities among the three programs. However, 4 of the 7 data collection priorities are shared. These include studies on (1) AIDS knowledge, attitudes, beliefs, and practices; (2) condom use and availability; (3) STD incidence; and (4) STD "points of first encounter."

With regard to academic resources, there is no central repository for research or reports on AIDS-related activities in Tanzania. The national AIDS control program recruited a young woman to maintain such a database, but at the time of our visit, she had been sent to England for 4 months for training, and it was unclear how complete this database was. There is also a library at Muhimbili University, but reports are not always available. Furthermore, there is little networking of researchers in Tanzania. As discussed in Chapter 7, local researchers often keep research results until an international conference, rather than publishing or distributing them locally.

Tanzania is unique in East Africa in having a department of social and behavioral science attached to a medical school. In the 1970s, Muhimbili Medical Center, now Muhimbili University College of the Health Sciences, established a Department of Behavioral Sciences with an applied focus. The department is a unique resource in East Africa, internationally known for its accomplished scientists. When funds were available in the 1970s, a cadre of young scientists was sent abroad for training. These behavioral scientists returned to Tanzania and became very active in child survival interventions, vector-borne disease control, and lately AIDS interventions. Unfortunately, most of these social and behavioral scientists are now senior and accomplished. Because the effort was not repeated, they are stretched very thinly across Tanzania's many health problems.

Most of the research projects at Muhimbili are determined by donor preferences. The university has not benefited to the extent it might have from its extensive collaboration with foreign affiliates. Buildings are in varying states of disrepair, and there are serious shortages of basic classroom equipment.

CAMEROON
FEBRUARY 6-10, 1995

Overview of Current HIV/AIDS Situation

The first cases of AIDS in Cameroon were reported in 1985. Through December 1994, a total of 3,067 AIDS cases had been reported to WHO (last reporting date December 1993).

The AIDS epidemic is at an earlier stage in Cameroon than in either Zambia or Tanzania, although it has experienced steady growth over the last decade. Currently, commercial sex workers in the large cities of Yaounde and Douala show infection rates of 20-35 percent. Studies of other populations at high risk include one of truck drivers in South West and Littoral provinces (HIV infection rate of 17 percent) and a national study of the military (HIV infection rate of 6 percent).

Studies among pregnant women in the large urban areas have found HIV prevalence rates of 2-5 percent. Sentinel data for this population group from five sites show 50-100 percent increases over data collected 15 months earlier, suggesting that the speed of the spread of the epidemic may be increasing. Surveys in other parts of the country show HIV infection rates among the general population ranging from less than 1 percent to over 10 percent.

History of AIDS-Prevention Efforts

Cameroon is in the middle of its second Medium-Term Plan. An external review of the plan was conducted in 1993. A sentinel surveillance system was established in 1989 and revised in 1992. Changes to the system included focusing on twice-yearly testing of pregnant women and using two rapid tests or two enzyme-linked immunosorbent assay (ELISA) tests rather than Western Blot confirmation.

A USAID-funded prevention program began activities in Cameroon in 1990, including a condom social marketing program. USAID-supported activities have continued with AIDSCAP since 1992. A number of other donors, including the German and the French governments' international aid agencies and CARE, are active in Cameroon, as discussed below.

The team met with several senior Cameroonian researchers working on AIDS issues in Cameroon, who questioned the real commitment of donors to help African populations and cited examples of linkages between foreign aid and political decisions to illustrate this point. This perceived lack of commitment extends to donor institutions, politics, and personnel.

As discussed earlier for Zambia and Tanzania, donors have their own priorities and do not fully take into account the needs of the country. In Cameroon, this is evidenced in an AIDS control program that is geographically fragmented, with donors operating programs that reflect their own priorities, each in a different geographic region of the country. If one local organization does not agree with the priorities or approach proposed by a donor, another organization is found to do the desired project. This raises the question of whether there is actually a *national* AIDS control program. One researcher suggested that there is not.

The researchers suggested that the way to address the threat of AIDS effectively in Cameroon is to build programs from the bottom up. Programs must consider relationships as the key to understanding behavior. The interface between program administrators at the top and the community needs to be the local government officers. A program needs to get them doing useful things at the local level by empowering them (including providing technical assistance and training) and encouraging demand for such services from the community, although, unfortunately, many at the top perceive such an approach as representing a loss of power and control. At the top, donors need to do the same with African policy makers and researchers.

Ongoing Prevention and Mitigation Efforts

Overview

AIDS control activities in Cameroon are divided among the various donors. There are four major donors currently active: USAID (AIDSCAP project), GTZ (Germany), FAC (France), and CARE. In addition, WHO/GPA provides some support. Donor activities tend to be divided either by region or by type of intervention. GTZ has a variety of programs in three of Cameroon's ten provinces—Littoral, Northwest, and Southwest provinces. It contributes about US $200,000 per year for these activities. FAC is active in three northern provinces, with an annual budget of US $1.3 million, much of which goes toward primary health-care programs. CARE is working in the eastern part of the country with a limited program. UNICEF will soon be starting a school-based HIV education program in Cameroon.

As discussed below, AIDSCAP has several specific interventions with commercial sex workers and university students and has a nationwide condom social marketing program (Population Services International). WHO/GPA supports purchase of blood screening reagents and some IEC activities, but its total contribution is about US $150,000 per year, which represents a significant drop in recent years.

Donor meetings have been held once or twice a year, but given the above description of activities, whether Cameroon has a national program or not is a legitimate question, as discussed earlier. Virtually all of the money spent on AIDS control activities in the country comes from external sources. The Cameroon government provides the (small) staff of the l'Unité du Lutte Contre le SIDA (ULS) (the national AIDS control program) and their office facilities. The ULS has six functional areas (IEC, counseling, laboratory, research, epidemiology, and STDs), each with a chief, but the chiefs seem to be serving in a part-time capacity, and there are no staffs in those functional areas. There is no support in other ministries for AIDS control activities, and most are doing nothing.

According to the director of the national AIDS control program, existing donor support funds about 50 to 60 percent of the current Medium-Term Plan, begun several years ago. The remainder of the plan is simply not being implemented. In addition, because donor funds are generally programmed, donors cannot be responsive to requests, for example from the ULS, for specific interventions or programs. The team found no evidence of a clear set of research and/or intervention priorities at the ULS that might help guide future donor activities.

AIDSCAP

Cameroon's AIDSCAP project, which succeeds AIDSTECH (1990-1992), began in September 1992. It includes the following five activities:

- Sentinel surveillance in antenatal clinics;
- IEC strategies with three high-risk target groups:
  - Military and police,
  - University students,
  - Commercial sex workers (a peer educator approach);
- A small grants program, which has supported the following:
  - Save the Children—for community-based strategies in the north,
  - CARE—for strategies targeting out-of-school youth in the east;
- Social marketing of condoms ("Prudence" brand) through Population Services International; and
- Research/STD studies conducted with graduate students at the university.

The military and university students have been targeted because they are frequent clients of commercial sex workers and because these groups are frequently single, male, and possessed of ready cash.

University Students The AIDSCAP-supported intervention program involves the use of peer educators in each university. Project planning began in May 1993, and the initial training of peer educators in Yaoundé was conducted in January 1994. The program has found working with students directly to be far more efficient than having to go through the major bureaucratic delays involved in contracting with the university per se for a project. Peer educators are drawn from various social groups at the university, including those involved with sports and the arts and those associated with particular ethnic groups.

The peer educators have developed their own educational materials and also are engaged in condom sales and promotion. They hold monthly meetings. However, their initial enthusiasm is beginning to wear off, and motivation is increasingly a problem. The project is not able to provide them with financial support, even to cover the cost of materials and transportation. As of our visit, only about half of those trained over the past year were attending the monthly meetings.

Commercial Sex Worker Project This project began as a pilot among Yaoundé commercial sex workers and their clients in 1988; STD clinic patients were also added as a target group. The project began with only 15 peer educators. As of our visit, it had 40 peer educators in Yaoundé and had expanded to other cities as well. The objectives of the project are as follows:

- To provide small-group and one-on-one peer education in locations that are high risk, such as bars, brothels, truckstops, hotels, and the "maisons du passage" (places where men can go for sex with a woman, not overnight accommodation).
- To conduct educational dramas.

The purpose of the project is to increase condom use among commercial sex workers and their clients; thus both men and women are being targeted. Project activities include (1) "health talks" given in small groups by the peer educators to commercial sex workers and their clients, (2) individual educational discussions and demonstrations on how to use condoms, (3) peer educator sales of condoms, and (4) drop-in HIV counseling and testing.

HIV Counseling Project In addition to the commercial sex worker project, AIDSCAP runs an HIV Counseling Center, which provides free and anonymous HIV counseling and testing and supportive counseling for those who are infected. There is also a home-visit program for people who cannot make it to the center for supportive services. About three-fourths of clients who come to the center accept testing after being counseled; approximately 50 percent come back for the results.

Condom Social Marketing—Population Services International With AIDSCAP support, Population Services International runs a condom social marketing program in Cameroon, marketing the "Prudence" brand. This activity was initiated under the earlier AIDSTECH project. Thus far, the program has achieved moderate success, selling about 0.6 condoms per capita in 1994. This places it about third among African condom social marketing programs.

The State of Social and Behavioral Research

Strengthening the capacity for social and behavioral research is a clear need in Cameroon. Not enough such research related to AIDS is being conducted, and the skills and experience of local researchers are consequently somewhat limited. In this light, the Cameroon experience with two local nongovernmental organizations composed of young social and behavioral scientists is encouraging and may serve as a model for the development of similar groups in other countries.

IRESCO

The Institute for Social and Behavior Research (IRESCO) is a nongovernmental organization composed of young social and behavioral scientists. Over the past several years, they have undertaken research and evaluation projects for donors such as AIDSCAP, WHO, and UNICEF. IRESCO maintains a core staff (secretariat) and can draw on other researchers in universities and elsewhere to conduct research projects.

FOCAP

The Cameroon Psychology Forum (FOCAP) is another local nongovernmental organization working in the area of social and behavioral research in Cameroon. Like IRESCO, FOCAP comprises an interdisciplinary team of young social and behavioral scientists. Initially begun as a professional association, over the past several years it has conducted a variety of studies in medical sociology, sociology of development, political sociology, community health, and anthropology. FOCAP has employed both qualitative (focus group) and quantitative (community-based survey) approaches in its work.

OVERALL THEMES

This section summarizes the main themes that arose from the panel's visits. The most significant themes (most of which are discussed in Chapter 5 of this report) were as follows: the real lack of solid evaluation research assessing behavior change due to the HIV-prevention strategies that have been tried; the lack of formative research, needs assessment, or tailoring of efforts in the development of HIV-prevention programs and a failure to utilize existing research findings; the paucity of information or strategies addressing the HIV-prevention needs of women and youth; and the questionable sustainability of the national AIDS control program infrastructures and their current gaps as a result of donor financial and technical assistance reductions and withdrawals, particularly the withdrawal of WHO/GPA advisers. Other overall themes are listed below.

1. A pervasive theme was a concern over the reduction or withdrawal of donor financial assistance and the consequent inability to sustain the HIV-prevention infrastructures that have been put in place. Some, maybe most, developing countries are going to need considerable donor assistance for HIV prevention and care for the foreseeable future. The costs of not providing this assistance in terms of both human and economic impact in Africa are staggering. Primary and secondary prevention programs are considerably more cost-effective than dealing with the costs of care and the indirect effects of the epidemic on the future of these countries. While government national AIDS control programs should be encouraged and helped to work toward sustainability, gradually reducing their dependency on foreign aid and introducing limited cost-recovery efforts, they are likely to need considerable financial and technical assistance for at least some 10-20 years.

2. The programs we visited were trying to recover from the major withdrawal of WHO/GPA technical advisers and the concomitant reduction in funds and guidance. According to the national AIDS control program managers, this GPA withdrawal was abrupt and not done in consultation with them; thus it has been very disruptive. All the managers with whom we spoke feel that there has been a real gap left in the wake of the GPA withdrawal. All of the national AIDS control program planning areas are having a difficult time coping with these losses.

3. Many national AIDS control program managers interviewed cited the need for change in certain social norms that are fueling the spread of HIV across Africa and the need for more sophisticated intervention strategies to address these norms (see Chapter 2). There was general agreement that what is needed is to (1) identify the specific practices that create an increased risk for spreading HIV (several of which are already well known, such as the low status of women and the general dislike of condoms); (2) identify the factors that influence or determine these practices; (3) conduct formative research to design interventions that address these determinants and specific risk behaviors, specifically targeting the social norm gatekeepers (e.g., elders, traditional healers, political and religious leaders), as well as the individuals involved in these practices; and (4) use indigenous people and strategies to implement these interventions on a large scale.

4. The surveillance systems that have been established (typically HIV surveillance in antenatal clinics) are often very limited, incomplete, and inconsistent and rarely measure behavioral variables. Thus there is still considerable need for basic monitoring information about HIV, STDs, sexual behavior, and other risks, and the strengthening of HIV and STD surveillance systems is a priority need for

most national AIDS control programs. Beyond the basic monitoring of the epidemic, there also needs to be more integration of behavioral and epidemiological research (see Chapter 3).

5. There are some good examples of national AIDS control programs using HIV behavioral research results in program planning. For example, the Zambian program used a situation analysis conducted by the Morehouse Project to inform significant policy changes concerning sexual inheritance practices. UNICEF's participatory model of program planning and qualitative assessment has been instrumental in evaluating Uganda's national AIDS control effort at the district level and has improved district-level program planning (UNICEF, 1993).

6. Behavioral research is needed on the types, frequency, and meaning of sexual practices that generate most individual risk of HIV infection (see Chapter 4). Information on practices such as the types and numbers of partners and condom use is seriously lacking. For example, social marketing data show that condoms are being sold in larger numbers than ever (in the millions); however, there are no good data showing that they are being used effectively, leaving everyone to rely on the implicit assumption that condom purchase equals effective condom use. It also appears that once social marketing of condoms takes hold, free distribution of condoms by the public sector subsides. The reasons for this need to be investigated further, since certain segments of African society will always require the availability of free condoms.

7. Programs and research projects are often launched without a sufficient period of formative research and pilot testing (see Chapter 5). These developmental activities are often not conducted because they are not funded. This is a short-sighted strategy: it may save funds in the short run, but will ultimately be costly because programs are less likely to be effective if they are not appropriately designed and tailored to local circumstances. In the worst case, untested strategies can waste time, money, and good will and possibly even do harm, as has been seen in a variety of misguided IEC campaigns.

8. In general, few rigorous impact evaluations of behavior change have been done in Africa (see Chapter 5). Evaluations that have been done often lack precision in their measurement of risk behaviors and thus are not very informative. As a result, few strategies have any real evidence of effectiveness. Consequently, even if program managers were to turn to the research literature for guidance, there would be little solid evidence of what works best or which strategies would be most appropriate for specific populations or conditions.

9. There is also a general absence of information about the costs of various interventions. Thus it is impossible to analyze the cost-effectiveness of various programs—one of the criteria that can be used to judge the usefulness of AIDS-prevention programs. Given the extreme scarcity of resources faced by most countries, implicit cost-effectiveness decisions are having to be made on a day-to-day basis. Consequently, there is a need to provide information that will allow countries to make more informed choices about where to spend their money.

10. There are many similar interventions being implemented across Africa—mostly information-based health education campaigns providing generic messages that are not personalized and do not address specific risk behaviors. Few if any intervention strategies are based on theory. Innovative approaches are few and far between.

11. Some innovative strategies are being tried, but they are very small scale and difficult to find. Examples are Saturday AIDS classes; youth-run health clubs and campaigns; and workshops for potential initiators of change, such as traditional healers. These strategies need to be evaluated to determine their effectiveness, and if they are found effective, operational research is needed to determine how to scale them up.

12. Reinterpretation of HIV-prevention messages is common as people seek to understand HIV in their own terms. The understanding of the epidemic is dynamic and evolving.

13. Economic, social, and political empowerment of women and youth, especially adolescent girls, was among the most frequently discussed issues and stated needs by the HIV professionals and policy makers interviewed (see Chapter 5). These are crucial HIV-prevention areas about which we know very little. There is an urgent need for substantial research that goes beyond traditional health education for commercial sex workers and creatively reaches women and youth in a variety of venues.

14. There was also a call for policy research to explore strategies for changing/developing policies so that they are more conducive to large-scale HIV-prevention efforts, condom promotion, and social norm change.

15. Research on the social and economic impact of the epidemic is also needed (see Chapter 6). Models of cost-effective strategies for the delivery of home-based care are needed. There are many issues uncovered in assessing the epidemic's impact that are now in need of operational research. Examples are issues surrounding care for AIDS orphans, inheritance and support for widows, and the increasingly compromised ability of kin-based groups to care for people with AIDS, as well as legal rights and antidiscrimination policy research.

16. In general, AIDS-prevention programs do not use research findings/data to target and design their efforts. Thus there is a great need to increase capacity to both conduct research and use research results in designing programs (see Chapter 7).

17. The USAID missions visited in Zambia, Tanzania, and Cameroon appear to have limited inclination to conduct research and limited capacity to synthesize or translate research findings.

18. Capacity for outcome research is limited in terms of human resources, expertise, fiscal resources, and equipment. Until this lack of resources for research is addressed, research studies cannot be expected to produce meaningful findings for program design and evaluation. However, basic program evaluation and some operational research should be feasible even in low-resource situations

and should be encouraged more by the donors as a requirement for any program implementation award.

19. Typically, donors develop HIV-prevention strategies on the basis of fundamental universal health principles and then dictate which interventions are implemented in particular settings. There is little community or stakeholder participation in program development and evaluation activities, with the exception of Uganda. Stakeholder and community participation in program design, implementation, and evaluation is essential to mounting an effective and sustainable HIV-prevention program in Africa (see Chapter 7).

20. Donor funding agendas and priorities often provide little opportunity to explore local needs. This means donor priorities may not match the priorities of national AIDS control programs. There is a need to consider introducing more flexibility into the process for directing funds to national AIDS control programs. There is also a need to shorten the bureaucratic delays in funding that can sometimes undermine effective strategies. As a result of such delays, it may be 2 or 3 years before a program approved for funding actually receives the funds and can be launched. Additionally, research funding decisions seem to be made on an ad hoc basis, with little attention paid to developing a thoughtful research agenda, building a portfolio that sets sound research priorities, and funding research based on these priorities.

21. In Africa, there is a serious lack of information sharing among AIDS professionals both within each country and among countries. Thus there are frequently duplication of effort and "reinventing-the-wheel" activities that waste time and limited resources (see Chapter 7). This lack of information sharing could be redressed if donors sponsored innovative information exchange activities both within and among countries. Examples are newsletters; electronic bulletin boards; national or regional clearinghouses for materials, articles, and relevant questionnaires; smaller local, national, or regional HIV-prevention conferences and training workshops; and traveling "road shows" that showcase model programs and experienced program managers, encouraging them to act as consultants to other HIV-prevention programs.

Sometimes information is not shared until it has been presented at an international conference. This practice ensures that timely information is not received by those who need it most—those fighting AIDS on the front lines who never go to international conferences. Incentives to share research findings in a timely and effective manner with those who can most use the results must be developed and encouraged by donors. A serious look at how best to synthesize research results and disseminate them to African HIV-prevention professionals is greatly needed. The development of a variety of dissemination systems, networks, and strategies would represent a meaningful contribution to HIV-prevention efforts in Africa.

22. There is a growing reliance on nongovernmental organizations to deliver HIV prevention and care services, rather than on the government. However, many of the small nongovernmental organizations depend totally on donor assis-

tance and appear to be unsustainable otherwise. Furthermore, exclusive reliance on such organizations by donors and government often leads to duplicate and uncoordinated efforts that frequently leave major geographical or substantive areas untouched. There are certainly examples of excellent nongovernmental organizations that are doing good work, but not all these organizations are local or effective, and many have a need for technical training and assistance from the government national AIDS control programs. The optimal roles of government, nongovernmental organizations, and donors in HIV prevention need further study.

REFERENCES

Barnett, T.
1994 The Effects of HIV/AIDS on Farming Systems and Rural Livelihoods in Uganda, Tanzania, and Zambia. Unpublished report prepared for the Food and Agriculture Organization. Overseas Development Group, University of East Anglia, Norwich, U.K.

Chela, C.M., R. Malska, T. Chava, A. Martin, A. Mwanza, B. Yamba, and E. van Prang
1994 Costing and evaluating home based care in Zambia. Abstract No. 099B/D, Volume 10(1):31. IXth International Conference on AIDS, August 7-12, Yokohama, Japan.

Social Policy Research Group
1993 *Orphans, Widows, and Widowers in Zambia: A Situation Analysis and Options for HIV/AIDS Survival Assistance.* Lusaka, Zambia: Institute for African Studies, University of Zambia.

UNICEF
1993 *Districts Speak Out: A Participatory Program Planning Workshop.* Kampala, Uganda: UNICEF.

World Bank
1992 *Tanzania: AIDS Assessment and Planning Study.* Washington, D.C.: The World Bank.

PEOPLE CONTACTED

Zambia

Dr. Stella Anyangwe, Morehouse School of Medicine
Dr. Mazuwa Banda, Churches Medical Association of Zambia
Ms. Heather Benoy, Private Consultant
Mrs. Given Daka, ZAMCOM
Dr. Knutt Flykesnes, World Health Organization
Mr. Paul H. Hartenberger, U.S. Agency for International Development
Professor Alan Haworth, University of Zambia
Father Michael T. Kelly, Director, Kara Counselling
Mr. Bradford Lucas, Population Service International
Dr. Roland Msiska, National AIDS Control Programme
Mr. Vincent Musowe, Chief Health Planner, Ministry of Health
Mr. Eli Nangawe, PHC Advisor, Ministry of Health
Dr. Masauso M. Nzima, Morehouse School of Medicine

Mr. Michael O'Dwyer, Overseas Development Administration
Mr. Leo O'Keeffe, UNICEF
Mr. Johnathon Phiri, Project Officer, UNICEF
Dr. Karen Romano, Morehouse School of Medicine
Ms. Birgitta Soccorsi, NORAD
Ms. Inger Teit, NORAD
Ms. Margareta Tullberg, Swedish Embassy
Mr. Joe Wiseman, Morehouse School of Medicine

Tanzania

Dr. B. Fimbo, IEC Director, National AIDS Control Programme
Mr. Khalid Hassan, Laboratory, National AIDS Control Programme
Dr. Susan Hunter, U.S. Agency for International Development
Dr. Saidi H. Kapiga, Muhimbili Medical Center
Theofrida A. Kapinga, Tanzanian Council for Social Development (TACOSODE)
Professor W.L. Kilama, National Institute for Medical Research
Dr. Japhet Z. J. Killewo, Muhimbili Medical Center
Kajab Kondo, TACOSODE
Dr. M.T. Leshabari Muhimbili Medical Center
Dr. George Lwihula, Muhimbili Medical Center
Tim Manchester, Population Services International
Immaculate Manyanda, Organization of Tanzanian Trade Unions (OTTU)
G. Mbonea, VIJANA
Professor Fred Mhalu, Muhimbili Medical Center
Siami Mohamed, Tanzania Girl Guide Association
Nuru S. Msangi, Tanzania Society for the Deaf
H. Mussa, VIJANA
Janeth Mziray, Tanzania Parents Association
Dr. E.F. Ndyetabura, clinical AIDS/STDs, National AIDS Control Programme
Justin Nguma, Tanzania AIDS Project
I.S. Ngunga, Tanzania Scouts Association
Penina Ochola, Tanzania AIDS Project
Dr. F. Owenya, Danish Red Cross
Abdul I.W. Pagali, Tanzania National Freedom From Hunger Campaign
Dr. R.O. Swai, Director, National AIDS Control Programme
Ms. Angela Trenton-Mbonde, World Health Organization Technical Advisor

Cameroon

Ms. Claude Cheta, Institut de Recherche et des Etudes de Comportements
Hortense M. Deffo, Institut de Recherche et des Etudes de Comportements
Jean Pierre Edjoa, Institut de Recherche et des Etudes de Comportements

Dr. Eleonare Seumo Fosso, CARE
Mr. P.L. Hougnoutou, Chief, IEC Section, Ministry of Health
Tchudjo Kamdem, Cameroon Psychology Forum
Charles Kamta, Cameroon Psychology Forum
Joseph Kemmegne, Cameroon Psychology Forum
Emmanuel Kiawi, Cameroon Psychology Forum
Mr. Alexis Boupda Kuate, AIDSCAP
Jean-Christophe Messina, Cameroon Psychology Forum
Dr. Ngole Eitel Mpoudi, Director, National AIDS Control Programme
Mr. Jopesh Betima Ndongo, Manager, CSWs project, Ministry of Health
Dr. Peter Ndumbe, Chief, Research Section, National AIDS Control Programme
Marc Ngwambe, Cameroon Psychology Forum
Zakariaou Njoumeni, Institut de Recherche et des Etudes de Comportements
Adonis Touko, Cameroon Psychology Forum

APPENDIX B
Biographical Sketches

JANE MENKEN *(Cochair)* is UPS Foundation professor in the social sciences at the University of Pennsylvania, where she was director of the Population Studies Center from 1989 to 1995. Her main area of research is fertility; she has developed mathematical models of reproduction and analytic techniques and has carried out studies of the increase in sterility as women age, of fertility determinants in Bangladesh, and of teenage pregnancy and childbearing in the United States. She has a B.A. in mathematics from the University of Pennsylvania (1960), an M.S. from the Harvard School of Public Health in biostatistics (1962), and a Ph.D. in sociology and demography from Princeton University (1975). She was elected to the National Academy of Sciences in 1989, the American Academy of Arts and Sciences in 1990, and the Institute of Medicine in 1995. She is a member of the board of directors of the Alan Guttmacher Institute and the advisory committee to the director of the National Institutes of Health. She has served on numerous committees of the National Research Council since 1977, including the Committee on Population and Demography; the Committee on Population; and the Committee on AIDS Research Needs in the Social, Behavioral, and Statistical Sciences. She is also a member of the Commission on Behavioral and Social Sciences and Education.

JAMES TRUSSELL *(Cochair)* is professor of economics and public affairs, director of the Office of Population Research, and associate dean of the Woodrow Wilson School of Public and International Affairs at Princeton University. He is the author or coauthor of more than 140 scientific publications, primarily in the areas of demographic methodology and reproductive health. He has a B.S. in mathematics from Davidson College (1971), a B.Phil. in economics from Oxford University (1973), and a Ph.D. in economics from Princeton University (1975). He is a research associate of the National Bureau of Economic Research and a member of the board of directors of the Population Association of American and the Alan Guttmacher Institute.

KOFI AWUSABO-ASARE is a senior lecturer in population and medical geography at the University of Cape Coast, Ghana. His research interests are in population policy formulation and implementation and the social dimensions of HIV/AIDS infection. His work in HIV/AIDS is part of the West African Research Network on Sexual Networking. He participated in the Ghana segment of the Agenda for Improving the Implementation of Population Programs in Africa in the early 1990s. He is currently a member of the Technical Committee on Population Policy of the Ghana National Population Council. He has a B.A. from the University of Cape Coast, an M.A. in demography from the Australian National University in Canberra, and a Ph.D. from the University of Liverpool.

JOHN G. CLELAND is professor of medical demography at the London School of Hygiene and Tropical Medicine. He has long-standing interests in fertility, family planning, and child survival in developing countries and has published widely on these subjects. He recently assisted the Global Programme on AIDS at the World Health Organization (WHO) in the design and analysis of surveys on sexual behavior and coedited a book on the main results. He currently serves on committees of WHO's Human Reproduction Programme, of Macro International's Demographic and Health Surveys Programme, and of the International Union for the Scientific Study of Population.

BARNEY COHEN is study director of the Panel on Data and Research Priorities for Arresting AIDS in Sub-Saharan Africa. Since 1992 he has served as program officer with the Committee on Population of the National Research Council/National Academy of Sciences, working on a variety of projects on adolescent fertility and overall population dynamics in sub-Saharan Africa, the demography of Senegal, the demography of North American Indians, and the relationship between infant and child mortality and fertility. Between 1982 and 1986 he lived and worked in The Sudan, and he has authored or coauthored a number of scientific papers on the functioning of urban labor markets in Khartoum. He has a B.Sc. (hons.) in pure mathematics and statistics from the University College of Wales (1980), an M.A. in economics from the University of Delaware (1987), and a Ph.D. in demography from the University of California, Berkeley (1991).

CARL KENDALL is associate professor in the Department of International Health and Development and director of the HIV/AIDS Track at the Tulane University School of Public Health and Tropical Medicine; he is also adjunct professor in the Department of International Health at The Johns Hopkins University. He was founding director of the Center for International Community-based Health Research at The Johns Hopkins University and served as chief of the Behavioral Science Unit's AIDS Control and Prevention Project from 1991 to 1993. He serves on the Commission on AIDS and Education of the American Anthropological Association. His research interests are in the methodology and conduct of health intervention research, particularly applications of qualitative methodologies, and in social network analysis. He has conducted several interventions and evaluations and is now involved in evaluations of a condom social marketing program in Louisiana, of the Zambia HIV/AIDS Project, and of a large health sector project that includes STD/HIV interventions in Honduras. He is a member of the American Anthropological Association and the Society for Medical Anthropology and a fellow of the Society for Applied Anthropology. He has a B.A. in sociology and anthropology from Swarthmore College and M.A. and Ph.D. degrees in social anthropology from the University of Rochester.

PETER R. LAMPTEY is senior vice president of AIDS programs at Family Health International in Arlington, Virginia. He is also director of the AIDSCAP project, which is funded by the U.S. Agency for International Development. A physician who has worked in public health positions in developing countries for 20 years, he has served as a lecturer in the Ghana Medical School for the past 10 years. He has been actively involved in AIDS prevention and was the director of the AIDSTECH project, funded by the U.S. Agency for International Development. He has an M.D. from the University of Ghana Medical School and received training in public health at the University of California, Los Angeles; Harvard University; and the Massachusetts Institute of Technology.

EUSTACE P.Y. MUHONDWA is host country social scientist and resident advisor with the Population Council in the Tanzania Office and associate professor of behavioral sciences at the Institute of Public Health of Muhimbili University College of Health Sciences in Dar es Salaam, Tanzania. Between 1992 and 1994, he was the director of the Institute of Public Health. Previously he served as head of the Behavioral Sciences Department in the Faculty of Medicine of the University of Dar es Salaam. His research interests are in health promotion, focusing on understanding the impediments to and seeking alternative approaches for health promotion; he has dealt with maternal and child health, primary health care, leprosy, and AIDS. He has served on the medical and public health committee of the Commission for Science and Technology in Tanzania and on the first and last steering committees on social and behavioral research of the World Health Organization's Global Programme on AIDS. He has B.A. and M.A. degrees in sociology from the University of Dar es Salaam and M.Med.Sci. and Ph.D. degrees in community medicine from the University of Nottingham, U.K.

A. MEAD OVER is senior economist in the Policy Research Department of The World Bank in Washington, D.C. After teaching econometrics and health economics at Williams College from 1975 to 1981 and at Boston University from 1981 to 1985, he joined The World Bank as a health economist in 1986. Since 1987 he has written and lectured on the economic impact of AIDS at both the micro and macro levels and on the costs and effects of alternative approaches to controlling HIV and other sexually transmitted diseases. He is the principal investigator of a research project on the impact of AIDS on households in Kagera, Tanzania. After receiving a B.A. degree from Dartmouth College in 1967, he spent 2 years in the Peace Corps in Burkina Faso and 1 year as a foreign scholar at the Institut National de la Récherche Agronomique in Paris. Subsequently he pursued doctoral studies in economics at the University of Wisconsin at Madison, obtaining a Ph.D. in 1978. He is a member of the American Economic Association and the Population Association of America.

THOMAS C. QUINN is professor of medicine in the Division of Infectious Diseases at The Johns Hopkins University School of Medicine and also senior investigator in the Laboratory of Immunoregulation at the National Institute of Allergy and Infectious Diseases. He has adjunct appointments as professor of international health and molecular microbiology and immunology at The Johns Hopkins School of Hygiene and Public Health. His research interests include international studies on the epidemiology, virology, and immunopathogenesis of HIV infection. He has conducted a number of studies in sub-Saharan Africa, Southeast Asia, and Latin America examining the factors related to heterosexual and perinatal transmission of HIV infection. He has B.S. and M.S. degrees in biology from the University of Notre Dame and an M.D. from Northwestern University School of Medicine. He is a fellow of the American College of Physicians and the Infectious Disease Society of America. He is a panel member of the Food and Drug Administration's Antiretroviral Review Committee and of the U.S.-Japan Cooperative Medical Science Program on AIDS and Related Retroviruses. He serves on the editorial board of a number of journals related to research on AIDS and other sexually transmitted diseases.

DEBORAH L. RUGG is a supervisory research psychologist in the Program Evaluation Branch of the Division of HIV/AIDS Prevention, which is within the National Center for HIV, STD, and TB Prevention of the U.S. Centers for Disease Control and Prevention in Atlanta. She has authored or coauthored more than 30 publications, primarily in the areas of evaluation methodology and HIV prevention with adolescents and HIV counseling and testing. She has a B.A. from the University of Wisconsin (1975) in physiological psychology; an M.A. from San Diego State University (1977) in experimental psychology; and a Ph.D. from the University of California, San Francisco, School of Medicine (1982) in health psychology. She was an assistant professor of health psychology at the

University of California, San Francisco, and San Diego State University for 5 years prior to joining the Centers for Disease Control and Prevention in 1987 as an epidemic intelligence service officer in the Division of HIV/STD Prevention. In 1991 she became the evaluation research section chief in the Division of Adolescent and School Health and focused her research on adolescent HIV, sexually transmitted diseases, and pregnancy prevention intervention development and evaluation. She continues to focus her research on evaluation methods in assessing the effectiveness of interventions targeting adolescent sexual risk behavior.

DANIEL TARANTOLA is director of the International AIDS Program at the François-Xavier Bagnoud Center of Health and Human Rights of the Harvard School of Public Health, where he has been a lecturer in population and international health since 1991. He has an M.D. from Paris University and did postgraduate training in nephrology and epidemiology. Over a period of 17 years through 1991, he participated in the launching of several global initiatives of the World Health Organization (WHO): childhood immunization; the prevention and control of diarrheal diseases and of acute respiratory infections; and, in 1987, the Global Programme on AIDS. He is a coeditor of *AIDS in the World*—the first global report on the HIV/AIDS pandemic, published in 1992—and is coeditor of the forthcoming second volume of this publication.

JUDITH WASSERHEIT is the director of the Division of STD Prevention in the National Center for HIV, STD, and TB Prevention of the Centers for Disease Control and Prevention (CDC) in Atlanta. She is responsible for developing and directing CDC's national STD prevention programs and related research in behavioral science, epidemiology and surveillance, health services, and program evaluation. Previously, she was the first chief of the STD Branch at the National Institute of Allergy and Infectious Diseases. She has a B.A. from Princeton University (1974), an M.D. from Harvard Medical School (1978), and an M.P.H. from The Johns Hopkins University School of Hygiene and Public Health (1989). She has published extensively on clinical and epidemiological aspects of sexually transmitted diseases and HIV prevention, particularly in relation to women's health, and is a member of the executive board of the American Venereal Disease Association and the Board of the International Society for STD Research.

MARIA J. WAWER is associate clinical professor of public health and director of the International Operations Research Program within the Center for Population and Family Health of the School of Public Health at Columbia University; she is also a faculty associate in the Department of Population Dynamics of the School of Hygiene and Public Health at The Johns Hopkins University. She is currently the principal investigator on a number of research projects on AIDS prevention and reproductive health, including a project on STD control for AIDS prevention in Rakai District, Uganda, supported principally by the National Institute of Allergy and Infectious Diseases of the National Institutes of Health. She has worked on family planning, AIDS, and reproductive health issues in more than 10 African countries, as well as in Latin America and Asia. She has a B.Sc. in biology from the University of New Brunswick (1974), an M.D. from McMaster University (1977), and an M.H.Sc. from the University of Toronto (1979). She is a fellow of the Royal College of Physicians of Canada.

PETER O. WAY is a senior research analyst in the International Programs Center of the U.S. Bureau of the Census in Washington, D.C. Currently he is involved in the analysis of HIV trends worldwide and in the estimation and projection of the current and future impact of AIDS epidemics. He was responsible for the development of the HIV/AIDS Surveillance Data Base and has collaborated in the development of a mathematical model of the AIDS epidemic, sponsored by the U.S. Department of State. He has given numerous presentations at major international AIDS meetings on worldwide HIV trends and on the demographic and economic impact of AIDS epidemics. His publications include chapters in several books, a monograph on the reliability of demographic estimates for Africa, and numerous articles on the current trends and projected impact of AIDS epidemics. He has a B.A. in sociology from St. Louis University (1971) and an M.A. (1973) and Ph.D. (1977) in sociology, both from the University of Chicago.

DEBREWORK ZEWDIE is reproductive health specialist and the AIDS/STD coordinator for the Human Development Department of The World Bank in Washington, D.C. Previously she held a number of public health positions in which she provided research and technical assistance on AIDS prevention and control, reproductive health, and sexually transmitted diseases. She was deputy regional director for the Africa Region of the AIDS Control and Prevention Project of Family Health International in Nairobi, Kenya; program manager of the AIDS/STD Prevention and Control Program of Ethiopia; deputy director of the National Research Institute of Health in Addis Ababa, Ethiopia; and head of the Referral Laboratory for AIDS in Addis Ababa. She consulted for the Global Programme on AIDS from 1989 to 1990 and has participated in the development of Medium-Term Plans and national serosurveillance in several countries in Africa. She has a B.Sc. in biology from Addis Ababa University and a Ph.D. in immunology from the University of London.

Index

B

C

G

H

I

N

O

P

R

S

T